Field Guide
to Bedside Diagnosis

David S. Smith, MD
Chief, Internal Medicine
Yale Health Plan
Associate Clinical Professor of Medicine
Yale University School of Medicine
New Haven, Connecticut

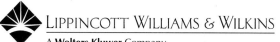

LIPPINCOTT WILLIAMS & WILKINS
A **Wolters Kluwer** Company

Philadelphia · Baltimore · New York · London
Buenos Aires · Hong Kong · Sydney · Tokyo

Editor: Richard Winters
Managing Editor: Mary Beth Murphy
Marketing Manager: Meg White
Production Editor: Lisa JC Franko
Design Coordinator: Mario Fernandez

351 West Camden Street
Baltimore, Maryland 21201-2436 USA

530 Walnut Street
Philadelphia, Pennsylvania 19106 USA

Printed in China

Library of Congress Cataloging-in-Publication Data

Smith, David S. (David Scott), 1954–
    Field guide to bedside diagnosis / David S. Smith.
        p.   cm.
    Includes bibliographical references and index.
    ISBN 0-7817-1630-6
        1. Diagnosis—Handbooks, manuals, etc. 2. Symptomatology—
Handbooks, manuals, etc. 3. Diagnosis, Differential—Handbooks,
manuals, etc. 4. Physical diagnosis—Handbooks, manuals, etc.
I. Title.
    [DNLM: 1. Diagnosis handbooks.   WB 39 S645f 1999]
RC71.S63   1999
616.07'5—dc21
DNLM/DLC
for Library of Congress   99-10808
                                                  CIP

00 01 02 03
3 4 5

To Sharon, Ryan, and Katie.

Preface

"Precise and intelligent recognition and appreciation of minor differences is the real essential factor in a successful medical diagnosis" wrote Sir Joseph Bell, Conan Doyle's medical professor at Edinburgh (and the model for Sherlock Holmes). "Eyes and ears which can see and hear, memory to record at once and to recall at pleasure the impressions of the senses, and an imagination capable of weaving a theory or piecing together a broken chain or unravelling a tangled clue, such are the implements of his trade to a successful diagnostician. To masters of [the] art there are myriad signs eloquent and instructive, but which need the educated eye to detect."

This *Field Guide to Bedside Diagnosis* is intended to be used as are the naturalist field guides. Observations of subtle clinical differences made at the bedside— the metaphorical field—are applied in diagnosis. Standard textbooks of medicine are oriented around specific diseases, for example, myocardial infarction. Unfortunately, patients do not come labeled as such but have undifferentiated symptoms and signs, such as chest pain, which may have many potential causes ranging from trivial to life-threatening. Standard physical diagnosis textbooks focus on techniques of physical examination rather than on the use of physical findings, integrated with history, in differential diagnosis. This book uniquely occupies that cognitive space between physical diagnostic skills and diseases, helping clinicians refine inchoate clinical presentations into working diagnoses. Although a clinical approach alone cannot entirely replace diagnostic technology, it can indicate which diseases are most likely, and in turn, which tests have the highest yield and are most cost-effective.

The text is organized to parallel the diagnostic reasoning process of a clinician. Patients present with a *chief complaint*, which focuses the diagnostic pursuit. These cardinal symptoms and physical findings, such as headache or diastolic murmur, form the central structure of the book. A *differential overview* for each problem allows a clinician to scan at a glance the causes, in rough order of probability (based on the biases of my own experience). The list focuses on the most common causes and rarer but serious diseases for which one must maintain an index of suspicion. A *diagnostic approach* follows, mapping the major diagnostic branch points for each differential. Finally, for each disease under consideration, *clinical findings* describe the findings on history and physical examination that most reliably point toward a particular diagnosis. They have been reduced to their most essential elements, what Osler called "burrs that stick in the memory," and polished smooth. This approach is based on research suggesting that clinical expertise is based on cognitive structures which describe clinical features as "illness scripts" of prototypical patients, containing rich detail about pathophysiology and contexts.

This field guide includes a comprehensive photographic atlas of classic observable phenomena and "field marks" that suggest underlying systemic disease processes. Images were chosen both as gold-standard prototypes and for their aesthetic qualities.

This book has a distinctly generalist approach. It is based on a synthesis of the literature filtered through my experience as a practicing general internist and teacher of medical students and residents at Yale, Dartmouth, and the University of Pennsylvania. Although primarily written for medical students and residents learning to make and analyze clinical observations, this book also contains many "clinical pearls" for the more experienced practitioner, to provide a critical edge in difficult cases. I hope that, above all, this book will be useful. By making the numerous physical signs more eloquent and instructive, I hope you will increase your mastery of the art of diagnosis.

New Haven, June 1998

Acknowledgments

The inspiration for this book came from many quarters. Brendan Reilly exemplified a clarity of thought about clinical diagnosis and inspired, advised, and encouraged me to write. Paul Gerber, a consummate clinician and teacher, modeled the consideration of the lush interconnections between manifest phenomena and deeper disease processes. Sankey Williams, Al Mushlin, Hal Sox, and David Sackett each had a role at a critical juncture in helping me to conceptualize a Bayesian approach to the science of the art of clinical diagnosis. Mark Berger introduced me to field guides and the art of field observation. Edward Tufte and Richard Winters gave me inspired advice on the design of this book.

Medical students and residents have contributed by challenging me to develop clear and justified diagnostic reasoning, thus refining the approach used in this book. My patients have been messengers from terra incognita, lands of illness to which I could never personally voyage and about which I now write. They have been astute observers and literate reporters.

The photographic atlas could not have been developed without the contributions of original images from the Yale Dermatology Residents' collection by Lisa Kugelman and Douglas Grossman, from the Dartmouth Dermatology collection by Stephen Spencer, and from the Yale and University of Iowa Ophthalmology collections by Peter Gloor.

How to Use This Guide

"See, and then reason and compare and control. But first see."

—Osler

General Design

This book follows the metaphor of the naturalist field guides, in which an un-known bird or wildflower can be identified through observation of key "field marks." It diverges in developing an approach that parallels that of clinical di-agnosis. The perspective begins with the manifest phenomena of disease, as they present to the clinician, which are then mapped inward to reveal the un-derlying disease structure. Mastery of bedside diagnosis requires an ability to translate the somatic language of symptoms, which evolution has developed to inform the organism about a problem. It also requires cultivation of the skills of activated observation, of engaging your mind, of discovering clues in find-ings on examination, and then of interpreting all within a cognitive framework built on deep knowledge of structure and pathophysiology.

The aim of this book is to be compact, colorful, aesthetic, and useful. It is designed to be as comprehensive as possible but still be portable. I have at-tempted to balance usefulness with the axiom that we cannot diagnose what we do not consider; therefore, I have focused on common or serious disorders. I have taken the approach of a generalist rather than a specialist. I have tried to take clinical observations to the edge of their ability to differentiate among competing diagnoses. Although these diagnostic hypotheses form the basis for the application and interpretation of diagnostic technology, such testing and treatment is beyond the intended scope of this book.

Chapters/Chief Complaints

The central organizing principle of this book revolves around the 147 symp-toms and physical findings that constitute the text chapters. David Eddy has de-scribed the first, and most critical, step in diagnosis as selection of a pivotal finding. These chapters represent the minimum set of such findings. They are derived from my extensive review of cases presenting to a walk-in clinic, as framed by the patient and clinician. Each is a razor's edge, representing a di-agnostic cluster that permits the clinician to gain traction and diagnostic lever-age.

Differential Overview

For each diagnostic problem, I developed a differential list focusing on com-mon causes and more unusual but serious diseases that must not be overlooked. The list is in rough order of prevalence, based on my clinical experience. Its prominence allows high-yield diagnoses to be scanned at a glance. Subgroups are used when possible to provide a first-pass refinement of the diagnostic problem.

Diagnostic Approach

This section structures the problem, indicates the major diagnostic branch points, and discusses the key findings and maneuvers to send your inquiry in one direction or another. When known, the likelihood ratios of findings in this problem/context are given, to suggest their diagnostic impact.

Clinical Findings

Remember that in bedside diagnosis, the diagnostician's task is one of inferring cause from observed effect. The main way this is accomplished is by comparing observations made about the patient before you with the clinical signature of each disease in the differential list. I have intentionally reduced descriptions of disease-specific phenomena to their most essential elements—those that are reliably useful and most diagnostic. Think of these as vignettes of archetypical patients. Your patient will usually represent a recognizable variation on the theme. When a phenomenon in the text is illustrated in the atlas of photographic plates, it is cross-referenced.

Color Atlas

The 240 color plates were selected to favor classic observable physical phenomena that mark underlying systemic disease processes. Each was chosen as an archetypical photographic representation of that finding. Each plate is labeled with the finding and often the underlying disease for that particular patient. A more detailed description can be found in the corresponding text. Frequently, more than one condition can cause the finding. Each plate is cross-referenced to the chapter(s) in which it is cited.

Bayesian Approach

A Bayesian approach is not about probability *per se* (a patient either has a disease or doesn't) but about uncertainty in decision making in real time. Probability is an expression of diagnostic certainty; that is, given the information available at that point in time, how certain are you that this patient has the disease under consideration? When known, and useful, the sensitivity, specificity, and likelihood ratio of findings are presented. The *sensitivity* (Se) is the frequency with which the finding appears in patients with the disease. The absence of a highly sensitive finding will rule out a diagnosis. The *specificity* (Sp) is the proportion of patients without the particular diagnosis in whom the finding is absent. A "pathognomonic finding" has a high specificity, often at the expense of sensitivity. Although not often seen, when it is present, the diagnosis is virtually certain. The ratio of the true positive rate (sensitivity) to the false positive rate (1-specificity) is the *likelihood ratio* (LR). The likelihood ratio indicates how much the presence of a finding ought to increase the odds of a given diagnosis (formally, prior odds × likelihood ratio = posterior odds), or increase your diagnostic certainty. For example, a LR of 2 doubles the odds of a diagnosis.

Case 1

A patient presents with an acute sore throat. You are considering obtaining a rapid strep test, but wonder how you will interpret the result. The rapid strep test has Se 0.78, Sp 0.96, and LR 19.5 for diagnosing streptococcal pharyngitis. Knowing only that the patient has a sore throat, with an *a priori* 10% chance of being caused by group A strep in your clinic, a positive test indicates a 68% chance that he has strep. However, with a negative result, he will still have a 2% chance of being infected, leaving considerable uncertainty. You should apply the observations found in chapter 144 and reexamine the patient. If he has fever, tonsillar exudate, and tender anterior cervical lymphadenopathy (LR 8.0), combined with a positive rapid test, there is a 93% probability of group A strep being present. If the patient has none of these clinical findings (LR 0.3) and a negative rapid test, he is quite likely to have a viral infection, with only a 0.2% probability of streptococcal infection. Clinical evaluation provides the infrastructure for sound diagnosis. Seldom will the clinical evaluation outperform technology, but often it will enhance the interpretation and extend the range of diagnostic tests.

Case 2

A patient with a history of mitral valve prolapse with mild mitral regurgitation presents acutely short of breath. On examination, he has a loud apical systolic murmur, bibasilar rales, and a third heart sound. You turn to chapter 32 on acute dyspnea, and find that the symmetrical dependent rales suggest left heart failure. You still do not know the cause of its acute appearance, however, so you turn to chapter 15 on congestive heart failure. You read that although a third heart sound usually suggests low cardiac output, acute mitral regurgitation, by augmenting early diastolic filling, can cause a third heart sound with a normal cardiac output. Endocarditis is listed in the differential, and remembering the loud murmur, you quickly turn to chapter 28 on systolic murmur. Finding mitral regurgitation, you read that in acute mitral regurgitation due to endocarditis, there is a grade 3/6 early systolic murmur. You are referred to plates 22–24, peripheral findings of endocarditis. Returning to your patient, everything is there: an early systolic murmur with a palpable thrill, an unmistakable Osler's node on his index finger, and even a history of a recent dental cleaning without prophylaxis.

Case 3

When my son signed up to play football, he failed to realize that it involved daily 2-hour practices during August. After a few weeks, he began to complain nightly of feeling tired and having a headache. I had him drink more water to avoid dehydration. When the complaints persisted, I concluded that he was using symptoms to get out of practice, and I gave him a pep talk about commitment and responsibility. At the end of the week, after a particularly hot and dusty practice, he took off his shirt to shower, thus revealing the answer: three red ovals with clearing centers on his back, classic erythema migrans of Lyme disease, as seen in plate 106.

Bedside diagnosis, grounded in history and physical examination, can be viewed from many vantage points. It is a portable, rapid, real-time method of hypothesis generation and testing, the doctor's "secret weapon." It is a low-tech guide to the intelligent selection of high-tech diagnostics. Probability estimates derived from clinical data form the basis of the Bayesian interpretation of test results—if in no other way than in semiquantitatively recognizing true versus false positive and negative results. Readily repeatable observations can be made over time to monitor the disease course and the effects of therapy, in a way not feasible with high-tech tools. The clinical examination is particularly effective in the ambulatory diagnostic environment, from the diagnosis of mundane conditions such as otitis media, which is defined by the observation of a red tympanic membrane, to the diagnostically sublime, such as the rapid assessment of critically ill patients, for whom management is time-sensitive.

The examination also has a therapeutic value via the "laying on of hands." The stethoscope allows you to connect not only your ears, but also your mind to the patient. Finally, making diagnoses based on finely tuned observations made with your unaided senses and interpreted using a richly interconnected matrix of knowledge and clinical experience produces the rare experience of intellectual pleasure: the application of the art of medicine in solving a mystery.

Contents

Part 1: Chief Complaints and Findings
Section I: General/Constitutional

Section II: Heart/Vascular

Section III: Lungs/Chest

Section VIII: Skin

Section IX: Head/Neck

Part 2. Color Plates

General/Constitutional

Chapter 1

Color Phenomena

Color can evoke a diagnosis.

Yellow   Jaundice can be deep yellow, or lemon-yellow with anemia. Pernicious anemia produces a bright yellow tint with a contrasting red tongue. Nephrotic syndrome produces the pallor of anemia that combines with increased carotene-binding globulin to produce a sallow-yellow cast. Red-brown lesions of cutaneous tuberculosis (lupus vulgaris) are yellow-brown, like apple jelly, on diascopy. Xanthelasma are waxy yellow lipid deposits. Lesions of pseudoxanthoma elasticum look like yellowish plucked chicken skin. Urate crystals produce a yellow translucence within tophi. Yellow nails occur with lymphedema or chronic lung disease. Bright yellow urine appears with phenacetin, quinacrine, riboflavin, and jaundice (in which the foam is also yellow). CMV retinitis has a yellowish retinal exudate, like "crumbled cheese." A yellow visual halo is characteristic of both digoxin intoxication and acute glaucoma (**Plates 46, 49, 53, 64, 69, 100, 175, 202**).

Orange   Carotenemia causes the skin to turn orange-yellow, but the sclera remain white. Orange urine can result from rhubarb, senna, Azulfidine (sulfasalazine), Pyridium (phenazopyridine), or rifampin (which can even cause orange tears). Patients with pityriasis rubra pilaris may develop a striking orange skin color, especially on their palms and soles. Tangier disease is marked by orange tonsils (**Plate 9**).

Blue/Gray   Blue-gray skin color can result from gold (chrysiasis), silver (argyria), metastatic melanoma, ochronosis, chloroquine, minocycline, and amiodarone (due to blue lipofuscin photodermatitis). Chlorpromazine produces a blue-purple "visage mauve." Blue sclera are typical for osteogenesis imperfecta. Cyanosis caused by reduced hemoglobin is purplish-blue to heliotrope. The skin in polycythemia is reddish-blue; in methemoglobinemia (a result of dapsone treatment), chocolate blue; in sulfhemoglobinemia, lead or mauve-blue. In Raynaud's syndrome, white blanching turns to slate-blue cyanosis to livid purple and finally to deep red. The rarity of phlegmasia cerulea dolens occurs with massive deep vein thrombosis (DVT). Distal embolism results in a blue toe. Gun-metal grey purpura is characteristic for meningococcemia. Blue urine may be a product of amitriptyline, triamterene, senna, or indigo blue. Blue nail lunulae are seen in argyria, Wilson's disease, and antimalarial treatment. A bluish cervix is a marker of pregnancy. The pharyngeal pseudomembrane of diphtheria is blue-white (to gray-green). Blue-tinted vision occurs with optic ischemia and Viagra treatment (**Plates 3, 5, 6, 25, 26, 27, 32, 36**).

Green   Green purulence indicates the presence of a copper-containing myeloperoxidase found in leukocytes. Pseudomonas infection tints the nails green. Green urine may result from urinary copper, Pseudomonas infection, biliverdin, Clorets, phenol, or gross hematuria in a patient with red–green color blindness. In iritis, a blue iris may become green due to vascular congestion. Anemia often produces a greenish waxy pallor (**Plates 1, 114**).

Gold/Copper/Silver   The golden iridic ring in Wilson's disease is a classic example, but desipramine also produces gold irises. Tuberculous peritonitis produces a bronzing of the skin, especially on the abdomen. Lesions of secondary syphilis are reminiscent of a copper penny in color and shape. Silver stools may rarely occur with ampullary carcinoma, resulting from acholic stools with bleeding. The mica scales of psoriasis are silver-colored (**Plates 2, 80, 105**).

Purple   The heliotrope eyelid rash of dermatomyositis may have a delicate lilac color. Purple striae are highly suggestive of Cushing's disease. Plum-colored nodules are found in cutaneous lymphoma. Currant jelly sputum is classic for klebsiella infection. Erysipeloid has a deep red-purple cast. Kaposi's sarcoma appears as deep purple papules. The coup de sabre lesion of localized scleroderma (morphea) is white and atrophic, with a violaceous edge. Amyloidosis causes waxy pink-purple periorbital patches. Ethionamide may cause a lilac brown photodermatitis. Purple urine may occur with porphobilinogen (**Plates 11, 94, 99, 147, 157, 159, 200**).

Black   A jet-black skin lesion is classic for melanoma. Velvety black patches of acanthosis nigricans suggest insulin resistance. Black, tarry stools indicate melena from upper gastrointestinal bleeding. Black urine occurs with alcaptonuria, tyrosinosis, methyldopa, methocarbamol, phenol, malaria (blackwater fever), methemoglobinemia and cascara (**Plates 160, 168**).

Diaphoresis Chapter 2

PLATES 4, 14, 19, 20, 22, 23, 24, 129

◤ DIFFERENTIAL OVERVIEW

- ❏ Fever
- ❏ Menopause
- ❏ Anxiety
- ❏ Drugs
- ❏ Gustatory
- ❏ Thyrotoxicosis
- ❏ Parkinson's disease
- ❏ Autonomic neuropathy
- ❏ Central neurologic injury
- ❏ Pheochromocytoma
- ❏ Carcinoid
- ❏ Acromegaly

DIAGNOSTIC APPROACH

Eccrine glands are concentrated on the palms, soles, face, and axilla. They function to cool the body through evaporation. They are under cholinergic control and may be stimulated by epinephrine. Apocrine glands are associated with hair follicles in the axilla and groin. Their secretions are viscid and produce an odor after acted on by bacteria.

Measuring the temperature during diaphoresis is important to determine whether a fever is present, which suggests infection.

Night sweats are distinguished as drenching sweats that require changing the bedclothes. They occur with conditions such as Hodgkin's or non-Hodgkin's lymphoma and tuberculosis.

Excessive sweating with vasoconstriction (cold and clammy skin) may be caused by insulin hypoglycemia, dumping syndrome, drug withdrawal, shock, vasovagal states, or intense pain.

CLINICAL FINDINGS

Fever Usually caused by infection, sweating occurs during defervescence, especially at night. Consider occult infections such as HIV, granulomatous disease, or endocarditis when localizing symptoms are not present **(Plates 22, 23, 24).**

Menopause Hot flashes usually produce objective flushing or at least a sensation of warmth. Irregularities in menstrual cycle length or flow are a key clue.

Anxiety Characteristically, sweating occurs on the palms and soles (eccrine).

Drugs Sweating occurs with antipyretics (fever lysis), insulin-induced hypoglycemia, tricyclic antidepressants, and withdrawal of addictive drugs (alcohol, opiates, depressants).

Gustatory Typically, sweating induced by spicy food occurs on the face, especially the upper lip.

Thyrotoxicosis Signs of a hypermetabolic state (e.g., tachycardia) are present with or without findings of Grave's disease (stare, lid lag, fine tremor, thyromegaly). The sweating will not be paroxysmal **(Plates 19, 20).**

Parkinson's disease There is an increase in both sweating and sebaceous activity, associated with masked facies, cyclical hand tremor, and shuffling gait with en-bloc movements.

Autonomic neuropathy Concomitant orthostatic hypotension is usually present.

Central neurologic injury A stroke or tumor underlies the sweating. Examine the eye grounds for papilledema, and look for focal neurological signs, which are usually obvious **(Plate 129).**

Pheochromocytoma Paroxysms of sympathetic hyperactivity (acute blood pressure elevation and flushing) occur in a patient with evidence of a hypermetabolic state (e.g., weight loss).

Carcinoid Episodic flushing, wheezing, and diarrhea are typical **(Plate 4).**

Acromegaly The handshake is characteristic: moist, warm, doughy. The hands, jaw, and tongue are enlarged, with frontal bossing. Compare the current appearance with old photographs **(Plate 14).**

Facial Appearances

◼ DIFFERENTIAL OVERVIEW

Phenomena
- ❏ Hyperthyroidism
- ❏ Parkinsonism
- ❏ Myxedema
- ❏ Pernicious anemia
- ❏ Systemic lupus erythematosus
- ❏ Renal failure
- ❏ Cushing's syndrome
- ❏ Addison's disease
- ❏ Acromegaly
- ❏ Polycythemia vera
- ❏ Dermatomyositis
- ❏ Myopathy
- ❏ Myasthenia gravis
- ❏ Mitral stenosis
- ❏ Congenital syphilis

Paresis
- ❏ Bell's palsy
- ❏ Lyme disease
- ❏ Trauma
- ❏ Parotid infection
- ❏ Central facial palsy
- ❏ Neurofibroma
- ❏ Ramsey-Hunt syndrome

DIAGNOSTIC APPROACH

The classic phenomena described here allow one to form a gestalt impression of the diagnosis.

With facial weakness, it is important to distinguish central from peripheral lesions by observing that central lesions preserve voluntary movements of the upper face and emotional movements of the mouth such as laughing and crying, due to crossed innervation.

CLINICAL FINDINGS

Hyperthyroidism This condition is marked by proptosis, a stare with sclera visible over the iris, and an unblinking gaze. The conjunctival surface appears unusually bright and glistening ("bright eye") **(Plates 19, 20).**

Parkinsonism The face is expressionless and motionless ("masked") with an absence of blinking.

Myxedema The features are thickened/coarsened; the skin is dry, sallow, pale, and waxy. There is periorbital edema, but the skin is doughy rather than edematous. The outer third of the eyebrows is often absent. The voice is a husky croak **(Plates 16, 17, 18).**

Pernicious anemia The face has a pale primrose yellow color, but there is no emaciation. The tongue is smooth and bright red **(Plate 69).**

Systemic lupus erythematosus A palpable "butterfly" rash over the cheeks and bridge of the nose is diagnostic **(Plates 91, 92).**

Renal failure The face is sallow with a half-bloated appearance. The ear lobes may enlarge, and facial features may coarsen to give a "leonine facies." Bronzed patchy hyperpigmentation may occur **(Plate 198).**

Cushing's syndrome It is characterized by a rosy-cheeked, hirsute "moon face." The cheeks may obscure the ears when the face is viewed from the front **(Plates 10, 11).**

Addison's disease The dark brown hyperpigmentation with gray pigmentation of the mucous membranes of the mouth is the most striking finding. Temporal wasting also occurs **(Plates 12, 13).**

Facial Appearances Chapter 3

Acromegaly Prominent arched brows; enlarged nose, lips, and tongue; and a projecting jaw are typical features. The changes are best appreciated by comparison with earlier photographs **(Plate 14).**

Polycythemia vera This appears as a ruddy or plum-colored cyanosis and weathered look of the nose, lips, ears, and palpebral conjunctivae **(Plates 26, 30).**

Dermatomyositis A dusky lilac hue ("heliotrope") may be found over the delicate skin of the eyelids. A dusky red eruption also appears on the cheeks, mottled or diffuse, intensely red or cyanotic **(Plate 94).**

Myopathy In fascioscapulohumeral dystrophy, there is a loose pout of the lips at rest and a "transverse" smile with inability to puff out the cheeks. The eyes may be prominent because of weakness of the levator palpebrae. In myotonic dystrophy, wasting of the sternomastoids and masseters occurs, giving a lean appearance. Frontal baldness is also common.

Myasthenia gravis The lids droop with fatigue, and the smile appears as a sneer **(Plate 219).**

Mitral stenosis A remarkable malar flush and dark crimson lips contrast with a yellowish pallor of the forehead, perioral, and perinasal skin **(Plate 28).**

Congenital syphilis A depressed nasal bridge, prominent forehead, and notched and widely-gapped "Hutchinson's" teeth create the distinctive appearance.

Bell's palsy Bell's phenomenon—upward movement of the eye during attempted bilateral eye closure—is present, along with tearing, facial numbness, altered taste, and hyperacusis (sounds are louder and brasher).

Lyme disease Weakness is often bilateral and associated with other cranial nerve abnormalities. An erythema migrans rash is usually present.

Trauma Weakness may result from a direct blow to the side of the head.

Parotid infection Swelling and tenderness appear at the angle of the jaw.

Central facial palsy Voluntary movements of the upper face and emotional movements of the mouth such as laughing and crying are preserved.

Neurofibroma A lesion of CN VIII (acoustic neuroma) is associated with decreased hearing, vertigo, tinnitus, decreased facial sensation, and decreased corneal reflex.

Ramsey-Hunt syndrome The key observation is vesicles in external auditory canal caused by zoster of the geniculate ganglion **(Plate 235).**

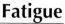

Chapter 4   Fatigue

PLATES 10, 11, 12, 13, 16, 17, 18, 22, 23, 24, 41, 63, 70, 71, 72, 130, 158, 159, 175, 188, 189, 198, 219, 229, 230

■ DIFFERENTIAL OVERVIEW

❏ Infectious mononucleosis
❏ Depression
❏ Diabetes
❏ Hypothyroidism
❏ Drugs
❏ Chronic sleep deprivation
❏ Congestive heart failure
❏ Occult infection
❏ Iron deficiency anemia
❏ Obstructive sleep apnea
❏ Renal failure
❏ Chronic fatigue syndrome
❏ Cushing's syndrome
❏ Occult cancer
❏ Addison's disease
❏ Myasthenia gravis

DIAGNOSTIC APPROACH

Organic causes of fatigue are characterized by physical weakness or exhaustion, which is exacerbated by activity and partially relieved by sleep, short duration (<2 months), unintentional weight loss of greater than 10%, and an ill appearance. Most organic causes have associated signs and symptoms, specific and few in number.

Psychological causes of fatigue are characterized by a primary inertia to initiation of physical activity, which when undertaken, can be performed. A protracted course, multiple and nonspecific associated symptoms, relation to stressful life events, and an anxious or depressed appearance are other clues. The sick role response to prior minor illness can indicate likely response to the current illness.

A diagnostic approach that involves careful history-taking and physical examination, assiduous avoidance of early closure, and a clear orientation to the reality of the patient's perceptions, whatever the cause (i.e., never implying "It's all in your head"), is most rewarding. The differential is wide, and identification of the unusual organic causes among the many psychophysiological ones takes great skill.

CLINICAL FINDINGS

Infectious mononucleosis   Acute onset of prominent fatigue in a young adult is accompanied by sore throat, fever, posterior cervical lymphadenopathy, and splenomegaly **(Plates 229, 230).**

Depression   Depressed mood is usually recognized by the patient, but the physical manifestations such as fatigue, sleep disturbance, anorexia, or anhedonia may obscure the depression.

Diabetes   It usually presents with concurrent weight loss and polyuria/nocturia.

Hypothyroidism   Fatigue is prominent, but other symptoms, including weight gain, dry skin, hoarseness, constipation, cold intolerance, periorbital edema, delayed relaxation phase to the ankle jerks, and thinning of the lateral third of the eyebrows, suggest the diagnosis. A goiter is usually present **(Plates 16, 17, 18).**

Drugs   Beta blockers, reserpine, diuretics (primarily via hypokalemia), antihistamines, antidepressants, tranquilizers, steroids, and alcohol can cause fatigue as a side effect.

Chronic sleep deprivation   This is a common cause of fatigue in workers who alter shifts, parents of young children, international travelers, and in patients with depression or fibromyalgia.

Congestive heart failure   Early disease may be suggested by paroxysmal nocturnal dyspnea and exertional fatigue. Fatigue represents reduced cardiac output **(Plate 41).**

Occult infection   The hallmark is fever. Endocarditis, tuberculosis, HIV, HBV, and occult abscess should be considered **(Plates 22, 23, 24, 175).**

Fatigue

Iron deficiency anemia   Fatigue may be associated with severe, but usually not mild, anemia. Menstrual blood loss and gastrointestinal blood loss are common causes **(Plates 188, 189).**

Obstructive sleep apnea   Excessive daytime somnolence is the prominent symptom. Obesity and the bedmate reporting heavy snoring and/or long periods of apnea at night are additional clues.

Renal failure   Edema and foamy urine are present if there is proteinuria. The skin is sallow **(Plates 41, 198).**

Chronic fatigue syndrome   CFS is defined as having a duration longer than 6 months at which the affected person has less than 50% physical capacity. Associated symptoms and findings include recurrent sore throat, lymphadenopathy, myalgia, headache, and sleep disorder. If tender trigger points are present, the fibromyalgia end of the diagnostic spectrum should be considered.

Cushing's syndrome   Indicators include hypertension, moon facies, purple striae, truncal obesity, and a "buffalo hump." Suspect this syndrome in patients taking steroids **(Plates 10, 11).**

Occult cancer   Leukemia, lymphoma, and pancreatic cancer commonly present with fatigue. Adenopathy, splenomegaly, and night sweats are helpful clues **(Plates 63, 70, 71, 72, 158, 159).**

Addison's disease   Look for hyperpigmentation, especially of the palmar creases and buccal mucosa. Suspect adrenal insufficiency in patients recently withdrawn from steroids. Concomitant symptoms include weakness, weight loss, anorexia, and hypotension **(Plates 12, 13).**

Myasthenia gravis   Muscle weakness characteristically increases with repeated use. Early disease involves cranial muscles with ptosis, diplopia, and chewing fatigue. Proximal limb weakness soon develops **(Plates 130, 219).**

Chapter 5

Fever of Unknown Origin

◼ DIFFERENTIAL OVERVIEW

Infection
- ❏ HIV
- ❏ Tuberculosis
- ❏ Endocarditis
- ❏ Osteomyelitis
- ❏ Malaria
- ❏ Syphilis
- ❏ Zoonoses
- ❏ Typhoid fever
- ❏ Chronic meningococcemia

Neoplasm
- ❏ Lymphoma
- ❏ Liver metastases
- ❏ Renal cell carcinoma
- ❏ Atrial myxoma

Connective Tissue Disease
- ❏ Giant cell arteritis
- ❏ Systemic lupus erythematosus
- ❏ Vasculitis
- ❏ Rheumatic fever
- ❏ Still's disease

Other
- ❏ Drugs
- ❏ Heat stroke
- ❏ Factitious
- ❏ Malignant hyperthermia
- ❏ Multiple pulmonary emboli

DIAGNOSTIC APPROACH

Fever of unknown origin (FUO), considered when a fever over 101°F (38.5°C) remains unexplained for longer than 3 weeks, is usually a result of infection (40%), neoplasm (20%), or connective tissue disease (20%). Before pursuing an FUO evaluation, always document the fever. It is usually caused by an atypical presentation of a common disease. Signs of sepsis such as systemic toxicity, hypotension, bands, and toxic granulations increase the tempo of the evaluation.

Consider relatively hidden (deep) sites: retroperitoneum (hematoma or infection), bone, dental, sinus, ovary, prostate, subphrenic (following abdominal surgery), renal, spleen, or prostheses. With FUO in a hospitalized patient, consider sequestered sites (sinuses in intubated patients, implanted hardware), indwelling lines, C. difficile, or drug reactions. With FUO in a neutropenic patient, consider catheters, perianal infections, Candida, and Aspergillus. Cardinal signs may be absent, e.g., meningitis with opportunistic pathogens without meningismus in 63%, and pneumonia without purulent sputum in 92%.

With FUO longer than 6 months, consider factitious fever, granulomatous hepatitis, neoplasm, Still's disease, infection, connective tissue disease, or exaggerated circadian rhythm. Patients who remain undiagnosed have a good prognosis (83% resolution in 1 year, 4% mortality) **(Plate 107).**

Examine carefully for clues:

- Petechial eruptions in meningococcemia and Rocky Mountain Spotted Fever **(Plate 139)**
- Pustular lesions in gonococcemia or staphylococcal sepsis **(Plate 75)**
- Ecthyma gangrenosum in Pseudomonas sepsis **(Plate 109)**

- Splinter hemorrhages, conjunctival hemorrhages, Roth spots, Osler's nodes, and Janeway lesions in endocarditis **(Plates 22, 23, 24)**
- Choroidal tubercles in miliary tuberculosis and candidemia
- Splenomegaly in endocarditis, lymphoma, and cirrhosis
- Hepatic bruit or friction rub in subphrenic abscess
- Temporal artery or scalp tenderness in giant cell arteritis
- Epitrochlear lymphadenopathy in syphilis

Extreme elevations of fever (>40°C) are found in heat stroke, hypothalamic dysfunction, meningitis, midbrain hemorrhage, falciparum malaria, Rocky Mountain Spotted Fever, typhus, sepsis, malignant hyperthermia, and hypernephroma.

Relative bradycardia occurs in salmonellosis (typhoid fever), meningitis with increased intracranial pressure, mycoplasma and legionella pneumonia, factitious fever, tularemia, brucellosis, mumps, hepatitis, and with concomitant beta blockers. Bradycardia in fever may also signal cardiac conduction abnormalities in acute rheumatic fever, Lyme disease, viral myocarditis, or endocarditis with valve ring abscess **(Plate 60).**

Relapsing fevers (days of fever alternating with days without) occur in brucellosis (fever with physical activity), Hodgkin's disease, extrapulmonary tuberculosis, malaria, and Lyme disease. Hectic fever (difference between peak and trough >1.5°C) suggests abscess, pyelonephritis, ascending cholangitis, tuberculosis, lymphoma, and drug reactions. Absence of diurnal variation suggests a central source. Reversal of the diurnal pattern ("typhus inversus") occurs with disseminated tuberculosis, typhoid fever, polyarteritis nodosa, and salicylate toxicity **(Plate 60).**

CLINICAL FINDINGS

HIV   Fever may be a prominent manifestation of acute or chronic HIV infection. It may be caused by the HIV infection itself, or it may be secondary to mycobacterium avian-complex, toxoplasmosis, cytomegalovirus, tuberculosis, pneumocystis, salmonellosis, cryptococcosis, histoplasmosis, non-Hodgkin's lymphoma, or drug fever.

Tuberculosis   Suspect tuberculosis in high-risk patients such as HIV-infected persons, homeless persons, recent Southeast Asian immigrants, or Native Americans. When FUO exists, tuberculosis is usually extrapulmonary (bones, nodes, renal, genital, or liver).

Endocarditis   Examine closely for splinter hemorrhages, splenomegaly, clubbing, conjunctival petechiae, or tender nodules on the hands (Osler's nodes) **(Plates 22, 23, 24).**

Osteomyelitis   Subacute in onset, there is dull, constant pain and soft tissue swelling/tenderness over the involved bone, with low-grade fever.

Malaria   Suspect malaria if the patient has a history of recent travel to the tropics. Tertian malaria, with fever every 2–3 days, occurs in vivax or ovale. Quartan malaria, in malariae, returns every fourth day. Falciparum malaria may have fever at irregular intervals. A palpable spleen and tender liver are often present in chronic malaria **(Plate 188).**

Syphilis   Secondary syphilis presents with a papulosquamous rash involving the palms and soles and generalized lymphadenopathy. A Jarisch-Herxheimer reaction, characterized by fever, increased rash, and malaise, may appear with treatment **(Plates 80, 81).**

Zoonoses   These should be considered in animal handlers, veterinarians, and butchers. Common syndromes include Lyme disease with erythema migrans at a deer tick bite site and arthritis, brucellosis with splenomegaly, lymphadenopathy, and hepatomegaly after drinking unpasteurized milk, and tularemia with fever and tender nodes in hunters and trappers **(Plates 106, 146).**

Typhoid fever   The fever progressively increases each night without tachycardia or rigors. Rose spots appear within the first week, as a rose-red 2–3 mm macule on the abdomen with blanching and a central punctum. Foul-smelling pea-soup diarrhea subsequently develops **(Plate 60).**

Chronic meningococcemia   The fever is intermittent with days during which the patient appears well. A maculopapular rash and arthralgias or arthritis wax and wane with the fever. Splenomegaly may be found in 20% **(Plate 32).**

Lymphoma   Fever is the presenting symptom (often with drenching night sweats), especially in Hodgkin's, with disease confined to the retroperitoneum or marrow. A Pel-Ebstein pattern, of relapsing fever of 3–10 days duration with a 3–10 day afebrile interlude, is seen in 16%. Non-Hodgkin's lymphoma often presents with fever, lymphadenopathy, hepatosplenomegaly and bone pain (especially sternal) **(Plate 159).**

Liver metastases   Fever is usually a late phenomenon in a patient with a known primary tumor. The liver contains hard palpable nodules.

Renal cell carcinoma   The classic triad of gross hematuria, flank pain, and a palpable abdominal mass occurs in only 10%. Systemic symptoms of fatigability, weight loss, and cachexia occur frequently. Renal vein involvement may produce a new left varicocele and lower extremity edema. Hormone secretion may produce hypertension, galactorrhea, feminization or masculinization, Cushing's, or symptomatic hypercalcemia **(Plates 10, 11, 15).**

Atrial myxoma   A changing murmur with tumor plop, embolic phenomena, and Raynaud's signal this rare phenomenon **(Plate 36).**

Giant cell arteritis   Consider when an elderly patient develops a new headache associated with a tender, ropy, or nodular temporal artery and/or fever. Polymyalgia rheumatica with proximal muscle pain and weakness is also part of the spectrum.

Systemic lupus erythematosus   Fever can be caused by the lupus itself or by a complicating infection. Malar rash, Raynaud's, serositis, and arthritis are important clues **(Plates 91, 92).**

Vasculitis   Consider vasculitis in a patient with systemic illness with glomerulonephritis, palpable purpura, necrotic skin lesions, mononeuritis multiplex, or pulse asymmetry **(Plate 110).**

Rheumatic fever   An antecedent sore throat, arthralgias or arthritis, carditis, and erythema marginatum are clues to diagnosis **(Plate 108).**

Still's disease   It occurs in a young adult with high fever, evanescent rash (coinciding with fever spikes), lymphadenopathy, hepatosplenomegaly, and arthralgias **(Plate 107).**

Drugs   Fever may be due to serum sickness, allergy, or immune-mediated vasculitis. A maculopapular rash, eosinophilia, and absence of chills are clues. Antibiotics (especially penicillin and sulfonamides), phenytoin, isoniazid, thiouracils, procainamide, quinidine, methyldopa, hydralazine, barbiturates, allopurinol, captopril, quinidine, and phenolthalein are notable causes. Drugs producing immediate fever include amphotericin, bleomycin, high dose cyclophosphamide, and antithymocyte globulin **(Plates 181, 182, 183).**

Heat stroke   Patients present with high fever, absence of sweating, delirium, or coma. Suspect in hot weather, with precipitants of exercise in high heat and humidity, or drugs such as anticholinergics, antiparkinson agents, diuretics, and phenothiazines.

Factitious   There are two types: manufactured fever and self-injection with foreign substances. Clues include medical training, failure to follow a normal diurnal curve, excessively high temperature (106–107°), lack of tachycardia or diaphoresis with fever, and normal temperature immediately after a (false) high reading.

Malignant hyperthermia   Extreme temperature elevations may occur in patients taking general anesthetics (halothane or succinylcholine), MAO inhibitors combined with meperidine, or neuroleptics, including phenothiazines, haloperidol, fluoxetine, tricyclic antidepressants, and metoclopramide (neuroleptic malignant syndrome). Rigidity is present.

Multiple pulmonary emboli   Consider in a patient with transient migratory pleuritic chest pain and shortness of breath **(Plate 42).**

Involuntary Weight Loss
Chapter 6

PLATES 6, 12, 13, 19, 20, 22, 23, 24, 57, 61, 63, 64, 67, 68, 69, 166, 167

◤ DIFFERENTIAL OVERVIEW

- ❏ Diabetes
- ❏ Depression
- ❏ Inadequate intake
- ❏ Drugs
- ❏ Hyperthyroidism
- ❏ Occult cancer
- ❏ Low cardiac output
- ❏ Anorexia nervosa
- ❏ Malabsorption
- ❏ Chronic infection
- ❏ Adrenal insufficiency

DIAGNOSTIC APPROACH

Most of the causes of weight loss will be evident, based on concurrent symptoms. If not, first document that weight loss has occurred by using prior records of measured weights or the discovery of loose-fitting clothes (tightening belt notches) or dentures. If the cause is not found on the first pass, document the weight and reexamine several weeks later.

Weight loss in patients with congestive heart failure, cirrhosis, and uremia may be masked by fluid retention, but temporalis and limb wasting will be prominent.

CLINICAL FINDINGS

Diabetes   At the onset, weight loss is primarily caused by osmotic diuresis with polyuria/nocturia. Later glycosuria produces caloric loss, combined with the increased catabolic state of insulin deficiency and glucagon excess **(Plates 166, 167).**

Depression   It is recognized by sadness, anhedonia, anorexia, and sleep disturbance.

Inadequate intake   Common causes include painful oral lesions (phenytoin gum hypertrophy, vitamin deficiency glossitis, heavy metal intoxication, candidiasis, poor dentition), solitary living in the elderly, early dementia, food fads, abnormal taste (hepatitis, zinc deficiency, drugs), or abdominal pain associated with eating (intestinal ischemia). With protein-calorie malnutrition, the skin is dry and baggy. There is weakness, tremor, polyuria, edema, and ascites **(Plates 61, 67, 68, 69).**

Drugs   Weight loss is associated with cholestyramine, digoxin, diuretics, oral hypoglycemics, cytotoxics, amphetamines, and sibutramine.

Hyperthyroidism   Despite an increased appetite, weight loss occurs. Tachycardia, fine tremor, silky skin, and eye signs (exophthalmos or lid lag) are useful clues. Apathetic hyperthyroidism can occur in elderly patients producing listlessness and tachycardia or atrial fibrillation **(Plates 19, 20).**

Occult cancer   Pancreatic cancer is the prototype, with aversion to food, and weight loss (20–40 lbs) that precedes visceral pain or jaundice, and is not proportional to size of the tumor. Weight loss is usually marked in gastric and pancreatic cancer, moderate in prostate, colon, and lung cancer, and mild in breast cancer **(Plates 63, 64).**

Low cardiac output   Easy fatigability, dyspnea on exertion, bibasilar rales, peripheral edema, third and/or fourth heart sounds, and jugular venous distension are found **(Plate 6).**

Anorexia nervosa   The patient is preoccupied with body weight, yet is unconcerned about being obviously very thin. There is usually overactivity, often the form of vigorous exercise, despite cachexia. Secretiveness leads to the false appearance of involuntary weight loss **(Plate 57).**

Malabsorption   Fat malabsorption produces sticky and greasy stools, borborygmi, abdominal distension, and vague abdominal pain. Malabsorption is also associated with loss of lipid-soluble vitamins, which sometimes produces peripheral neuropathy, anemia, dermatitis, or bleeding. Sprue causes a malabsorption syndrome, bone pain with compression deformities, and anxiety/depression.

Chronic infection   Fever is the key sign. Common occult causes include bacterial endocarditis, osteomyelitis, tuberculosis, and HIV **(Plates 22, 23, 24).**

Adrenal insufficiency   Fatigue, hypotension, and hyperpigmentation—especially when seen in the palmar creases or buccal mucosa—are important findings **(Plates 12, 13).**

Lymphadenopathy

PLATES 80, 81, 88, 89, 169, 170, 171, 172, 173, 174, 179, 181, 182, 183, 204, 206, 229, 230

◼ DIFFERENTIAL OVERVIEW

Generalized
- ❏ Infectious mononucleosis
- ❏ Drugs
- ❏ Connective tissue disease
- ❏ HIV infection
- ❏ Sarcoidosis
- ❏ Serum sickness
- ❏ Toxoplasmosis
- ❏ Secondary syphilis

Localized
- ❏ Regional infection
- ❏ Lymphadenitis
- ❏ Hodgkin's disease
- ❏ Cat-scratch disease

DIAGNOSTIC APPROACH

Palpable adenopathy is present in half of healthy young adults. Red flags for malignancy include a node larger than 2 cm in size and enlarging, age older than 40 years (LR 5), weight loss greater than 10% (LR 3), and a supraclavicular node (LR 10). On occasion, reactive lymphadenopathy may persist for months, but observation for enlargement over time is a useful tool to select which patients need biopsy. Nodes with an irregular shape and rubbery consistency suggest malignancy. Matted nodes can be found with inflammation or malignancy.

Coexistence of splenomegaly implies a systemic illness such as lymphoma/leukemia, lupus, EBV, sarcoidosis, toxoplasmosis, or cat-scratch disease.

Structures that may be mistaken for cervical lymph nodes include the parotid gland, thyroglossal and branchial cysts, an abscess, a lipoma, thyroid nodules, submaxillary infections, or dental infections.

Suppuration occurs with tuberculosis, streptococcal infections, anthrax, cat-scratch disease, plague, tularemia, chancroid, lymphogranuloma venereum, or sporotrichosis.

The location of adenopathy often narrows the differential:

- **Anterior cervical** Unilateral: pharyngitis, thyroid cancer, nasopharyngeal cancer, or buccal infection. Bilateral: pharyngitis, mononucleosis, sarcoidosis, or toxoplasmosis.
- **Preauricular** They are common in oculoglandular fevers such as adenoviral conjunctivitis, rubella, tularemia, and leptospirosis. These are also commonly found in infection in the cheek, eyelid, ear, or temporal scalp. If a source is not evident, look for a retinal melanoma.
- **Posterior auricular** Consider infectious mononucleosis, rubella, or otitis media.
- **Right supraclavicular** Consider an intrathoracic (pulmonary, mediastinal, or esophageal) malignancy.
- **Left supraclavicular** A sentinel or Virchow's node, via the thoracic duct, suggests intraabdominal, renal, testicular, or ovarian malignancy and tuberculous peritonitis.
- **Axillary** Consider breast malignancy, upper extremity infection, and Hodgkin's disease.
- **Epitrochlear** Consider syphilis (bilateral), hand infection (unilateral), and rheumatoid arthritis (helps differentiate from osteoarthritis).
- **Inguinal** Consider syphilis, genital herpes, chancroid, lymphogranuloma venereum, and lower extremity infection. A femoral hernia can be confused with adenopathy.
- **Occipital** Consider scalp infection (especially pediculosis capitis), secondary syphilis, Hodgkin's disease, and tuberculosis.
- **Periumbilical** Consider abdominal malignancy.

Lymphadenopathy

CLINICAL FINDINGS

Infectious mononucleosis   The typical presentation is in an adolescent or young adult with prominent fatigue, fever, and sore throat with exudative tonsillitis. Posterior cervical adenopathy and splenomegaly (50%) may be found. Petechiae can often be seen at the junction of the soft and hard palate **(Plates 229, 230)**.

Drugs   Lymphadenopathy can be caused by phenytoin, allopurinol, hydralazine, carbamazepine, antithyroid medications, and isoniazid.

Connective tissue disease   In rheumatoid arthritis, adenopathy occurs in areas draining the involved joints. Felty's syndrome (with neutropenia) is marked by splenomegaly and generalized lymphadenopathy. Mixed connective tissue disease, lupus, and Sjogren's are also associated with lymphadenopathy **(Plates 88, 89)**.

HIV infection   Lymphadenopathy occurs in 75% of patients with acute HIV syndrome. Consider this in a patient with fever; widespread diffuse maculopapular rash, including the palms and mucocutaneous ulceration; and a recent high-risk exposure. Chronic undiagnosed HIV infection can be recognized by noting weight loss, thrush, fever, and HIV risk factors **(Plate 206)**.

Sarcoidosis   Parotid or lacrimal gland enlargement is common. Skin lesions are waxy and reddish-brown or deeply indurated. Scalp lesions with scarring alopecia may also occur **(Plates 169, 170, 171)**.

Serum sickness   Consider when fever, rash, and acute polyarthritis occur in a patient who is taking a new medication **(Plates 181, 182, 183)**.

Toxoplasmosis   Look for exposure to cats or turtles **(Plate 204)**.

Secondary syphilis   A generalized scaling rash including the palms and soles is characteristic. Painless silver-gray erosions on the oral or genital mucosa may also be found **(Plates 80, 81)**.

Regional infection   Infection may be subtle, such as dermatophytes or scabies. Gardening scrapes may be infected with sporotrichosis **(Plates 172, 173, 179)**.

Lymphadenitis   A tender, warm, red, rapidly enlarging node reflects acute pyogenic infection of the node itself.

Hodgkin's disease   A chain of large, rubbery, nontender nodes; a palpable spleen; and lymphoma B symptoms of night sweats and fever are helpful clues. Alcohol consumption may produce pain in the nodes.

Cat-scratch disease   The primary lesion is similar to a furuncle, associated with unilateral regional lymphadenopathy. Lymphangitis is absent, but constitutional symptoms are present **(Plate 174)**.

Multiple Somatic Complaints

Chapter 8

PLATES 16, 17, 18

◼ DIFFERENTIAL OVERVIEW

❑ Anxiety
❑ Depression
❑ Hypothyroidism
❑ Premenstrual syndrome
❑ Hypochondriasis
❑ Somatization disorder
❑ Chronic fatigue syndrome
❑ Fibromyalgia
❑ Panic disorder
❑ Malingering
❑ Conversion reaction

DIAGNOSTIC APPROACH

This presentation is marked by multiple vague complaints, symptoms out of proportion to the physical findings or anticipated spectrum of physical illness, and symptoms that do not follow anatomic distributions. The patient is often more concerned with the physician accepting authenticity of symptoms than relieving them. Vague, diffuse descriptions or overly detailed vivid and elaborate ones are suggestive. The patient often seems to be amplifying normal bodily sensations. Psychological factors may be revealed in the symbolic choice of words (e.g., "pain in the neck").

"Stress" for most patients is an acceptable framework within which to obtain psychological information. Care must be taken during the interview *not* to suggest that the symptoms are "all in the head."

A thorough and thoughtful history and physical examination are preferred to a battery of tests, but somatization remains a diagnosis of exclusion.

CLINICAL FINDINGS

Anxiety   Chronic anxiety presents with a pattern of the patient focusing on and becoming alarmed by normal bodily sensations. Patients will often suspect the most dire cause. Acute anxiety may present with physical symptoms, such as palpitations, chest pain, tachycardia, shortness of breath, diarrhea, or lightheadedness.

Depression   Although multiple vague somatic symptoms are often the presenting finding, vegetative signs of depression such as change in weight and appetite, sleep disorder, fatigue, and decreased libido are usually present if searched for. Finding depressed affect, anhedonia, and abnormal cognition is also helpful. Typical patterns may be unusual worry and preoccupation with the body, a "positive review of systems," chronic pain, symptoms related to multiple organ systems, and "complaints" that are difficult to characterize pathophysiologically.

Hypothyroidism   Sluggishness, constipation, impaired concentration, cold intolerance, and edema are typical of the vague symptoms caused by this condition **(Plates 16, 17, 18).**

Premenopausal syndrome   This occurs cyclically with the menses and is characterized by irritability, fatigue, depressed mood, and waxing and waning somatic symptoms. The pathophysiology is unknown.

Hypochondriasis   Chronically preoccupied with their bodies and health, patients are convinced that they have a serious occult disease. Symptoms shift and fluctuate, but worry is constant and is not assuaged by reasonable reassurance. The patient uses language that is often very "medicalized." Many symptoms are recited in boring detail—a process known as the "organ recital." The patient's chart becomes quite thick with trivial diagnoses unless he or she changes doctors frequently, searching for "answers."

Somatization disorder   This is characterized by multiple symptoms in multiple organ systems, medically unexplained, and severe enough to lead the patient to take treatment or see a physician. The onset is usually before age 30 and is associated with depression and with chaotic interpersonal relationships.

Chronic fatigue syndrome   This syndrome is recognized by prominent persistent fatigue that interferes with role function and other somatic complaints such as impaired concentration and short-term memory, low-grade fevers, arthralgias, and adenopathy. It may be a subset of the aforementioned diagnoses; however, it is suspected by some (especially sufferers) to be viral in origin.

Fibromyalgia   Fatigue and poorly referent periarticular pain and stiffness are found. Exquisite tenderness at 11 or more of the 18 specific trigger points is the most helpful finding. Paired sites include the base of the skull, the neck at C5-7, the midtrapezius, the upper medial scapula, the second costochondral junction, the lateral epicondyle, the upper outer buttock, the posterior greater trochanter, and the medial fat pad of the knee.

Panic disorder   It presents with discrete unprovoked attacks of anxiety and a sense of impending doom, accompanied by symptoms of dyspnea, palpitations, dizziness, tremors, sweating, choking, nausea, paresthesias, and/or chest pain.

Malingering   Consider this explanation when obvious secondary gain (often litigation) is pending and the patient has exaggerated symptoms, demonstrates suggestibility, and varies his or her description of symptoms. A self-limited form of this is seen in persons required by their jobs to have a medical excuse for a day off.

Conversion reaction   Symptoms are either sensory or neuromuscular, such as weakness, paralysis, ataxia, blindness, anesthesia, seizures, or aphasia. Clues include short-lived symptoms, a prior history of similar reactions, major emotional stress prior to the onset of symptoms, symbolic meaning to the symptoms, inappropriate lack of concern about the symptoms ("la belle indifference"), secondary gain contingent upon illness, or the presence of other psychopathology.

Obesity

Chapter 9

PLATES 10, 11, 16, 17, 18

◤ DIFFERENTIAL OVERVIEW

❑ Caloric excess
❑ Depression
❑ Drugs
❑ Hypothyroidism
❑ Hypogonadism
❑ Cushing's syndrome
❑ Polycystic ovary syndrome
❑ Hypothalamic
❑ Insulinoma

DIAGNOSTIC APPROACH

Abdominal obesity (apple shape) is associated with an increased incidence of adverse outcomes (waist–hip ratio >0.95 in men and >0.85 in women). A body mass index (BMI) kg/m^2 greater than 30 also correlates with increased risk. Important complications of obesity include type II diabetes, sleep apnea syndrome, steatohepatitis, gallstones, gout, degenerative joint disease, and accelerated atherogenesis.

Less than 1% of obesity has an endocrine or other secondary cause.

CLINICAL FINDINGS

Caloric excess   Weight gain is commonly caused by an imbalance between energy intake and use, either voluntary or via an altered hypothalamic "set point." A familial form occurs in childhood or with onset of puberty and is characterized by peripheral as well as central obesity.

Depression   Diagnostic clues include depressed mood, anhedonia, and an altered sleep pattern, especially with early morning awakening.

Drugs   Glucocorticoids, oral contraceptives, phenothiazines, cyproheptadine, and tricyclic antidepressants all cause weight gain.

Hypothyroidism   Cold intolerance (obese individuals are usually heat intolerant), dry waxy skin, constipation, delayed deep-tendon relaxation phase, and goiter are helpful clues **(Plates 16, 17, 18).**

Hypogonadism   This is a common cause of modest weight gain in the perimenopausal period.

Cushing's syndrome   Truncal obesity with thin limbs is typical. Purple striae, plethoric moon facies, and a buffalo hump are usually found to some degree **(Plates 10, 11).**

Polycystic ovary syndrome   It is associated with hirsutism, acne, irregular menses/oligomenorrhea, and infertility.

Hypothalamic   This is characterized by marked and uncontrollable hyperphagia. Other manifestations of hypothalamic and pituitary dysfunction are usually present. Causes may include craniopharyngioma, sarcoidosis, cyst, or tuberculous encephalitis.

Insulinoma   Modest weight gain occurs with a history of episodic hyperepinepherinemic and hypoglycemic symptoms.

Chapter 10

Prevention Phenomena

◪ DIFFERENTIAL OVERVIEW

Cancer Screening
❏ Prostate cancer
❏ Breast cancer
❏ Ovarian cancer
❏ Colon cancer
❏ Thyroid cancer
❏ Testicular cancer

Cardiovascular Screening
❏ Cardiovascular risk
❏ Carotid stenosis
❏ Renal artery stenosis
❏ Abdominal aortic aneurysm

Other
❏ Osteoporosis
❏ HIV

CLINICAL FINDINGS

Prostate cancer   Digital rectal exam screening for the findings of nodule, induration, or asymmetry has Se 0.58, Sp 0.96, and LR 14.5.

Breast cancer   Clinical breast examination has Se 0.83, Sp 0.88, and LR 6.9 when used in the screening setting. Characteristics such as stony hardness, fixation to underlying tissues, and indistinct borders help differentiate cancer from benign lesions.

Ovarian cancer   A pelvic/ovarian mass on exam has Se 0.93, Sp 0.63, and LR 2.0 for cancer. Although the presence of a mass is not very indicative of cancer, the absence of a mass reduces the likelihood of cancer tenfold.

Colon cancer   Optimistic estimates for occult blood screening are Se 0.80, Sp 0.85, and LR 5.3. Screening patients older than 45 years results in 3–5% positive, of which 10–15% have cancer and 20–30% have polyps. Colonoscopy should be pursued if any one of three tests is positive. Most cancers found will be Duke's A or B with a 5-year survival of 80% or more.

Thyroid cancer   A palpable nodule may be detected in 4–7% of adults, of which only 5% are cancer. Findings suggesting high risk are rapid growth, very firm consistency, fixation, vocal cord paralysis, enlarged regional lymph nodes, or family history of medullary cancer.

Testicular cancer   It presents in a young man as a firm, heavy nontender mass, which does not transilluminate. An enlarged left supraclavicular node, adherence to the scrotum, or gynecomastia increase the likelihood of cancer.

Cardiovascular risk   An ankle/brachial index of less than 0.9 predicts a fivefold increase in cardiovascular mortality whereas a waist/hip ratio of greater than 0.9 indicates that mortality is increased by 3.4 times. A blood pressure of 140/95 in men and 160/95 in women is associated with a 50% increase in cardiovascular mortality.

Carotid stenosis   A carotid bruit is a moderately good marker for high-grade carotid stenosis (>70%), with Se 0.63–0.71, Sp 0.61–0.79, and LR 1.6–3.4. Bruit is most predictive of outcome in the presence of ipsilateral transient ischemic symptoms.

Renal artery stenosis   An abdominal or flank bruit has Se 0.49, Sp 0.93, and LR 7.0 for renal artery stenosis. A systolic/diastolic bruit is rare, but highly specific with Se 0.39, Sp 0.99, and LR 39.

Abdominal aortic aneurysm   A pulsatile upper abdominal mass is very specific for abdominal aortic aneurysm (0.97), but the sensitivity is low (0.28–0.34). If a pulsatile mass is felt, a workup should be conducted.

Osteoporosis   Premature graying, especially salt-and-pepper hair, has an Se 0.50, Sp 0.81, and LR 2.6 for osteoporosis.

HIV   Ability to recognize the acute retroviral syndrome has import for the early use of antiretroviral therapy. The combination of fever (Se 0.96), lymphadenopathy (0.74), pharyngitis (0.70), and rash (0.70) in a patient with potential exposures should raise suspicion. Rash characteristics may be helpful: an erythematous maculopapular rash including the palms and soles, or mucocutaneous ulceration involving the mouth, esophagus, or genitals.

Section II
Heart/Vascular

Acute Chest Pain

PLATES 25, 36, 42, 43, 44, 45, 91, 92, 141, 198, 211

◪ DIFFERENTIAL OVERVIEW

Nonpleuritic
❏ Chest wall pain
❏ Angina
❏ Unstable angina
❏ Myocardial infarction
❏ Esophageal spasm
❏ Herpes zoster
❏ Thoracic root compression
❏ Panic disorder
❏ Aortic dissection
❏ Mediastinal mass
❏ Biliary disease

Pleuritic
❏ Costochondritis
❏ Pneumonia
❏ Rib fracture
❏ Pulmonary embolism
❏ Pleurisy
❏ Pneumothorax
❏ Pericarditis
❏ Lung cancer
❏ Pneumomediastinum
❏ Splenic infarction

DIAGNOSTIC APPROACH

It is essential to maintain a high index of suspicion (low threshold for investigation) for critical problems; however, most chest pain has a benign cause. *Pleuritic* chest pain, intensified by a deep breath, usually has a pulmonary or chest wall origin. Recurrent episodic pain or persistent pain lasting days is unlikely to represent a critical problem. Pain lasting a few seconds or pain that is sharp or stabbing in quality is almost never ischemic.

"Angor anomie," a sense of impending doom, is found in serious conditions such as myocardial infarction, pulmonary embolism, aortic dissection, and to a lesser extent, panic disorder.

Sternal pain may be caused by xiphoidalgia, myelomatosis, ankylosing spondylitis, osteomyelitis, or traumatic fracture.

CLINICAL FINDINGS

Chest wall pain   Pain is characteristically aggravated by deep inspiration or movement, and exactly reproduced or heightened by direct pressure. Press on the contralateral side as a control. Coughing and repetitive motion of the shoulder girdle are the usual precipitants.

Angina   Substernal chest pressure caused by exertion or emotion and relieved by rest or nitroglycerin is typical. Patients will often be reluctant to call the symptom pain, referring to it as pressure, heaviness, or tightness, and they often attribute it to indigestion. A closed fist held to the sternum is commonly used to explain the symptoms. Pain is predominantly left-sided and may radiate to the jaw, neck, or shoulder, with left arm numbness. A fourth heart sound may accompany the pain.

Unstable angina   This form of ischemia may be difficult to diagnose, as it may not have a clear relationship to exertion. A *high risk* for subsequent myocardial infarction is characterized by prolonged ongoing chest pain, pulmonary edema, or angina with a new or worsening S3, mitral regurgitation, or hypotension. An *intermediate risk* of MI is signaled by prolonged (>20 minutes) chest pain with a high likelihood of CAD, rest angina (>20 minutes) now resolved with nitroglycerin, nocturnal angina, and new NYHA

Acute Chest Pain

Class III or IV angina within 2 weeks. *Low-risk* unstable angina includes increased frequency, severity, or duration; angina provoked at a lower exertional threshold; and new-onset angina within 2 weeks. Vasospastic angina is a variant that occurs at rest in patients with a vasospastic substrate (e.g., Raynaud's or migraine) **(Plate 36).**

Myocardial infarction Prolonged, crushing substernal pain is the prototype. The pain is similar to established angina but more intense and prolonged. The episode is often preceded by an unstable angina pattern. Diaphoresis and hypotension are common. Nausea and bradycardia should suggest inferior ischemia but can be distractors when the pain is epigastric in location. Pain radiating to the arm, neck, or jaw has a likelihood ratio of 3:4 for MI. On occasion, the pain is only perceived in the distal radiation, as a toothache or tennis elbow pain.

Esophageal spasm A sharp substernal pain occurs on a substrate of heartburn. It is precipitated by swallowing and referred substernally to the level of the lesion.

Herpes zoster Pain may occur as a prodrome preceding development of lesions. There will be a unilateral dermatomal distribution of a sharp, burning, or numb dysesthesia **(Plate 141).**

Thoracic root compression Thoracic radiculopathy is unusual because of the splinting provided by the ribs. When it occurs, one must consider an expanding lesion (e.g., infection or cancer).

Panic disorder Symptoms occur in paroxysms of substernal heaviness, accompanied by lightheadedness, palpitations, nervousness, and weakness. The patient feels a strong sense of panic and impending catastrophe. The patient's anxiety is notable even after the symptoms resolve.

Aortic dissection Dissection presents as a tearing pain with a sudden onset at maximal severity. It travels in location with the progression of the dissection, and it often radiates between the scapulae. The patient will appear quite restless, constantly in motion in an attempt to find a comfortable position. Asymmetry of pulses is a critical clue, as is a new aortic insufficiency murmur. Blood pressure may be normal in the presence of gray cyanosis. There may be a history of hypertension, blunt chest trauma, or Marfan's with high arched palate and long limbs **(Plates 25, 43, 44, 45).**

Mediastinal mass Symptoms begin with a vague sense of central pressure, accompanied by dyspnea and cough, which becomes increasingly severe over time.

Biliary disease The epicenter of the pain is in the epigastrium. Biliary colic may be relieved by nitroglycerin.

Costochondritis Pain is localized over the costochondral junctions, which will be exquisitely tender with palpation.

Pneumonia Pleuritic pain, fever, and cough that produces colored sputum are the hallmarks of pneumonia.

Rib fracture Pain is usually preceded by a history of chest wall trauma or malignancy although vigorous cough may precipitate it. There is exquisite tenderness focally over a rib.

Pulmonary embolism High suspicion must be maintained for pulmonary embolism. Pleuritic pain occurs in only 10% of cases of pulmonary embolism, and when present, suggests pulmonary infarction. Look for associated signs of acute dyspnea, hemoptysis, and an embolic source (e.g., leg swelling) **(Plate 42).**

Pleurisy Pain is worsened by deep inspiration or cough but is not affected by palpation. There is often a friction rub and low-grade fever. This may be caused by bacterial pneumonia or primary viral infection (e.g., coxsackievirus), pulmonary infarction, neoplasm, uremia, or connective tissue disease (lupus) **(Plates 91, 92, 211).**

Pneumothorax Acute pleuritic chest pain and dyspnea are the principal symptoms. With a large pneumothorax, there may be unilateral diminished or distant breath sounds, increased tympany, and decreased chest movement on the affected side. It commonly occurs in a young asthenic patient or in one with emphysema. A tension pneumothorax produces rapidly developing shock with chest tympany and a tracheal shift.

Pericarditis Pain is usually sharp and pleuritic, increased with twisting, coughing, breathing deeply, swallowing, and lying supine. It is characteristically relieved by sitting up and leaning forward. A two-component or three-component friction rub with a to-and-fro cadence is a key finding. Inflammation of the diaphragmatic pleura may cause radiation to the trapezius, costal margin, or shoulder. Inflammation may arise from underlying causes such as a recent myocardial infarction, viral infection, uremia, tuberculosis, or connective tissue disease. Noninflammatory causes such as uremia may progress to tamponade with little pain **(Plate 198).**

Lung cancer   Pain occurs when there is pleural involvement and is often accompanied by a unilateral effusion, marked by dullness to percussion.

Pneumomediastinum   It presents with a retrosternal "crunch" on exam, central chest pain, and dyspnea.

Splenic infarction   It appears with low left anterior chest pain and a friction rub.

Anemia

Chapter 12

PLATES 64, 69, 134, 188, 189

 DIFFERENTIAL OVERVIEW

- ❏ Iron deficiency
- ❏ Chronic disease
- ❏ Vitamin B12 deficiency
- ❏ Subacute blood loss
- ❏ Thalassemia trait
- ❏ Folate deficiency
- ❏ Sickle cell trait
- ❏ Immune hemolytic anemia
- ❏ Aplastic anemia
- ❏ Sideroblastic anemia

DIAGNOSTIC APPROACH

Symptoms include dyspnea on exertion, fatigue, headache, palpitations, difficulty concentrating, and tinnitus. There are few symptoms when the anemia is gradual in onset and the patient is otherwise healthy.

Tachycardia and a systolic flow murmur occur when hemoglobin is less than 7.5. Pallor is found in the conjunctivae and notably in the palmar creases with hand extension (they normally flush). Press the base of the nail to observe blanching and flushing, comparing with the color of your own nailbeds. Always test for orthostatic blood pressure changes to assess acuteness of blood loss. Check stools for occult blood. Splenomegaly is found in hemolysis, pernicious anemia, liver diseases, infection, and thalassemia. In chronic anemia, there will be strong pulses with a wide pulse pressure and a midsystolic murmur.

Heavy menses are recognized by clots and gushing of blood with tampon removal. A family history of anemia suggests hemoglobinopathy (e.g., sickle cell anemia or thalassemia). Drug or toxin exposure suggests aplastic anemia, myelodysplasia, or G6PD hemolysis. Glossitis is seen with iron, folate, or vitamin B12 deficiency. Lymphadenopathy is seen with marrow infiltration or infection.

CLINICAL FINDINGS

Iron deficiency Specific symptoms include paresthesias, burning tongue, and dysphagia. Pica, which is a craving for dirt, clay, or other substances not fit as food, or more commonly, ice craving may be seen in 50%. Findings include atrophic glossitis and angular cheilitis. Spoon nails with thinning and ridging are fairly specific. The most common cause is blood loss, either menstrual in young women or GI in older patients. Occult blood will usually be found concurrently in the stool if it is the source **(Plates 188, 189)**.

Chronic disease Chronic inflammatory diseases, chronic infections, neoplasms, cirrhosis, and renal failure are the common causes, and these causes are usually evident although they may be occult (e.g., pancreatic cancer).

Vitamin B12 deficiency This deficiency is usually caused by pernicious anemia, which may be associated with immune thyroiditis or vitiligo, or to blind loop syndrome. Symptoms include numbness in the extremities (the earliest sign), sore tongue, anorexia, diarrhea, memory impairment, and depression. Physical findings of glossitis, cheilitis, and loss of position and vibratory sense are common on exam. The skin is lemon-yellow, which is caused by a mild increase in bilirubin combined with the pallor of anemia. Premature graying of the hair occurs **(Plate 69)**.

Subacute blood loss Although presenting with anemia, subacute blood loss will usually have an evident source, such as black, sticky stools or a history of heavy menses.

Thalassemia trait Consider this in patients with microcytic anemia and Mediterranean ancestry.

Folate deficiency No neurological deficits are present. Folate deficiency is recognized by the setting: dietary (alcohol abuse, no fruits or vegetables), increased metabolic demand (pregnancy, psoriasis, cancer), malabsorption (sprue, phenytoin), and direct antagonism (methotrexate, trimethoprim, triamterene). Sprue is recognized by weight loss, steatorrhea, hyperpigmentation, and circumoral fissuring.

Sickle cell trait   Sickle crisis with abdominal pain may first occur with low oxygen tension, such as on an airplane flight. The patient is usually of African descent.

Immune hemolytic anemia   It is usually drug-related, with quinidine, penicillin, or methyldopa the most common agents. Splenomegaly is a hallmark. Jaundice with dark urine is also present **(Plate 64).**

Aplastic anemia   Fatigue and bleeding are the initial symptoms. There is no splenomegaly. Chloramphenicol and propylthiouracil are classic causes.

Sideroblastic anemia   A preleukemic type occurs in elderly patients. The liver and spleen are palpable in more than 50% of cases. A secondary type is associated with rheumatoid arthritis, polyarteritis, malabsorption, alcoholism, porphyria, lead poisoning, and pyridoxine deficiency **(Plate 134).**

Arterial Pulse Variants

PLATES 19, 31, 33, 144

◼ DIFFERENTIAL OVERVIEW

Phenomena
- ❏ Irregularly irregular pulse
- ❏ Asymmetric pulses
- ❏ Bounding pulse
- ❏ Bisferiens pulse
- ❏ Bigeminal pulse
- ❏ Pulsus alternans
- ❏ Pulsus paradoxus
- ❏ Thready pulse
- ❏ Pulsus parvus et tardus
- ❏ Narrow pulse pressure

DIAGNOSTIC APPROACH

Examine the pulse using the method of trisection: apply pressure until the pulse is maximal, and then vary pressure while concentrating on phases of the pulse.

Early Chinese medicine based diagnosis primarily on careful examination of the pulse. There were six sets of pulses, each connected with a certain part of the body and each able to register even the subtlest physiological changes within it. The principal pulses were *Fu*, a light-flowing pulse like a piece of wood floating on water; *Ch'en*, a deeply impressed pulse like a stone thrown into water; *Ch'ih*, a pulse with three beats to one cycle of respiration; and *Shu*, a pulse with six beats to one cycle of respiration.

CLINICAL FINDINGS

Irregularly irregular pulse   A hallmark of atrial fibrillation, the amplitude of each beat varies with the filling interval. It can also be found with PVCs, PACs, and multifocal atrial tachycardia. PVCs are recognized by a regular rhythm with a dropped beat followed by a compensatory pause, then a beat of increased amplitude. PACs throw the rhythm out of synchrony.

Asymmetric pulses   Consider subclavian artery atherosclerosis, arterial thrombosis (especially with atrial fibrillation), thoracic outlet compression, or aortic dissection.

Bounding pulse   A hyperkinetic pulse with a rapid large-amplitude upstroke and rapid collapse is associated with increased stroke volume or decreased arterial compliance. The classic "collapsing pulse" is found in aortic regurgitation, along with the manifestations of diastolic murmur, pulsating retinal arteries, and nailbed pulsations (Quincke's pulses). It also occurs in thyrotoxicosis (a rapid and snapping pulse), pregnancy, fever, anemia, patent ductus arteriosus, and arteriovenous fistula. A slow, bounding pulse, which is caused by a prolonged ventricular filling time, may be found in complete heart block **(Plate 19).**

Bisferiens pulse   The pattern is a tapping percussion wave with a rapid early rise, a decline, then a second tidal wave. This pulse is classically found in hypertrophic cardiomyopathy and in combined aortic stenosis and regurgitation.

Bigeminal pulse   It is palpable as a strong pulse alternating with a weak one, the second beat caused by decreased ventricular filling with an early contraction. Occasionally, the alternate beat is so weak as to be nonpalpable, in which case the auscultated heart rate is twice the palpated pulse. It is found in ventricular bigeminy and digoxin overdose.

Pulsus alternans   The amplitude varies with each pulse and is accentuated after a premature contraction. A loud S3 gallop is usually present. Although usually owing to severe left ventricular dysfunction, a decreased pulse after a premature contraction suggests hypertrophic obstructive cardiomyopathy.

Pulsus paradoxus   The easiest way to obtain this measurement is to start above systole, deflating the cuff until the first sounds are heard, with the pulse disappearing during inspiration. Continue to deflate the cuff until the heart sounds are rapid and regular. A difference between these measures of more than 10 mm Hg is abnormal. Increased pulsus

Chapter 13   **Arterial Pulse Variants**

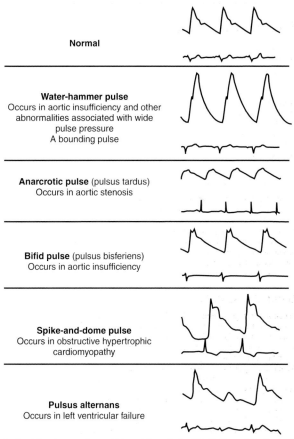

Normal

Water-hammer pulse
Occurs in aortic insufficiency and other
abnormalities associated with wide
pulse pressure
A bounding pulse

Anarcrotic pulse (pulsus tardus)
Occurs in aortic stenosis

Bifid pulse (pulsus bisferiens)
Occurs in aortic insufficiency

Spike-and-dome pulse
Occurs in obstructive hypertrophic
cardiomyopathy

Pulsus alternans
Occurs in left ventricular failure

Figure 1. Arterial pulse waveforms. (Adapted from: Judge RD, Zuidema GD, Fitzgerald
FT. Clinical Diagnosis. 5th ed. Boston: Little, Brown, 1989, p. 258.)

paradoxus may be observed in severe asthma (FEV1<0.5 L, Se 0.80), pericardial tamponade (Se 0.70–1.0), pulmonary embolism (Se 0.30), and hypovolemic shock (Se
0.50). It does not occur with constrictive pericarditis, severe CHF, or right ventricular
failure.
Thready pulse   A low-volume thready pulse is found in hypovolemic or septic shock, severe aortic stenosis, and severe left ventricular dysfunction. Intense vasoconstriction
may produce a diminished pulse with normal stroke volumes (**Plates 31, 33, 144**).
Pulsus parvus et tardus   The classic finding in hemodynamically significant aortic
stenosis, the carotid pulse is low in volume and has a slowly rising upstroke with a prolonged plateau. A "shudder" may also be felt.
Narrow pulse pressure   Defined as (systolic−diastolic)/systolic <0.25, it may be found
with pericardial tamponade, constrictive pericarditis, or aortic stenosis.

Bradycardia

Chapter 14

PLATES 16, 17, 18, 106, 108, 169, 171

◼ DIFFERENTIAL OVERVIEW

Sinus Bradycardia
❑ Hypothyroidism
❑ Hypervagotonia
❑ Hypersensitive carotid sinus
❑ Hypothermia
❑ Acute increased intracranial pressure

Complete Heart Block
❑ Inferior myocardial infarction
❑ Drugs
❑ Viral myocarditis
❑ Acute rheumatic fever
❑ Lyme disease
❑ Sarcoidosis
❑ Sick sinus syndrome

DIAGNOSTIC APPROACH

Symptoms include paroxysmal dizziness, fatigue, presyncopal lightheadedness, and syncope. Sinus bradycardia is manifest as a regular slow rhythm. Complete heart block is usually accompanied by a very slow escape rhythm and a symptomatic reduction in cardiac output.

Relative bradycardia—that is, failure to respond to fever with tachycardia—suggests typhoid fever, mycoplasma pneumonia, factitious fever, or concomitant beta blockers.

CLINICAL FINDINGS

Hypothyroidism   Cardinal findings include weight gain, dry skin, coarse hair, hoarseness, delayed relaxation phase of the ankle jerks, and thyroid enlargement **(Plates 16, 17, 18).**

Hypervagotonia   Most often observed in aerobically trained athletes, it is also found in patients with vasovagal syncope, if examined while experiencing symptoms.

Hypersensitive carotid sinus   Carotid massage produces a prolonged pause (>5 seconds), correlated with symptoms.

Hypothermia   Bradycardia occurs with environmental cold exposure, especially in near drowning, due to the diving reflex. Hypothermia can be underestimated unless the core temperature is measured with a special hypothermia thermometer.

Acute increased intracranial pressure   The Cushing reflex, with bradycardia, occurs in patients with intracerebral hemorrhage, malignant hypertension, or brain edema.

Inferior myocardial infarction   Nausea and diaphoresis are prominent in the setting of protracted substernal chest pressure.

Drugs   Digoxin, beta blockers, and calcium channel blockers are the usual causal agents. A junctional rhythm at a rate of 60 appears in digoxin toxicity.

Viral myocarditis   Although it begins with fever, tachycardia, congestive heart failure, and vague chest pains, development of heart block is marked by bradyarrhythmia.

Acute rheumatic fever   A recent sore throat, fever, polyarthritis, and erythema marginatum are key clues **(Plate 108).**

Lyme disease   Other manifestations of Lyme disease, such as erythema marginatum and arthritis, precede it **(Plate 106).**

Sarcoidosis   Bradycardia may occur in the setting of a granulomatous cardiomyopathy. Adenopathy is a clue **(Plates 169, 171).**

Sick sinus syndrome   Sinus node dysfunction may be first manifest as failure to cardioaccelerate with fever or exercise, or with excessive bradycardia when given a beta blocker or calcium channel blocker. Symptoms of dizziness, confusion, fatigue, syncope, and congestive heart failure occur in association with bradycardia and long pauses.

Cardiomegaly/Congestive Heart Failure

◼ DIFFERENTIAL OVERVIEW

❑ Hypertensive left ventricular hypertrophy
❑ Congestive heart failure
❑ Anterior myocardial ischemia
❑ Athlete's heart
❑ Mitral regurgitation
❑ Aortic stenosis
❑ High output
❑ Hypertrophic obstructive cardiomyopathy
❑ Pulmonary hypertension
❑ Cor pulmonale
❑ Dilated cardiomyopathy
❑ Endocarditis
❑ Pericardial effusion
❑ Left ventricular aneurysm
❑ Mitral stenosis

DIAGNOSTIC APPROACH

The Framingham criteria for congestive heart failure are a good reference point. Major criteria include paroxysmal nocturnal dyspnea, rales, cardiomegaly, acute pulmonary edema, third heart sound, jugular pressure greater than 16 cm, and positive abdominojugular reflex. Minor criteria include edema, night cough, dyspnea on exertion, hepatomegaly, pleural effusion, and pulse rate slower than 120.

Findings suggesting left ventricular hypertrophy include a sustained forceful apical thrust, a double apical impulse, an apical impulse larger than 3 cm, and a fourth heart sound on auscultation. Left ventricular enlargement will cause the apical impulse (PMJ) to be displaced downward and to the left. An apical impulse more than 10 cm from the midclavicular line has Se 0.92, Sp 0.88, and LR 7.7 for cardiomegaly.

Systolic heart failure is marked by decreased cardiac output, with manifestations such as weakness, fatigue, and decreased exercise tolerance. A third heart sound (S3) has Se 0.31, Sp 0.95, and LR 6.2 for LVEF less than 40%. Mitral regurgitation, especially when acute, augments early diastolic inflow and may produce an S3 with normal systolic function. Diastolic heart failure has reduced ventricular compliance and increased filling pressures with manifestations of dyspnea and rales. Rales have Se 0.24, Sp 1.0, and LR greater than 12 for LVEDP greater than 18 mm Hg.

Right ventricular hypertrophy will cause a sustained right parasternal lift. It is seen with pulmonary hypertension, pulmonic stenosis, and volume overload with tricuspid regurgitation or atrial septal defect. Right ventricular failure is recognized by edema, jugular venous distension, and abdominojugular reflux (sustained elevation of jugular pressure greater than 4 cm for longer than 10 seconds with abdominal pressure has Se 0.90, Sp 0.89, and LR 8.2 for RVEDP more than 12 mm Hg).

CLINICAL FINDINGS

Hypertensive left ventricular hypertrophy   The PMI is discrete, brisk, and brief. A fourth heart sound is usually prominent. Inadequately controlled hypertension is present.

Congestive heart failure   Signs of left or right heart failure such as symmetric bibasilar rales, edema, and a third heart sound are present **(Plate 41).**

Anterior myocardial ischemia   A systolic bulge in the left third and fourth interspace that is medial to the PMI occurs transiently during episodes of chest pain and corresponds to anterior dyskinesia.

Athlete's heart   Isometric training, such as weight lifting, will produce the greatest degree of enlargement although enlargement can also be seen in persons with expanded aerobic capacity.

Cardiomegaly/Congestive Heart Failure

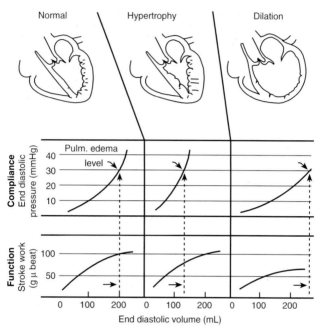

Figure 2. Starling relationships in left heart diastolic failure (hypertrophy) and systolic failure (dilation). (Adapted from: Fauci AS, Braunwald E, Isselbacher KJ, et al., eds. Harrison's Principles of Internal Medicine. 4th ed. New York: McGraw-Hill, 1998, p. 1285.)

Mitral regurgitation The PMI is diffuse, rolling, and displaced downward to the left. There will be a holosystolic murmur at the apex, radiating toward the axilla. Atrial fibrillation is often present with severe mitral regurgitation.

Aortic stenosis A crescendo-decrescendo murmur is loudest at the upper right sternal border, radiating into the carotids.

High output A systolic flow murmur will be detected. Causes include hyperthyroidism, anemia, pregnancy, arteriovenous fistula, and Paget's disease **(Plate 19).**

Hypertrophic obstructive cardiomyopathy An aortic outflow murmur changes dramatically in loudness with changes in position (intensifying with standing).

Pulmonary hypertension This is marked by a right parasternal lift and accentuated P2.

Cor pulmonale Vasodilation, large volume pulses, warm extremities, and throbbing fingers are signs. The cardiac apex may be hidden by the expanded lung volume. Causes include massive or recurrent pulmonary embolism, primary pulmonary hypertension, or emphysema.

Dilated cardiomyopathy The PMI is diffuse, displaced, and sluggish.

Endocarditis Valvular damage with acute regurgitation (aortic or mitral), fever, myocarditis, and anemia all contribute to the heart failure. Clues include underlying valvular heart disease with a change in character or intensity of the murmur and embolic stigmata such as splinter hemorrhages, Osler's nodes, and conjunctival or retinal petechiae (Roth spots) **(Plates 22, 23, 24).**

Pericardial effusion The heart sounds are muffled. There may be a pericardial friction rub or chest pain that is partially relieved by sitting forward. Signs of hemodynamic

Cardiomegaly/Congestive Heart Failure

compromise (pericardial tamponade) include hypotension, jugular venous distension with Kussmaul's sign (filling an inspiration), and pulsus paradoxus. Uremia, hypothyroidism, lupus, or acute myocardial infarction are frequent underlying causes (**Plates 16, 17, 18, 91, 92, 198**).

Left ventricular aneurysm   A systolic bulge is palpable, similar to anterior ischemia, but presents continuously. There is a history of prior anterior myocardial infarction.

Mitral stenosis   The PMI is normally located, but the impulse is snapping in quality. There is a right ventricular lift. A low-pitched apical diastolic murmur can be heard with the bell of the stethoscope. A malar flush, cold blue fingers, and small volume pulses are other features (**Plate 28**).

Carotid Bruit

Chapter 16

PLATES 16, 19

◼ DIFFERENTIAL OVERVIEW

- ❏ Carotid artery stenosis
- ❏ Carotid artery ruptured plaque
- ❏ Transmitted valvular murmur
- ❏ Carotid tortuosity
- ❏ Carotid compression
- ❏ Jugular venous hum
- ❏ Thyrotoxicosis

DIAGNOSTIC APPROACH

At increased flow rates, laminar flow becomes turbulent and produces a bruit. A rule of thumb is that at 50% reduction in diameter (70% cross-sectional area), a soft bruit may be heard. At 60% reduction, the bruit becomes high-pitched, intense, and holosystolic. At 80%, a systolic–diastolic bruit is heard. At near occlusion, the bruit disappears as does the pulse. High-output conditions can produce bruits at lesser degrees of stenosis.

CLINICAL FINDINGS

Carotid artery stenosis   The bruit becomes higher pitched and longer in duration as the stenosis tightens. Bruits are considered clinically significant if associated with ipsilateral transient cerebral ischemia. In patients with anterior circulation TIAs, a carotid bruit has an Se 0.62, Sp 0.61, and LR 1.6 in predicting high-grade (>70%) stenosis. Such a bruit predicts a threefold in increased risk of stroke and cardiovascular mortality.

Carotid artery ruptured plaque   Plaque rupture produces a bruit associated with a sudden shower of anterior circulation ischemic symptoms (unstable TIAs or amaurosis fugax). The carotid pulse is usually normal.

Transmitted valvular murmur   Aortic stenosis produces a murmur that can be heard equally at the upper right sternal border and both carotids. A murmur produced by mitral regurgitation from a ruptured chordae tendineae or mitral valve prolapse may also radiate to the neck.

Carotid tortuosity   In an elderly patient, the carotid may become palpably tortuous with prominent pulsations in addition to a bruit.

Carotid compression   False creation of a carotid bruit by stethoscope compression is easily recognized by varying the pressure of the stethoscope.

Jugular venous hum   It occurs most prominently in adults with high cardiac output states and can be confirmed by disappearance with compression of the internal jugular vein.

Thyrotoxicosis   A systolic bruit, which is produced by enhanced flow, can be heard directly over an enlarged thyroid **(Plates 16, 19)**.

Chapter 17

Claudication

◪ DIFFERENTIAL OVERVIEW

- ❏ Atherosclerotic occlusion
- ❏ Lumbar radiculopathy
- ❏ Muscular strain
- ❏ Deep vein thrombosis
- ❏ Arterial embolism
- ❏ Spinal stenosis
- ❏ Aortic dissection
- ❏ Aortic coarctation
- ❏ Erythromelalgia

DIAGNOSTIC APPROACH

Claudication—muscle pain and fatigue occurring after sustained exertion and relieved by rest—usually represents muscle ischemia because energy demand outstrips the arterial blood supply. Several other conditions present with leg pain increased with use, however, so a careful history and examination is required to differentiate among them.

The level of the arterial occlusion can be determined by the location of the symptoms. Superficial femoral artery occlusion produces calf pain. Iliofemoral occlusion produces thigh and calf pain. Aortoiliac occlusion produces buttock pain and erectile dysfunction (Leriche's syndrome). Rapid worsening of symptoms suggests occlusion at multiple levels.

CLINICAL FINDINGS

Atherosclerotic occlusion   Classic exertional pain is gradually progressive in a patient with a substrate of hypertension, diabetes, smoking, or evidence of vascular disease at other sites (angina, renal insufficiency). The pulse distal to the occlusion is reduced or absent. The severity of symptoms (latency and amount of pain) corresponds to the degree of obstruction. Severe arterial insufficiency is associated with rest pain, and the findings of dependent rubor, a cool foot with poor capillary refill when supine, and waxy pallor of the sole of the foot upon elevation. An ankle-brachial systolic blood pressure ratio of less than 1.0 is found in arterial disease, and a ratio less than 0.5 is consistent with severe ischemia **(Plate 152)**.

Lumbar radiculopathy   Pain begins in the back and radiates down a dermatome into the foot. It may be worsened by walking, and has an electrical or burning character. The pulses are normal, but the deep tendon reflexes may be absent.

Muscular strain   Such a strain presents with pain and tenderness in the large muscle groups (hamstrings, quadriceps, gastrocnemius), increased by specific use. There is localized tenderness, and passive stretching can reproduce the pain.

Deep vein thrombosis   The pain is not related to exertion although standing often worsens it. The affected limb is usually asymmetrically swollen, with calf tenderness. Extension into the inferior vena cava may produce phlegmasia cerulea dolens, with massive (often bilateral) swelling, pallor/cyanosis, and pain **(Plate 27, 42)**.

Arterial embolism   It presents acutely with numbness, weakness, and excruciating leg pain at rest. Predisposing factors such as atrial fibrillation or recent myocardial infarction are present along with showers of small peripheral emboli (e.g., to the toes). The limb will be cold with waxy pallor, distal cyanosis, and an absent pulse. The location of obstruction can be surmised from the level of coldness. Obstruction at the aortic bifurcation will cause coldness bilaterally below the groin; common iliac obstruction, in one leg below the groin; common femoral, below the knee; and popliteal, in one foot **(Plate 25)**.

Spinal stenosis   Compression produces "pseudoclaudication," or bilateral vaguely localized gluteal and lower extremity pain worsened by standing or walking and relieved by sitting or lying with the hip and spine flexed. The patient will assume a "simian stance" to alleviate pain. Weakness and numbness may accompany the pain in the legs.

Aortic dissection In the context of tearing, traveling back pain, the patient develops a pulseless, cold, painful extremity. There may also be flaccid paralysis of the limb if unilateral spinal arteries are affected.

Aortic coarctation Consider coarctation when there is hypertension and symmetric diminished distal leg pulses in a young adult.

Erythromelalgia Characterized by severe burning hyperesthetic pain with rubor of the feet, it occurs in polycythemia, gout, and frostbite **(Plate 26).**

Continuous Murmur

PLATE 55

◼ DIFFERENTIAL OVERVIEW

❑ Aortic stenosis/aortic insufficiency
❑ Pericardial friction rub
❑ Pulmonary arteriovenous fistula
❑ Venous hum
❑ Mammary souffle
❑ Aortic coarctation
❑ Mediastinal air dissection
❑ Patent ductus arteriosis
❑ Ruptured sinus of Valsalva

CLINICAL FINDINGS

Aortic stenosis/aortic insufficiency   A to-and-fro murmur radiates into the carotids.

Pericardial friction rub   Discrete harsh/scratching sounds are heard, synchronized with the heartbeat, composed of one, two, or three components.

Pulmonary arteriovenous fistula   The murmur is localized over one area of the chest. Telangiectasias can usually be found cutaneously in patients with cirrhosis and on the lips and tongue in those with hereditary hemorrhagic telangiectasia **(Plate 55).**

Venous hum   The murmur occurs over the base of the heart, increases with sitting, and decreases with compression of the jugular.

Mammary souffle   Increased blood flow with engorged breasts late in pregnancy or with breast-feeding produces a shuffling sound.

Aortic coarctation   The murmur is caused by enhanced flow within enlarged intercostal arteries. The blood pressure in the legs will be low compared with the arms.

Mediastinal air dissection   Usually a complication of mechanical ventilation, it produces a continuous crunching sound and is associated with subcutaneous emphysema.

Patent ductus arteriosis   A "machinery" murmur with late systolic accentuation is best heard in the pulmonic area and is loudest at S2. A thrill is present. If right-to-left shunting has developed, cyanosis will be observed.

Ruptured sinus of Valsalva   Marked by sudden development of a continuous murmur with a thrill over the base of the heart, it is caused by a ruptured aneurysm, usually as a complication of endocarditis.

Cyanosis

Chapter 19

PLATES 5, 6, 26, 29, 30, 36, 42, 55, 130, 132, 152, 219

⬛ DIFFERENTIAL OVERVIEW

- ❏ Asthma
- ❏ Chronic obstructive pulmonary disease
- ❏ Hypoventilation
- ❏ Pulmonary embolism
- ❏ Cardiac right-to-left shunt
- ❏ Pulmonary edema
- ❏ Low cardiac output/shock
- ❏ Polycythemia vera
- ❏ Arterial insufficiency
- ❏ Intrapulmonary shunts
- ❏ Tracheal obstruction
- ❏ Tricuspid insufficiency
- ❏ Superior vena cava obstruction
- ❏ Pneumonitis
- ❏ Methemoglobinemia
- ❏ Patent ductus arteriosus
- ❏ Pseudocyanosis

DIAGNOSTIC APPROACH

Central cyanosis is best seen in the nailbeds or mucous membranes in good natural light. Peripheral cyanosis (due to increased capillary oxygen extraction) is seen in exposed areas such as the fingers, earlobes, and the tip of the nose. Massage or heat, which increase blood flow, will abolish peripheral but not central cyanosis.

Cyanosis becomes clinically apparent when there is 5 gm/dL of unsaturated hemoglobin. With a normal hemoglobin count, this corresponds to a pAO2 of less than 50 torr or SaO2 less than 85%. Cyanosis depends on the absolute concentration of deoxyhemoglobin and may not be apparent if anemia exists concurrently.

Cyanosis Type	Color
Reduced hemoglobin	Purplish-blue to heliotrope
Oxyhemoglobin	Red
Polycythemia	Reddish-blue
Methemoglobinemia	Chocolate blue
Sulfhemoglobinemia	Lead or mauve-blue
Carboxyhemoglobinemia	Bright red
Cyanohemoglobinemia	Bright red

"Harlequin cyanosis" with one arm pink and the other blue can occur with aortic dissection, embolic arterial occlusion, or patent ductus arteriosis with pulmonary hypertension. Blue fingers and pink toes suggest complete transposition of the great vessels, preductal coarctation with a patent ductus arteriosis, or pulmonary hypertension with reversed flow through a patent ductus.

CLINICAL FINDINGS

Asthma Episodic wheezing and a prolonged expiratory time are observed. By the time cyanosis is apparent, there will be marked retractions, a large pulsus paradoxus, and a rapidly failing patient. Acute worsening with a localized wheeze may be caused by an inspissated mucous plug.

Chronic obstructive pulmonary disease There may be chronic hypoxemia and cor pulmonale in "blue bloaters." Acute bronchospastic exacerbations can also cause cyanosis.

Hypoventilation Hypoventilation can occur as a consequence of narcotic overdose, anterior horn cell disease (amyotrophic lateral sclerosis, polio), neuromuscular junction disease (myasthenia gravis, botulism), muscle weakness (muscular dystrophy, fatigue), or kyphoscoliosis **(Plates 130, 132, 219).**

Pulmonary embolism   It is acute in onset and associated with pleuritic chest pain or hemoptysis. The cyanosis is caused by a combination of ventilation-perfusion mismatches and low cardiac output occurring with major hemodynamic compromise **(Plate 42).**

Cardiac right-to-left shunt   In adults, shunts occur with congenital or acquired atrial or ventricular septal defects, which are recognized by their prominent murmurs. Cyanosis occurs when more than one-third of the blood is shunted. There is little reduction in cyanosis with oxygen administration **(Plate 29).**

Pulmonary edema   Labored breathing, moist rales, and a third heart sound are observed. There may be pink-tinged frothy sputum, especially with "flash" pulmonary edema.

Low cardiac output/shock   Cyanosis is caused by excessive oxygen extraction with a prolonged circulatory time and can occur regardless of the shock mechanism. Other signs of low output are present such as hypotension, vasoconstriction with cool skin, oliguria, and confusion.

Polycythemia vera   Ruddy plethora occurs with cyanosis due to slow flow with high viscosity. Heat-induced pruritus is common **(Plates 26, 30).**

Arterial insufficiency   In Raynaud's, the cyanosis is transient, usually triggered by cold exposure. In severe atherosclerotic vascular disease, the distal pulses are thready or absent and the limb has dusky rubor when dependent and a waxy paleness when elevated **(Plates 36, 152).**

Intrapulmonary shunts   Cyanosis due to intrapulmonary shunts can occur in cirrhosis and can be suspected when numerous cutaneous telangiectasias exist. With congenital pulmonary arteriovenous malformation, there will also be cutaneous telangiectasias and a continuous murmur over the AVM **(Plate 55).**

Tracheal obstruction   The patient presents acutely with stridor caused by foreign body aspiration or epiglottitis. The latter produces a severe sore throat out of proportion to pharyngeal findings. Cyanosis develops rapidly.

Tricuspid insufficiency   Advanced tricuspid insufficiency may produce icterocyanosis owing to elevated venous pressure.

Superior vena cava obstruction   Facial plethora/cyanosis, swelling, and elevated jugular veins are telltale signs.

Pneumonitis   Alveolar hypoxemia may be caused by infectious (lobar pneumonia or Pneumocystis carinii), inflammatory (sarcoidosis or desquamative interstitial pneumonitis), or allergic (Loeffler's) causes. Cyanosis may first appear on exertion. Cough is prominent.

Methemoglobinemia   Deoxyhemoglobin may be converted to methemoglobin by nitrates, sulfonamides, chlorates, aniline dyes, and phenacetin. The skin color is leaden.

Patent ductus arteriosus   Cyanosis and clubbing in the lower but not upper extremities is seen when reversed flow is present, due to severe pulmonary artery hypertension. At this point, the machinery murmur is usually absent.

Pseudocyanosis   Silver causes a blue discoloration in sun-exposed skin. Amiodarone deposits blue lipofuscin in the skin. Polymers of chlorpromazine oxidation give a blue-purple color **(Plates 5, 6).**

Diastolic Murmur

Chapter 20

PLATES 28, 29, 52

◤ DIFFERENTIAL OVERVIEW

- ❏ Aortic insufficiency
- ❏ Pulmonic insufficiency
- ❏ Mitral stenosis
- ❏ Tricuspid stenosis
- ❏ Atrial septal defect

DIAGNOSTIC APPROACH

A diastolic murmur is always abnormal. An early diastolic murmur, caused by aortic or pulmonic insufficiency, is high-pitched and decrescendo. The duration of the murmur is an index of severity. A mid-diastolic murmur is caused by mitral and tricuspid stenosis.

The murmur of mitral stenosis decreases or does not change with inspiration whereas the murmur of tricuspid stenosis increases.

CLINICAL FINDINGS

Aortic insufficiency A blowing decrescendo diastolic murmur begins with the aortic closure sound. This may be best heard with the diaphragm in the aortic area, with the patient leaning forward, holding his breath at end-expiration. With severe insufficiency, a low-pitched diastolic rumble may be heard at the apex, like distant thunder; this is known as the Austin Flint murmur. The apical impulse is hyperdynamic, there is a wide pulse pressure with a bounding pulse, and there may be a systolic thrill in the URSB and

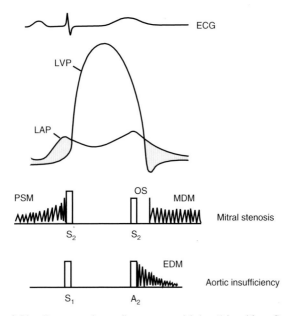

Figure 3. Diastolic murmurs: intracardiac pressures and timing. (Adapted from: Crawford MH, O'Rourke RA. A systemic approach to the bedside differentiation of cardiac murmurs and abnormal sounds. Curr Prob Cardiol 1979;1:1.)

neck. Other clues include a systolic/diastolic bruit when the femoral artery is compressed (Duroziez's sign), visible nailbed pulsations (Quincke's sign), and head bobbing with each pulse (Musset's sign). Acute aortic regurgitation (caused by endocarditis, aortic dissection, or trauma) produces acute pulmonary edema and low cardiac output.

Pulmonic insufficiency   Regurgitation begins with pulmonic closure, but because closure is delayed beyond A2 due to a prolonged right ventricular ejection time, the murmur appears to start in midsystole. The second heart sound will be single. Pulmonic insufficiency associated with pulmonary hypertension produces a Graham Steell murmur at the left sternal border, which is difficult to distinguish from aortic insufficiency.

Mitral stenosis   A diastolic rumble is loud early in diastole, softens in mid-diastole, and is accentuated in late diastole. This latter phase, resulting from flow produced by atrial contraction, is lost in atrial fibrillation. The murmur is best heard at the apex, with the bell, in the left lateral decubitus position. Concurrent findings include dyspnea, hemoptysis, and a malar flush. Atrial myxoma can mimic this but is accompanied by systemic emboli **(Plate 28).**

Tricuspid stenosis   It has the same characteristics as mitral stenosis but is of lower frequency due to lower flow. The sound should become louder with inspiration and increased stroke volume. A prominent jugular a wave and edema, ascites, and hepatomegaly are useful clues to severe stenosis.

Atrial septal defect   A low-pitched rumbling is found at the mid-left sternal border. There is a prominent right ventricular impulse with a palpable pulmonary artery pulsation. When pulmonary vascular resistance rises, the left-to-right shunt decreases, and a single S2 with a murmur of pulmonic insufficiency develops. Cyanosis and clubbing are usually present at this point **(Plates 29, 52).**

Discrete Heart Sounds

◼ DIFFERENTIAL OVERVIEW

Phenomena
- ❏ S4 gallop
- ❏ Midsystolic click
- ❏ Loud S2
- ❏ S3 gallop
- ❏ Widely split S1
- ❏ Widely split S2
- ❏ Ejection click
- ❏ Variable S1
- ❏ Paradoxical splitting of S2
- ❏ Loud S1
- ❏ Fixed splitting of S2
- ❏ Opening snap
- ❏ Pericardial knock
- ❏ Tumor plop
- ❏ Sail sound

DIAGNOSTIC APPROACH

The A2-P2 interval increases normally with inspiration due to decreased intrathoracic pressure and increased venous return, which leads to increased stroke volume.

The cadence of S3 gallop matches that of the word Tennessee, and S4, Kentucky. Mentally say this while listening to the heart sounds.

CLINICAL FINDINGS

S4 gallop   It is a low-pitched presystolic heart sound (heard best with the bell) and may be palpable at the left heart border. Caused by atrial contraction into a noncompliant ventricle, a fourth heart sound is often heard in hypertension with left ventricular hypertrophy, and in aortic stenosis, ischemic heart disease, and acute mitral regurgitation. Increased ventricular filling during atrial contraction, caused by anemia, thyrotoxicosis, or prolonged PR interval, can also produce an S4.

Midsystolic click   Heard in mitral valve prolapse, it may be a single click or multiple midsystolic clicks, often followed by a mitral regurgitant murmur. It is mobile with maneuvers that change ventricular volume, such as positional change.

Loud S2   A2 is increased in systemic hypertension. P2 is increased in pulmonary hypertension.

S3 gallop   The third heart sound is a low-pitched early diastolic sound heard best at the apex with the bell. It is associated with the rapid ventricular filling phase of the cardiac cycle, and its presence correlates with left ventricular dysfunction in congestive heart failure (ischemia, cardiomyopathy, myocarditis, cor pulmonale) or overload (acute valvular regurgitation, high output state, left-to-right shunt, complete heart block). In young adults, an S3 may be a normal finding due to a hyperkinetic heart or increased filling volume with mitral regurgitation. This filling sound has the same auscultatory quality as an S3.

Widely split S1   Splitting may be produced by electrical delay of atrioventricular conduction in right bundle branch block, ventricular tachycardia, or left ventricular pacing.

Widely split S2   If splitting is present both recumbent and standing and is increased with inspiration, it suggests right bundle branch block, preexcitation, atrial septal defect, right ventricular pressure overload (pulmonary hypertension with right ventricular failure, severe pulmonary stenosis, or massive pulmonary embolism), or decreased resistance to left ventricular outflow (mitral regurgitation) **(Plate 42).**

Ejection click   A sharp, high-pitched early systolic sound, it is associated with a bicuspid aortic valve (a predictor of development of aortic stenosis later in life), pulmonic stenosis, and aortic dilation.

Discrete Heart Sounds

Variable S1   Beat-to-beat variation in intensity occurs with a variable PQ interval, such as occurs in Wenckebach, complete heart block, or atrial fibrillation.

Paradoxical splitting of S2   Splitting decreases with inspiration, due to delayed aortic valve closure with left bundle branch block, severe aortic stenosis, hypertrophic cardiomyopathy, or severe left ventricular dysfunction, especially early in myocardial infarction. Differentiate A2-P2 from A2-OS by having the patient stand. A2-OS widens, while A2-P2 narrows or is unchanged.

Loud S1   An accentuated first heart sound occurs in hemodynamically significant mitral stenosis, hyperadrenergic states, and left atrial myxoma.

Fixed splitting of S2   Splitting is not affected by Valsalva. It is found in atrial septal defect and severe right heart failure.

Opening snap   It is a high-pitched sound occurring shortly after the second heard sound. Usually associated with mitral stenosis, it is also heard in tricuspid stenosis. The greater the degree of stenosis, the closer the snap moves toward the second heart sound. It can be distinguished from a split S2 by audibility over the sternal notch.

Pericardial knock   Caused by sudden restriction of ventricular filling by a thickened nondistensible pericardium, it occurs earlier in diastole than an S3.

Tumor plop   The hallmark of an atrial myxoma, it occurs in the same part of the cardiac cycle as an S3, but has varying timing.

Sail sound   This loud sound is produced by delayed tricuspid valve closure in Ebstein's anomaly.

Edema

Chapter 22

PLATES 16, 17, 18, 38, 40, 41, 42, 59, 61, 62, 63, 64, 151, 198

◪ DIFFERENTIAL OVERVIEW

- ❏ Congestive heart failure
- ❏ Venous insufficiency
- ❏ Hypoalbuminemia
- ❏ Drugs
- ❏ Cirrhosis
- ❏ Deep vein thrombosis
- ❏ Inferior vena cava obstruction
- ❏ Lymphatic obstruction
- ❏ Glomerular injury
- ❏ Idiopathic edema
- ❏ Myxedema
- ❏ Lipedema
- ❏ Toxemia
- ❏ Cyclical edema
- ❏ Refeeding
- ❏ Filariasis
- ❏ Milroy's

DIAGNOSTIC APPROACH

The degree of edema is influenced by membrane permeability, hydrostatic pressure, and/or oncotic pressure. Edema implies an increase in interstitial volume of several liters. Low protein fluids (hypoalbuminemia, cardiac, and venous edema) pit easily and recover quickly on release. High protein fluids (cellulitis, lymphedema) resist pitting and recover slowly.

Anasarca suggests cardiac, renal, or hepatic disease. Splenomegaly is found more often in patients with cirrhosis than those with congestive heart failure.

CLINICAL FINDINGS

Congestive heart failure   The edema is pitting and responds readily to changes in position. The mechanism involves excessive fluid and sodium retention, decreased right ventricular pump function, and increased central venous pressure. Usually, other signs of right-sided heart failure are present, such as jugular venous distension and hepato-jugular reflux **(Plate 41).**

Venous insufficiency   Superficial varicosities and brownish discoloration of the skin will be clues to this condition. Swelling will be worse after prolonged dependency on the leg, and there may be a sensation of heaviness in the leg **(Plate 151).**

Hypoalbuminemia   The edema pits and is often accompanied by morning periorbital edema and ascites. With the albumin less than 2.5 gm/dL, there will be decreased oncotic pressure, and the kidneys will overcompensate by retaining sodium. Underlying causes include malnutrition, nephrotic syndrome (dipstick proteinuria will be present), cirrhosis, and protein-losing enteropathy **(Plates 41, 59, 61, 198).**

Drugs   Antihypertensives such as calcium channel blockers, methyldopa, or minoxidil can produce edema through fluid retention and/or negative inotropy. Anabolic steroids, NSAIDs, and danazol can also cause edema.

Cirrhosis   Suspect cirrhosis when there are collateral venous channels visible on the abdominal surface, ascites, jaundice, and spider angiomata. Cirrhosis is caused by a combination of hypoalbuminemia, blockage of hepatic venous outflow, and activation of the renin-angiotensin-aldosterone axis with sodium and volume retention **(Plates 62, 64).**

Deep vein thrombosis   Edema is usually unilateral or at least asymmetric. Homan's sign (calf pain with dorsiflexion of the foot), calf tenderness, or palpable cords are variably present **(Plate 42).**

Inferior vena cava obstruction   Lower extremity swelling is massive. Veins on the abdominal wall are dilated, and flow below the umbilicus is reversed so that the veins fill from below when stripped.

Lymphatic obstruction   The edema is brawny and nonpitting and has overlying hypertrophic skin changes. Palpable lymphadenopathy or splenomegaly and signs of a primary cancer should be sought. This obstruction occurs with primary retroperitoneal tumors or tumors that have metastasized to the retroperitoneal lymph nodes (prostate cancer in men, lymphoma in women) **(Plates 40, 63).**

Glomerular injury   Caused by proteinuria (recognized by foamy urine), edema is present, with concurrent hematuria and hypertension.

Idiopathic edema   It presents as periodic nonmenstrual edema with abdominal distension.

Myxedema   There is brawny edema in the legs and periorbital edema. Usually the patient has signs of profound hypothyroidism, such as lethargy and coarse hair and facial features **(Plates 16, 17, 18).**

Lipedema   There is disproportionate fat accumulation in the legs and buttocks. This pseudoedema does not pit and spares the feet.

Toxemia   Edema is an early sign in patients in their third trimester of pregnancy. Hypertension and proteinuria also occur **(Plate 38).**

Cyclical edema   Occurring in women, cyclical edema is often synchronous with menstrual periodicity. Transient abdominal distension and rapid weight fluctuations are common, accompanied by headache, fatigue, or anxiety.

Refeeding   Edema occurs especially in patients with protein–calorie malnutrition.

Filariasis   Suspect in persons with geographic exposure risk and massive nonpitting lymphedema.

Milroy's   A benign form of edema in young adults, Milroy's is characterized by swelling that is sharply demarcated at a joint (e.g., sparing the toes).

Hypertension

PLATES 10, 11, 37, 38, 129

◼ DIFFERENTIAL OVERVIEW

- ❏ Essential hypertension
- ❏ "White coat" hypertension
- ❏ Renal artery stenosis
- ❏ Drug-induced hypertension
- ❏ Atherosclerotic vascular noncompliance
- ❏ Pheochromocytoma
- ❏ Cushing's syndrome
- ❏ Hyperaldosteronism
- ❏ Aortic coarctation
- ❏ Acute renal artery obstruction
- ❏ Toxemia

DIAGNOSTIC APPROACH

The level of blood pressure associated with 50% increase in cardiovascular mortality: men younger than 45 years old, 130/90; men older than 45 years, 140/95; women, 160/95. An ankle-brachial systolic blood pressure ratio of less than 0.9 predicts a fourfold increase in cardiovascular mortality.

Clues to secondary hypertension include onset at a young age (<35), abrupt onset of hypertension, blood pressure difficult to control that requires high dosages of two or more drugs, and very high or labile blood pressure. Hypertension with relative tachycardia may be a clue to sympathetic effect or diastolic dysfunction. Headaches with severe hypertension will be occipital and worse in the morning.

Hypertensive end organ damage must be searched for when the BP is greater than 130 diastolic and the patient exhibits confusion, dyspnea, restlessness, or blurred vision. Perform fundoscopy looking for papilledema or retinal hemorrhages and cardiopulmonary exam for third heart sound or bibasilar rales. Clues to hypertension-associated left ventricular hypertrophy include a fourth heart sound, an apical impulse greater than two intercostal spaces (LR 2.2), a holosystolic sustained apical impulse (LR 7.8), and a hypertensive response to exercise (>210 systolic). Left ventricular hypertrophy multiplies the risk of cardiovascular endpoints. Cotton wool spots, which are caused by anoxic edema with axon degeneration, are seen in advanced hypertension (also in diabetes, dysproteinemia, and fat emboli).

Grading hypertensive retinopathy provides a marker of end-organ damage, which is tied to prognosis **(Plates 37, 38, 129)**:

Grade	AV Ratio	Hem/Exu	Papilledema	Arteriole	AV Cross
Normal	3:4	None	Absent	Fine yellow line Red blood column	None
Gr I	1:2	None	Absent	Broad yellow line	Mild
Gr II	1:3	None	Absent	Copper wire	Vein depression
Gr III	1:4	Present	Absent	Silver wire vein under arteriole	Tapering, disappearing
Gr IV	Fibrous cord	Present	Present	Fibrous cord	Same

CLINICAL FINDINGS

Essential hypertension   Gradual onset, an increase in diastolic blood pressure with standing, and a family history of hypertension are clues.

Hypertension

"White coat" hypertension   High blood pressure readings occur when measured by the physician but not when the patient is at home. Evidence of anxiety-induced sympathetic stimulation such as tachycardia, perspiration, cold hands, tremor, and/or pupil enlargement will usually be present.

Renal artery stenosis   A bruit is heard in the upper abdomen over the kidneys in 40 to 50% of patients and is more specific with a diastolic component (Sp 0.99, LR 39). Evidence of widespread arterial disease is usually present.

Drug-induced hypertension   Hypertension can be caused by amphetamines, steroids, licorice, L-thyroxine, cocaine, and oral contraceptives.

Atherosclerotic vascular noncompliance   Systolic hypertension with a wide pulse pressure is found. Osler's maneuver is positive: The radial arterial pulse remains palpable with the blood pressure cuff inflated.

Pheochromocytoma   Systemic sympathetic symptoms such as severe paroxysmal headache, anxiety, perspiration, palpitation, postural hypotension, and weight loss are seen. Blood pressure is often normal between paroxysms, but orthostatic hypotension may be found without medications. Abdominal palpation may reveal a suprarenal mass or cause a rise in blood pressure.

Cushing's syndrome   The usual precipitant is chronic steroid use. The patient has truncal obesity with thin limbs, a plethoric moon face, easy bruising, purple striae, and hirsutism **(Plates 10, 11).**

Hyperaldosteronism   Hypokalemia may cause muscle weakness, polyuria, and polydipsia.

Aortic coarctation   Simultaneous palpation of radial and femoral pulses reveal a pulse delay and volume and blood pressure decrement. An interscapular bruit can be heard. The feet will be cold, and there will often be bilateral lower extremity claudication.

Acute renal artery obstruction   The onset of hypertension will be acute, with high, labile blood pressure readings. There is usually evidence of atherosclerotic disease or atrial fibrillation.

Toxemia   Accelerated hypertension, edema, and proteinuria occur at the end of pregnancy **(Plate 129).**

Jugular Pulse Variants Chapter 24

■ DIFFERENTIAL OVERVIEW

Phenomena
- ❏ Elevated jugular venous pressure
- ❏ Kussmaul's sign
- ❏ Giant a waves
- ❏ Cannon a waves
- ❏ Prominent v wave
- ❏ Flutter waves
- ❏ Precipitous x descent
- ❏ Prominent y descent
- ❏ Slow y descent

DIAGNOSTIC APPROACH

Tangential light and the patient at a 45° angle facilitate observation of the meniscus of the undulating internal jugular pulse. Uncertainty may be reduced by light pressure over the base of the neck, which will obliterate the jugular but not carotid pulse, and by stripping the external jugular veins from below. The sternomanubrial angle is 5–10 cm above the mid-right atrium.

The *a wave* is the dominant waveform, caused by right atrial contraction, preceding the carotid impulse. It is absent in atrial fibrillation. The *c wave* is simultaneous to the carotid pulse, caused by bulging of the tricuspid into the right atrium or by transmission of a carotid pulse. The *v wave* occurs during systole until the tricuspid valve opens, and is due to passive increase in right ventricle pressure with filling in late systole and early diastole. The *x descent* is caused by atrial relaxation and downward displacement of the tricuspid valve during ventricular systole. The *y descent* results from the opening of the tricuspid valve and rapid inflow of blood into the right ventricle.

Engorged veins over the thoracic outlet may be caused by retrosternal goiter or superior venal cava obstruction. Unilateral JVD may be due to supraclavicular occlusion caused by enlarged lymph nodes, neoplasm, or subclavian neoplasm.

CLINICAL FINDINGS

Elevated jugular venous pressure   Elevated JVP is associated with right heart failure, constrictive pericarditis, and tamponade. Acute left ventricular failure (as in acute myocardial infarction) may raise the pulmonary artery pressure without increasing the mean right atrial pressure. Pulmonary hypertension or tricuspid insufficiency may cause JVD without left heart failure. Abdominojugular reflex (sustained elevation of the jugular vein with abdominal pressure due to augmented venous return) suggests right ventricular dysfunction. It correlates with LVEDP greater than 15 with Se 0.93, Sp 0.86, and LR 6.6.

Kussmaul's sign   JVP paradoxically rises rather than collapses during inspiration. It occurs in constrictive pericarditis (40% of cases) but is uncommon in acute tamponade. It is also commonly seen in acute right ventricular infarction and severe congestive heart failure.

Giant a waves   The jugular pulse appears to be leaping, caused by the right atrium contracting against a noncompliant right ventricle (pulmonic stenosis, cor pulmonale, or restrictive cardiomyopathy), tricuspid stenosis, or a right ventricular mass (presenting with syncope).

Cannon a waves   These waves are variable in height and appearance. They occur when the atrium contracts against a closed tricuspid valve. Irregular cannon a waves occur with atrioventricular dissociation (complete heart block or ventricular tachycardia) whereas regular cannon a waves can occur with junctional tachycardia.

Prominent v wave   The v wave may be as prominent as the a wave in atrial septal defect or tricuspid regurgitation. Severe tricuspid regurgitation may cause earlobe or liver pulsation.

Flutter waves   In atrial flutter, they appear as rapid low amplitude jugular waves.

Chapter 24

Jugular Pulse Variants

Precipitous x descent   It may occur in pericardial constriction and tamponade but not in right heart failure.

Prominent y descent   Associated with an S3 or pericardial knock, it suggests constrictive pericarditis.

Slow y descent   Due to delayed right atrial emptying, it is caused by tricuspid stenosis or right atrial myxoma.

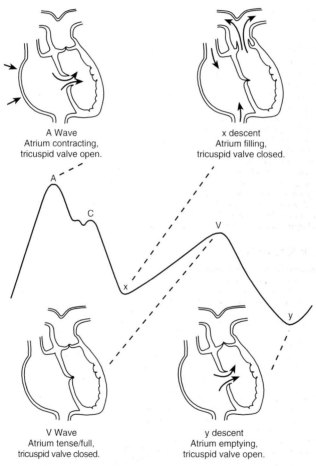

A Wave
Atrium contracting,
tricuspid valve open.

x descent
Atrium filling,
tricuspid valve closed.

V Wave
Atrium tense/full,
tricuspid valve closed.

y descent
Atrium emptying,
tricuspid valve open.

Figure 4. Jugular venous waveforms. (Adapted from: Judge RD, Zuidema GD, Fitzgerald FT. Clinical Diagnosis. 5th ed. Boston: Little, Brown, 1989, p. 269.)

Orthostatic Hypotension   Chapter 25

PLATES 12, 13, 69, 131, 145, 157, 166

◼ DIFFERENTIAL OVERVIEW

Dysautonomia
❑ Diabetes
❑ Drugs
❑ Pernicious anemia
❑ Amyloidosis
❑ Guillain-Barré syndrome
❑ Wernicke's syndrome

Other
❑ Dehydration
❑ Prolonged standing
❑ Hemorrhage
❑ Thermodilation
❑ Vasovagal response
❑ Pregnancy
❑ Addison's disease

DIAGNOSTIC APPROACH

Dysautonomia is characterized by orthostatic hypotension (postural lightheadedness, faint-ing, dim vision, weakness, unsteady gait), urinary dysfunction (frequency, urgency, stress incontinence), sexual dysfunction (impotence, retrograde ejaculation), bowel dysfunction (nocturnal diarrhea, incontinence), and decreased sweating. It is most easily recognized by the presence of orthostatic hypotension without reflex tachycardia.

With gastrointestinal hemorrhage, an orthostatic blood pressure change of 10 mm Hg suggests a loss of at least 20% of intravascular volume.

CLINICAL FINDINGS

Diabetes   Early in the course, orthostatic hypotension with a preserved cardioaccelerator mechanism develops, along with gastroparesis with early satiety and vomiting, noctur-nal diarrhea, and retrograde ejaculation. A common finding is a bilateral symmetric neu-ropathy with decreased vibration sensation and absent ankle jerks **(Plate 166).**

Drugs   Dysautonomia can be caused by methyldopa, barbiturates, clonidine, isoniazid, L-dopa, MAO inhibitors, phenothiazines, tricyclic antidepressants, prazocin, quinidine, procainamide, reserpine, and vincristine. Volume depletion may occur with diuretics, al-cohol, and nitrates.

Pernicious anemia   Lower limb paresthesias and distal areflexia are early findings, fol-lowed by pallor with anemia; either of these may contribute to orthostasis **(Plate 69).**

Amyloidosis   It often presents as a sensory neuropathy with autonomic dysfunction, oc-curring in the setting of a chronic inflammatory disease (cancer or infection). Associated findings include edema caused by congestive heart failure or nephrotic syndrome, an en-larged tongue, and waxy purpuric periorbital plaques **(Plates 131, 157).**

Guillain-Barré syndrome   The onset is subacute but rapid. Classically, the patient re-ports tingling in the hands and feet, an ascending motor weakness manifesting as a gait disorder, a mild distal sensory loss, and areflexia. Bilateral facial weakness, if present, is an important clue.

Wernicke's syndrome   Autonomic dysfunction is a late finding in a patient with ab-ducens gaze palsy, ataxia, and confusion.

Dehydration   Mucous membranes are dry, there is decreased skin turgor (tenting), and eyes appear sunken. A precipitating cause such as diarrhea or vomiting is usually evi-dent.

Prolonged standing   Orthostatic fainting occurs with prolonged motionless standing, es-pecially in combination with cutaneous vasodilation produced by a hot day.

Hemorrhage   The source is usually acute gastrointestinal blood loss or trauma, but sig-nificant volume loss may occur with retroperitoneal hemorrhage (renal trauma, hemorrhagic pancreatitis, or aortic rupture), in which localization is more obscure **(Plate 145)**.

Thermodilation   The skin will be flushed and perspiring.

Vasovagal response   It occurs most often in the setting of psychological stress. The pulse will be slow, and orthostatic changes will disappear when symptomatic recovery occurs.

Pregnancy   Impaired venous return causes blood pooling and an orthostatic drop in blood pressure.

Addison's disease   The patient will complain of asthenia and vague abdominal pains. Hyperpigmentation, especially in the palmar creases and mucous membranes, is a critical clue **(Plates 12, 13)**.

Palpitations/Tachycardia

Chapter 26

PLATES 19, 28, 188

◼ DIFFERENTIAL OVERVIEW

- ❏ Sinus tachycardia
- ❏ Paroxysmal supraventricular tachycardia
- ❏ Atrial fibrillation
- ❏ Atrial flutter
- ❏ AV nodal reentrant tachycardia
- ❏ Ventricular premature beats
- ❏ Anxiety
- ❏ Drugs
- ❏ Anemia
- ❏ Multifocal atrial tachycardia
- ❏ Ventricular tachycardia

DIAGNOSTIC APPROACH

A disquieting awareness of the heartbeat described as pounding, skipping, racing, flopping, or fluttering is usually due to an arrhythmia, or a change in rhythm, rate, or contractility.

Arrhythmia should be approached both from the standpoint of determining the specific rhythm disturbance and recognizing it as a marker for other potentially serious disorders. Signs of underlying heart disease such as ischemia (exertional chest pain), cardiomyopathy (rales, S3 gallop, diffuse PMI), or syncope must be searched for because they alter the prognostic implications of the rhythm disorder.

A jugular cannon a wave implies atrial contraction and can rule out atrial fibrillation. Regular cannon waves characterize supraventricular tachycardia. Intermittent cannon a waves result from atrioventricular dissociation.

With atrial flutter, carotid massage will suddenly halve the rate, but there is a gradual slowing of the pulse with sinus tachycardia. Supraventricular tachycardia either continues or terminates abruptly.

CLINICAL FINDINGS

Sinus tachycardia   There is a gradual onset and decline of the tachycardia, and the rate fluctuates with physiological stimuli. A primary cause such as fever, intravascular volume depletion, anxiety, hyperthyroidism, or congestive heart failure is usually evident.

Paroxysmal supraventricular tachycardia   The onset and termination are sudden (an "alarm clock heart"), the rhythm is regular, and symptoms last minutes to hours. The patient may be dizzy, feel anxious, and have chest pressure. Termination with vagal stimulation (vomiting, Valsalva, or carotid massage) is an important clue. PSVT usually occurs in an otherwise healthy heart.

Atrial fibrillation   The pulse will be rapid and irregular in rhythm and volume. Jugular a waves will be absent. The peripheral pulse may vary in intensity due to variable ventricular filling with varying cycle lengths. There will often be a precipitating cause, such as underlying mitral regurgitation, new-onset congestive heart failure, pulmonary embolism, hyperthyroidism, or myocardial ischemia.

Atrial flutter   A regular tachycardia at a rate of 150/minute suggests flutter. A precipitating cause, such as pericarditis, ischemia, hyperthyroidism, or mitral stenosis, usually exists **(Plates 19, 28).**

AV nodal reentrant tachycardia   There is a sudden-onset regular tachycardia at a rate of 120–250/minute. There may be hypotension due to the loss of atrial filling, acute pulmonary edema caused by sudden increases in atrial pressure, or cannon a waves with A-V dyssynchrony.

Ventricular premature beats   A compensatory pause is often felt as a cessation of the heartbeat because of the increased stroke volume of the beat after the pause due to increased filling time. VPBs will usually decrease in frequency with exertion unless they are caused by ischemia.

Anxiety   Awareness of palpitations will be increased at rest and suppressed with exertion. Symptoms occur despite the heart's regular rate and rhythm.

52

Drugs   Symptomatic tachycardia/palpitations may be caused by insulin, cocaine, caffeine, sympathomimetics, theophylline, MAO inhibitors, alcohol, and tricyclic antidepressants.

Anemia   When anemia is mild, palpitations are present on exertion. When it is severe, they are present at rest **(Plate 188).**

Multifocal atrial tachycardia   There is an irregular rhythm caused by varying A-V conduction, but there will not be cannon a waves. It is usually secondary to severe cardiac or pulmonary disease, digitalis or theophylline intoxication, or hypokalemia.

Ventricular tachycardia   When there is A-V dissociation, cannon a waves may occur at irregular intervals, a helpful clue in deciding between ventricular tachycardia (VT) and supraventricular tachycardia (SVT) with aberrant conduction. There is usually subtle beat-beat variability, and S1 varies in intensity and quality. It usually accompanies ischemic heart disease, cardiomyopathy, or metabolic disorders and is more likely to be associated with hypotension.

Shock

 DIFFERENTIAL OVERVIEW

Cardiogenic
❑ Anterior myocardial infarction
❑ Arrhythmia
❑ Dilated cardiomyopathy
❑ Aortic stenosis
❑ Hypertrophic obstructive cardiomyopathy
❑ Acute mitral regurgitation

Obstructive
❑ Massive pulmonary embolism
❑ Pericardial tamponade
❑ Constrictive pericarditis
❑ Tension pneumothorax

Hypovolemic
❑ Hemorrhage
❑ Fluid depletion

Distributive
❑ Sepsis
❑ Anaphylaxis
❑ Adrenal insufficiency
❑ Neurogenic

DIAGNOSTIC APPROACH

A patient in shock will lie still, paying little attention to events around him. If agitated, he will answer in a weak voice. His pupils are dilated and react slowly to light. The coloration is gray and pale. There is marbling of the skin on the back or the hands and legs, with cyanosis of the lips. The pulse is rapid and thready; temperature and blood pressure are low.

CLINICAL FINDINGS

Anterior myocardial infarction   Shock ensues following an episode of prolonged chest pain, when there is loss of greater than or equal to 40% of left ventricular mass. In cardiogenic shock, pulmonary edema and a gallop rhythm are usually evident, the patient is frequently obtunded, there is oliguria, and the extremities are cold and cyanotic.

Arrhythmia   A rapid, slow, or irregular pulse will be felt. Acute atrial fibrillation, with a 25% decrease in ventricular filling, may produce hypotension in the presence of preexisting left ventricular dysfunction.

Dilated cardiomyopathy   The patient presents with a gradual worsening of congestive heart failure, except in the setting of acute myocarditis, which can be recognized by the fever it produces.

Aortic stenosis   There is usually a loud upper right sternal border murmur that radiates into the carotids, but it may decrease in volume with a reduction in flow. The carotid upstroke will be delayed and small in volume (pulsus parvus et tardus). A2 will be absent.

Hypertrophic obstructive cardiomyopathy   The systolic murmur will increase with maneuvers that decrease left ventricular filling, such as standing.

Acute mitral regurgitation   There will be a new loud apical systolic murmur with radiation to the axilla. This usually occurs with a ruptured papillary muscle caused by acute ischemia or myxomatous degeneration.

Massive pulmonary embolism   Acute-onset dyspnea, pleuritic chest pain, hemoptysis, and swollen legs are all good clues, but these symptoms are variably present **(Plate 42).**

Pericardial tamponade   An exaggerated pulsus paradoxus, muffled heart sounds, and distended neck veins with Kussmaul's sign (inspiratory filling) are present if the tamponade is advanced enough to cause hypotension.

Constrictive pericarditis   The findings are similar to pericardial tamponade, but there is no pulsus paradoxus.

Tension pneumothorax   Findings include an enlarged hemithorax with absent breath sounds, tympany to percussion, and a contralateral tracheal shift. It should be suspected in patients with trauma or mechanical ventilation.

Hemorrhage   Massive gastrointestinal hemorrhage with bright red blood or melena is usually evident, but occult bleeding, such as retroperitoneal hemorrhage or aortic dissection, may make the diagnosis more difficult **(Plate 145).**

Fluid depletion   Occurring in the setting of vomiting, diarrhea, burns, or dehydration in conditions such as diabetic ketoacidosis, fluid depletion can be recognized by such findings as decreased skin turgor and dry mucous membranes. The face is drawn, the eyes sunken, and the tongue dry and coated. The urine is decreased in volume and dark in color.

Sepsis   Spiking fever, rigors, and warm, mottled extremities are clues **(Plates 31, 32, 33).**

Anaphylaxis   Shock occurs cataclysmically after contact with allergens such as penicillin, sulfonamides, iodinated contrast, or hymenoptera venom. Additional findings include flushing, urticaria, angioedema, dyspnea, vomiting, diarrhea, and abdominal cramps **(Plates 182, 185).**

Adrenal insufficiency   It should be considered in patients who chronically take steroids and in those with hyperpigmentation and orthostatic hypotension without evident cause **(Plates 11, 12).**

Neurogenic   Spinal shock occurs in acute spinal cord transection, trauma with cord edema, or with a space-occupying spinal lesion. Acute cerebral hemorrhage can also cause hypotension.

Systolic Murmur

PLATES 22, 23, 24

◼ DIFFERENTIAL OVERVIEW

- ❑ Systolic ejection murmur
- ❑ Mitral regurgitation
- ❑ Mitral valve prolapse
- ❑ Hypertrophic obstructive cardiomyopathy
- ❑ Aortic stenosis
- ❑ Aortic valve sclerosis
- ❑ Atrial septal defect
- ❑ Pulmonic stenosis
- ❑ Tricuspid regurgitation
- ❑ Ventricular septal defect
- ❑ Aortic coarctation

DIAGNOSTIC APPROACH

The *intensity* of the murmur is proportional to the degree of stenosis until flow decreases markedly. Intensity can be expressed semiquantitatively, from grade 1/6, heard only with concentration, to grade 4/6, a loud murmur associated with a palpable thrill, to grade 6/6 with a thrill and murmur heard with the stethoscope off the chest. The *duration* of the murmur is proportional to the pressure differential between the two chambers.

An *early systolic* murmur, decrescendo at the apex, occurs in acute, severe MR with a papillary muscle rupture, endocarditis, a ruptured chordae tendineae, or blunt chest trauma. A *midsystolic* murmur is typical of AS. It can also be found with HOC and with hyperdynamic states. A *late systolic* murmur is usually heard with MVP in association with a midsystolic click. A *holosystolic* murmur can be produced by severe MR or TR, or by a VSD. Holosystolic murmurs are almost never innocent.

Handgrip decreases AS and ASH murmurs but increases MR, AR, VSD, and MS. Transient arterial occlusion by a blood pressure cuff 20 mm above systolic increases left-sided murmurs. Valsalva decreases most murmurs (decreased RV and LV filling), except HOC and MVP, which increase. Augmentation of the murmur with inspiration has Se 1.0, Sp 0.88, and LR 8.3 for a right-sided murmur.

Problem	Maneuver	Result	
MS vs. TS	Inspiration	TS incr	MS decr
S2/OS vs. widely split S2	Standing	S2-OS widens	Split S2 narrows
MR vs. TR	Inspiration	TR incr	MR decr
AS vs. MVP	Squatting	AS incr	MVP decr and delayed
AS vs. HOC	Squatting	AS incr	HOC decr
MVP vs. HOC	Valsalva	MVP decr	HOC incr
MR vs. AS		AS murmur increases with long cycle length	

CINICAL FINDINGS

Systolic ejection murmur   This is appreciated as a soft, pure, early or midsystolic murmur, heard best at the base without radiation and decreased by Valsalva or standing. S2 varies normally with respiration. In young adults, these originate in the pulmonary outflow tract. Physiologic murmurs caused by hyperdynamic blood flow may be heard with anemia, fever, pregnancy, and thyrotoxicosis.

Mitral regurgitation   It is a holosystolic murmur, often musical or honking in quality. It is heard best at the apex and radiates to the axilla; the intensity varies little with respiration. Atrial fibrillation often accompanies it. Acute mitral regurgitation, due to a papillary muscle rupture or endocarditis, is characterized by an early systolic murmur because the atrium is normal-sized and less distensible. The murmur is harsh, low-pitched, and grade 3/6 or louder. With a flail posterior leaflet, the murmur will radiate to the base,

Systolic Murmur

Auscultation areas

AO Aortic area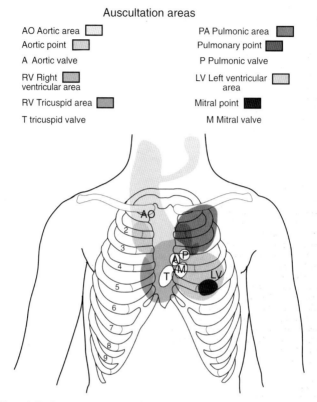
Aortic point
A Aortic valve

RV Right ventricular area

RV Tricuspid area

T tricuspid valve

PA Pulmonic area
Pulmonary point
P Pulmonic valve

LV Left ventricular area

Mitral point

M Mitral valve

Figure 5. Cardiac auscultation areas. (Adapted from: Droste C, von Planta M. Memorix Clinical Medicine. London: Chapman & Hall, 1997, p. 51.)

and with a flail anterior leaflet, to the axilla and back. Hypotension and acute pulmonary edema are often present **(Plates 22, 23, 24).**

Mitral valve prolapse   It produces a midsystolic click accompanied by a late or holosystolic murmur, which is heard over the apex without radiation. Maneuvers that decrease left ventricular volume move the click earlier. Those that increase volume increase the intensity of the murmur. Findings may vary from exam to exam.

Hypertrophic obstructive cardiomyopathy   It is characterized by a midsystolic ejection murmur that changes in intensity with changes in left ventricular stroke volume. Maneuvers that decrease the volume, such as Valsalva and standing, increase the relative obstruction and increase the intensity of the murmur. The murmur is maximal at the apex and lower left sternal border and does not radiate well into the carotids. There may be a double or triple apical impulse with a thrill. A fourth heart sound is common. The carotid impulse may be brisk and bisferiens.

Aortic stenosis   Typically, a loud, harsh, and low-pitched crescendo-decrescendo murmur is heard maximally at the upper right sternal border, and the murmur radiates to the carotids. As the severity of obstruction increases, the murmur peaks later in the cycle. At that point, the murmur is usually loud, and a thrill may be felt, corresponding to a

Systolic Murmur **Chapter 28**

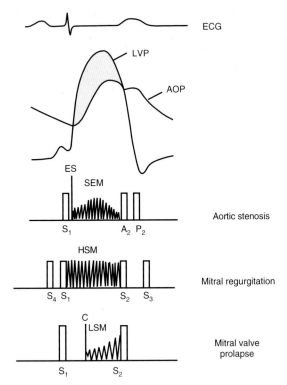

Figure 6. Systolic murmurs: intracardiac pressures and timing. (Adapted from: Crawford MN, O'Rourke RA. A systematic approach to the bedside differentiation of cardiac murmurs and abnormal sounds. Curr Prob Cardiol 1979;1:1.)

peak gradient of 50–60 mm Hg. As flow decreases, the murmur may decrease in intensity. Other signs of hemodynamically significant obstruction include absence of A2 (S2 is often obscured by the murmur) and a carotid impulse that has a weak, rounded rise rather than a brisk upstroke.

Aortic valve sclerosis It has an acoustic signature similar to aortic stenosis but with a normal S2 and carotid impulse.

Atrial septal defect A widely fixed splitting of S2 is characteristic as is a pulmonic midsystolic murmur.

Pulmonic stenosis A loud and long murmur, widely split or absent P2, and an ejection click heard during expiration are diagnostic signs. In Tetralogy of Fallot, the PS murmur varies widely in intensity in relation to fluctuations in the volume of the veno-arterial shunt.

Tricuspid regurgitation It appears as a soft, high-pitched holosystolic murmur, maximal at the lower left sternal border and subxiphoid region. Large tricuspid waves may be seen in the jugular venous pulsations. If pulmonary hypertension is the cause, a pulmonary ejection click will often be audible, with the murmur increasing with inspiration (Carvallo's sign). Severe tricuspid regurgitation is associated with a right ventricular S3, jaundice, an enlarged pulsatile liver with positive abdominojugular reflex, pulsatile ear lobes, edema, ascites, a right ventricular heave at the right lower sternal border, and prominent v waves.

Systolic Murmur

Ventricular septal defect   The murmur is high-pitched, holosystolic, usually grade 3/6 or louder, and maximal over the mid-left sternal border but heard widely over the precordium. A thrill and third heart sound are often present as is a delayed P2. If pulmonary hypertension produces reversal of shunting (Eisenmenger's physiology), the murmur becomes early peaking, associated with a loud P2, pulmonary ejection click, early diastolic Graham Steel murmur, and a right-sided Austin Flint murmur.

Aortic coarctation   A late systolic murmur heard in the back medial to the left scapula is associated with a blood pressure decrement in the legs.

◼ DIFFERENTIAL OVERVIEW

- ❏ Deep vein thrombosis
- ❏ Venous insufficiency
- ❏ Calf muscle strain/hematoma
- ❏ Cellulitis
- ❏ Superficial thrombophlebitis
- ❏ Ruptured Baker's cyst
- ❏ Postphlebitic syndrome
- ❏ Calf muscle infarction
- ❏ Lymphatic obstruction

DIAGNOSTIC APPROACH

Because the clinical findings alone are not sufficient to differentiate benign causes from deep vein thrombosis, a high index of suspicion must be maintained. All patients with new unilateral leg swelling must be imaged with venous duplex or venogram. Occasionally, bilateral edema with asymmetry may occur. Most often, this will not be due to a new deep vein thrombosis although the conditions that cause edema increase the risk of thrombosis.

One must be alert for signs of compartment syndrome, especially in the setting of trauma. Early clues to this include numbness over the foot and weakness of muscles within the compartment. The distal pulses are often preserved.

The circumference difference in normals (95% CI) is 1.5 cm between the thighs and 1.7 cm between the calves.

CLINICAL FINDINGS

Deep vein thrombosis   Asymmetric swelling may be the only sign. Other signs include Homan's (calf pain upon dorsiflexion of the foot), tenderness over the medial aspect of the thigh, and the presence of dilated "sentinel veins" over the anterior tibia, which do not collapse with leg elevation. None of these signs are specific **(Plate 42).**

Venous insufficiency   The swelling is more chronic and is accompanied by findings such as varicosities and hemosiderin hyperpigmentation over the shin. Stasis ulcers may also occur **(Plate 151).**

Calf muscle strain/hematoma   Strain occurs following vigorous exercise. The muscle body is tender to lateral compression. Although there will be no ecchymosis if the hematoma is beneath the muscle fascia, a telltale purple crescent will later appear under the malleolus.

Cellulitis   Although thrombophlebitis and Baker's cyst can both cause erythema, cellulitis will have sharply demarcated and advancing borders. Fever, chills, lymphangitis, and tender adenopathy in the ipsilateral groin when present suggest cellulitis.

Superficial thrombophlebitis   It can be recognized as superficial erythema and tenderness, often with a superficial palpable cord.

Ruptured Baker's cyst   A palpable fluid-filled bursa in the popliteal space can often be felt in patients with rheumatoid arthritis.

Postphlebitic syndrome   This presents as chronic unilateral swelling and aching pain in a leg previously affected by deep vein thrombosis. Acute changes in the degree of swelling make differentiation from a recurrent thrombosis difficult.

Calf muscle infarction   There is usually an embolic source (e.g., atrial fibrillation or aortoiliac atherosclerosis). The muscle becomes tender, then swollen and tense. The distal pulse may be preserved. Numbness over the foot is an early sign of compartment syndrome.

Lymphatic obstruction   The edema is chronic and brawny, with little pitting or change with elevation **(Plate 40).**

Chapter 30

Venous Variants

PLATES 42, 62, 64

▧ DIFFERENTIAL OVERVIEW

- ❏ Varicose veins
- ❏ Venous stars
- ❏ Jugular vein distension
- ❏ Deep vein thrombophlebitis
- ❏ Superficial thrombophlebitis
- ❏ Migratory thrombophlebitis
- ❏ Caput medusa

CLINICAL FINDINGS

Varicose veins   They usually occur with venous valve incompetence, which can be demonstrated by the Trendelenburg test. Raise the leg and occlude the proximal saphenous vein. Have the patient stand, and then release the vein. Immediate filling will be seen with incompetence. Incompetence of the lowest perforators will give a "flare sign" with dilation of the veins over the posterior ankle with calf contraction.

Venous stars   They appear as a cluster of fine, purplish dilated veins, usually located over the medial thigh above the knee and above the ankle. They become more prominent with pregnancy and IVC obstruction.

Jugular vein distension   An undulating internal jugular meniscus observed above the clavicle with the patient at 45° indicates pathologic right heart volume overload or failure. The hepatojugular reflux, a persistent elevation of the jugular meniscus when pressure is applied to the upper abdomen for 60 seconds, indicates latent right heart failure.

Deep vein thrombophlebitis   The most common presentation is a unilateral swollen lower leg. There may be a deep palpable cord—or prominent "sentinel" veins over the proximal third of the shin—which remain filled with leg elevation **(Plate 42).**

Superficial thrombophlebitis   The hallmark is a superficial palpable cord, which may be red or tender.

Migratory thrombophlebitis   When observed in otherwise normal superficial veins without precipitant, and at several sites, they may be associated with adenocarcinomas such as pancreatic or gastric cancer (Trousseau's syndrome).

Caput medusa   Dilated veins on the abdominal surface can occur with inferior vena caval obstruction or with portal hypertension. Both produce leg swelling, but the latter usually has ascites, jaundice, and spider angiomata **(Plates 62, 64).**

Section III
Lungs/Chest

Chapter 31

Acute Cough

◤ DIFFERENTIAL OVERVIEW

- ❏ Viral upper respiratory infection
- ❏ Asthma
- ❏ Sinusitis
- ❏ Mycoplasma bronchitis
- ❏ Pneumonia
- ❏ Gastroesophageal reflux
- ❏ Congestive heart failure
- ❏ ACE inhibitor
- ❏ Aspiration
- ❏ Cough in HIV
- ❏ Thermal
- ❏ Fume inhalation
- ❏ Pertussis
- ❏ Lung abscess

DIAGNOSTIC APPROACH

Respiratory viruses cause most acute cough. The main issue in diagnosis is to detect bacterial infection (especially pneumonia), which would benefit from treatment with antibiotics. Unfortunately, the spectrum of viral bronchitis and that of bacterial bronchitis overlap considerably, making accurate diagnosis difficult.

Detection of induced bronchial hyperreactivity (reactive airways disease), which benefits from bronchodilator treatment, is also important. Wheezing, shortness of breath, and a predisposition (atopy or smoker) are helpful clinical clues.

A cough appearing mostly at night suggests congestive heart failure or reflux.

CLINICAL FINDINGS

Viral upper respiratory infection Concurrent nasal congestion, scratchy sore throat, or laryngitis is usually found. The cough is often "irritative." Wheezing may occur especially in smokers and atopic individuals.

Asthma Bilateral expiratory wheezing with prolonged expiratory phase is diagnostic of asthma. Occasionally cough without wheezing can also be caused by bronchospasm ("cough-variant asthma").

Sinusitis There is usually a sensation of postnasal drainage and of the cough originating in the throat rather than in the lungs. Mucous can often be observed in the pharynx. Local symptoms of sinusitis, such as nasal congestion and facial fullness/pressure/pain, are also present.

Mycoplasma bronchitis Mycoplasma is difficult to distinguish from viral bronchitis, as it produces a fever and a dry, hacking cough that progresses to one productive of purulent sputum. Epidemiologic data is helpful, i.e., spread among family contacts with a 2-3-week latency. Bullous myringitis is unusual, but if seen strongly suggests mycoplasma. Chlamydia pneumoniae produces a similar clinical picture **(Plate 232).**

Pneumonia Sudden onset, spiking fever with rigors, cough producing purulent sputum, dyspnea, pleuritic chest pain, systemic toxicity, and localized consolidative lung findings (rales) all point to pneumonia. Rusty sputum is classic for pneumococcus.

Gastroesophageal reflux It occurs more often at night and is accompanied by heartburn.

Congestive heart failure Left heart failure is suggested by a dry cough awakening the patient, in the presence of unexplained tachycardia, S3 gallop, fine bibasilar rales, exertional dyspnea, and/or orthopnea.

ACE inhibitor An irritative, nonproductive cough coincides temporally with the use of the drug.

Aspiration Foreign body aspiration can produce a prominent expulsive cough and unilateral or focal wheezing.

Cough in HIV Productive cough suggests bacterial pneumonia. Pneumocystis produces a dry cough and dyspnea that is subacute and progressive. Pleuritic chest pain can occur

65

with spontaneous pneumothorax in Pneumocystis or Kaposi's. Tuberculosis is suggested by hemoptysis **(Plate 200).**

Thermal   Inhalation of cold air, especially in patients who have reactive airways and in those who are exercising, may cause coughing or wheezing.

Fume inhalation   Tobacco, smoke, and volatile chemical inhalation are obvious, but ambient air pollutants can be more subtle causes.

Pertussis   Paroxysms of cough end in a loud inspiratory "whoop" with expectoration of a mucous plug. A frenulum ulcer may appear due to tongue protrusion with dental abrasion.

Lung abscess   It is marked by the sudden appearance of a large amount of purulent, foul-smelling sputum.

Acute Dyspnea

◼ DIFFERENTIAL OVERVIEW

- ❏ Asthma
- ❏ COPD exacerbation
- ❏ Left heart failure
- ❏ Pneumonia
- ❏ Pulmonary embolism
- ❏ Pneumothorax
- ❏ Hyperventilation
- ❏ Pleural effusion
- ❏ Pericardial tamponade
- ❏ Upper airway obstruction
- ❏ Pulmonary hypertension
- ❏ Lung cancer
- ❏ Noncardiogenic pulmonary edema
- ❏ Bilateral diaphragmatic paralysis

DIAGNOSTIC APPROACH

Dyspnea is a sensation of inability to take in enough air, which causes anxiety and discomfort. It may not correlate reliably with arterial oxygen saturation, being caused by factors including tissue hypoxia, reduced lung compliance, and activation of J receptors.

Paroxysmal nocturnal dyspnea occurs in those with congestive heart failure (CHF) when patients awaken with a sense of suffocation and wheezing. Patients with chronic bronchitis may also awaken with shortness of breath and wheezing caused by mucous plugging. This clears with a cough. Orthopnea is seen in CHF, asthma, and bilateral diaphragmatic paralysis. Sudden onset suggests pneumothorax, pulmonary embolism, or "flash" pulmonary edema.

CLINICAL FINDINGS

Asthma Diffuse wheezing occurs without fever or localizing findings. There will usually be a history of prior asthma, croup, or atopy. Mild bronchospasm may present with vague dyspnea (especially exertional) and cough. An acute increase in shortness of breath can occur with plugging of tenacious mucous.

COPD exacerbation Diffuse wheezing with productive cough occurs in smokers with chronic bronchitis, usually when an upper respiratory infection develops.

Left heart failure Orthopnea, paroxysmal nocturnal dyspnea, and S3 gallop are helpful clues. Interstitial edema is marked by tachypnea and rales, which are inspiratory and dependent. Alveolar edema produces wet rales/rhonchi, anxiety, and frothy, blood-tinged sputum.

Pneumonia Fever, productive cough, and consolidative findings (localized rales, egophony, and diminished breath sounds) are characteristic. Subacute onset of dyspnea in an HIV-positive patient suggests Pneumocystis.

Pulmonary embolism It is recognized by acute pleuritic chest pain, hemoptysis (with pulmonary infarction), an embolic source in the legs, or at least factors predisposing to deep venous thrombosis. A pleural friction rub occurs in 20% **(Plate 42).**

Pneumothorax The onset is acute, with unilateral diminished breath sounds and hyperresonance to percussion. It usually occurs in thin, young adults or older patients with bullous disease. A tracheal shift suggests tension pneumothorax.

Hyperventilation It is recognized by the concurrence of perioral and acral paresthesias, the stressful setting in which it occurs, and perceived anxiety.

Pleural effusion Unilateral diminished breath sounds and percussive dullness are found.

Pericardial tamponade Findings of jugular venous distension with Kussmaul's sign (veins fill with inspiration), exaggerated pulsus paradoxus, and hypotension are key clues.

Upper airway obstruction   Stridor and a tracheal wheeze are characteristic. Sudden aphonia while eating occurs with tracheal obstruction by a food bolus. Other causes include severe laryngitis, diphtheria, and allergic laryngeal edema **(Plate 185).**

Pulmonary hypertension   An accentuated pulmonary component of the second heart sound and right ventricular lift are suggestive.

Lung cancer   Acute dyspnea can occur with bronchial obstruction and lobar collapse. A unilateral wheeze and absent segmental breath sounds are found. The patient is most frequently a smoker.

Noncardiogenic pulmonary edema   This occurs in the setting of infection, aspiration, shock, narcotic or salicylate overdose, high-altitude, or CNS events. With salicylate intoxication, central hyperventilation occurs.

Bilateral diaphragmatic paralysis   This is a cause of acute dyspnea in neurologic or myopathic disorder, recent thoracic trauma, or surgery.

Breast Discharge

◼ DIFFERENTIAL OVERVIEW

- ❑ Drugs
- ❑ Postpartum
- ❑ Prolactin-secreting pituitary adenoma
- ❑ Intraductal papilloma
- ❑ Fibrocystic disease
- ❑ Breast cancer
- ❑ Mammary duct ectasia
- ❑ Repeated nipple stimulation

DIAGNOSTIC APPROACH

Galactorrhea occurs when high levels of prolactin act upon a breast primed by estrogen and progesterone. Therefore, it is extremely rare in men unless there is a feminizing state. It can usually be visually differentiated from serous or bloody discharge. If confirmation is needed, microscopic examination for oval fat bodies (or use of Sudan stain) can be performed. Breast secretions can be found in up to one-fourth of women previously pregnant.

Watery, serous, serosanguinous, and bloody discharges can be caused by intraductal papilloma (50%), fibrocystic disease (31%), breast cancer (14%), or duct ectasia (5%).

CLINICAL FINDINGS

Drugs Oral contraceptives, phenothiazines, tricyclic antidepressants, benzodiazepines, verapamil, reserpine, methyldopa, isoniazid, and opiates have all been associated with galactorrhea, through inhibition of dopamine secretion by the hypothalamus, thus increasing prolactin production.

Postpartum Normal lactation.

Prolactin-secreting pituitary adenoma Galactorrhea occurring concurrently with amenorrhea and persistent galactorrhea after childbirth is a common scenario. Visual field defect and headache may be additional clues **(Plate 15).**

Intraductal papilloma Unilateral discharge is found with an areolar mass.

Fibrocystic disease The breasts are symmetrically nodular, and the nodules enlarge before the menses.

Breast cancer A hard, fixed mass may be found in association with a blood-tinged discharge **(Plate 51).**

Mammary duct ectasia It presents as bilateral discharge in a perimenopausal woman, associated with pain, itching, and swelling of the nipple. A tubular "bag of worms" structure is felt on palpation of the areola. The discharge is gray-green.

Repeated nipple stimulation Galactorrhea may occur in a woman previously pregnant, the wet-nurse phenomenon. Prolactin levels are normal **(Plate 15).**

◼ DIFFERENTIAL OVERVIEW

❑ Fibrocystic disease
❑ Fibroadenoma
❑ Breast cancer
❑ Intraductal papilloma
❑ Mastitis
❑ Hematoma
❑ Thrombophlebitis
❑ Galactocele

DIAGNOSTIC APPROACH

Breast lumps should be approached with a high index of suspicion for breast cancer. Approximately 20% of solitary or dominant breast masses are breast cancers. A biopsy is always necessary with the exception of a cystic mass that disappears after aspiration, with negative cytology and mammogram. Equivocal or nonsuspicious masses should be reexamined during the follicular phase of the menstrual cycle (days 5–7).

Cyclical pain and tenderness are usually due to fibrocystic disease. Although breast cancer can present with pain, it is often atypical and there is usually no tenderness. Characteristics of pain with alternative diagnoses include the following: heavy or full of milk (fibrocystic), sharp and radiating (radiculitis), itching, burning, drawing (duct ectasia), burning and stinging (mastodynia), sore, bruised, stabbing (trauma), throbbing (infectious), aching, and locally tender (costochondritis).

CLINICAL FINDINGS

Fibrocystic disease   There is an underlying substrate of lumpy breasts with radially arranged fine nodular cysts. A mobile, rubbery (feels fluid-filled) nodule will be present, which will be similar in consistency to the other smaller nodules. It usually increases in size just before the period or after breast trauma. It may be painful or tender. Two diagnostic strategies include needle aspiration of thick yellow-green fluid, which should make a cyst disappear or reexamination after the menses, at which time the nodule should be smaller.

Fibroadenoma   The mass is highly mobile, rubbery, firm, well-demarcated, nontender, and may have a kidney-like notch. It may increase in size with adolescence, pregnancy, menopause, or hormonal treatment.

Breast cancer   Classically, the mass is as hard as a stone, fixed to the underlying tissue, and has indistinct borders. These findings are not reliable, however, because 60% of cancers are freely mobile, 40% are soft or cystic, and 40% have regular borders. Additional findings, usually at more advanced stages of disease, include peau d'orange (orange peel) changes of the overlying skin and axillary adenopathy. Infiltrating ductal carcinoma is stony hard. Papillary cancer is multicentric. Infiltrating lobular cancer produces a vague thickening. Inflammatory carcinoma produces erythema and edema of the skin of the breast. Paget's disease produces eczematous skin changes of the nipple or discharge **(Plate 51).**

Intraductal papilloma   This presents with unilateral serous or serosanguinous discharge and a rounded subareolar mass.

Mastitis   There is a radial mass, which is quite tender, red, and warm, localized to one quadrant. It is usually caused by an obstructed duct.

Hematoma   It is usually posttraumatic and tender.

Thrombophlebitis   Superficial tenderness over the inferolateral breast and a palpable cord are found.

Galactocele   It occurs only during lactation **(Plate 15).**

Chronic Cough

PLATE 52

◤ DIFFERENTIAL OVERVIEW

- ❑ Upper respiratory infection
- ❑ Allergy
- ❑ Chronic bronchitis
- ❑ Cough-variant asthma
- ❑ Chronic sinusitis
- ❑ Esophageal reflux
- ❑ ACE inhibitor
- ❑ Pollutants
- ❑ Psychogenic
- ❑ Foreign body
- ❑ Congestive heart failure
- ❑ Lung cancer
- ❑ Tuberculosis
- ❑ Mediastinal mass
- ❑ Bronchiectasis
- ❑ Pulmonary fibrosis
- ❑ Cystic fibrosis
- ❑ Aspergillosis

DIAGNOSTIC APPROACH

Green color in the sputum may be caused by either polymorphonuclear leukocytes or eosinophils.

Hoarseness suggests tumor with involvement of the vocal cords or recurrent laryngeal nerve, or it may suggest chronic esophageal reflux.

CLINICAL FINDINGS

Upper respiratory infection Prolonged cough (and bronchial hyperreactivity) following a URI is common. One-fourth of patients still have cough 1 month after the onset of symptoms, usually those with a history of asthma or atopy (i.e., allergic rhinitis or hay fever).

Allergy The patient will relate a sensation of chronic drainage of postnasal mucous, prompting chronic coughing, or throat-clearing.

Chronic bronchitis A prominent morning cough, productive of mucoid sputum with occasional blood streaks, develops in a cigarette smoker.

Cough-variant asthma Recurrent cough may be the predominant symptom, sometimes without apparent wheeze. The patient's breathing usually feels tight.

Chronic sinusitis Facial fullness or pain, associated with a purulent postnasal drainage (which may be seen in the pharynx), produces an "irritated" cough and a sensation that the throat needs to be cleared.

Esophageal reflux Reflux is recognized by nocturnal cough, concurrent with heartburn, an acid taste in the throat, and hoarseness.

ACE inhibitor A dry, irritative cough occurs in 15–20% of patients taking any ACE inhibitor and will resolve soon after discontinuing use of the drug.

Pollutants Heavy smog, sulphur dioxide, and nitrous oxide are typical causes. Dusts and particulate matter may potentiate the problem.

Psychogenic Cough occurs at times of emotional stress and ceases during the night. Cough suppressants are not effective.

Foreign body Beginning after a choking episode, a localized wheeze occurs.

Congestive heart failure Typically the cough is nocturnal, with orthopnea and paroxysmal nocturnal dyspnea. An S3 gallop and dependent rales are often present.

Lung cancer Cough is an early manifestation with an endobronchial lesion, suggested by a change in the pattern of a smoker's cough. Hemoptysis may be found early in 10–15% of cases. Other clues are clubbing, localized wheezing, and an unexplained minor weight loss (Plate 52).

Chronic Cough

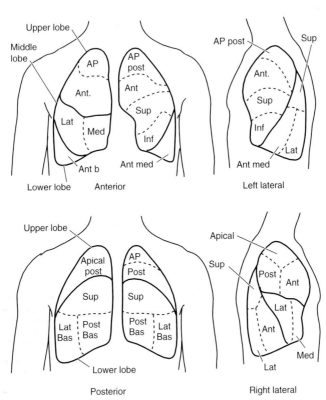

Figure 7. Surface projection of lung segments. (Adapted from: Reilly BR. Practical Strategies in Outpatient Medicine. 2nd ed. Philadelphia: W.B. Saunders, 1991, p. 328.)

Tuberculosis   Night sweats, hemoptysis, fever, and recent immigrant status are clues. Apical lung findings are present occasionally.

Mediastinal mass   Extrinsic compression produces a dry, "brassy" cough, which may be positional. Hoarseness caused by recurrent laryngeal compression is an additional clue.

Bronchiectasis   This is characterized by copious amounts of mucopurulent sputum and repeated bouts of hemoptysis and pneumonia. Focal rhonchi and wheezes are often found on exam. The sputum will characteristically separate upon sitting into a foamy top layer, a serous middle layer, and pus and debris in the bottom layer.

Pulmonary fibrosis   The cough is nonproductive and associated with dyspnea on exertion. Fine, dry, "Velcro" rales are fixed in location. Clubbing is often found (**Plate 52**).

Cystic fibrosis   Infrequently it is first recognized in adulthood, manifest as a chronic cough since childhood, progressive dyspnea, hemoptysis, malabsorption with low weight and diarrhea, and a swallowing disorder with choking when ingesting food or drink.

Aspergillosis   Atopic asthmatics cough up tough, spindle-shaped plugs, 1–2 cm in length.

Chapter 36

Chronic Dyspnea

PLATES 28, 36, 41, 52, 219

◼ DIFFERENTIAL OVERVIEW

- ❏ Chronic obstructive pulmonary disease
- ❏ Congestive heart failure
- ❏ Asthma
- ❏ Recurrent pulmonary embolism
- ❏ Interstitial lung disease
- ❏ Lung cancer
- ❏ Chronic pleural effusion
- ❏ Primary pulmonary hypertension
- ❏ Cystic fibrosis
- ❏ Kyphoscoliosis
- ❏ Myasthenia gravis
- ❏ Tracheal stenosis
- ❏ Mitral stenosis

DIAGNOSTIC APPROACH

Nonproductive cough may be a "dyspnea equivalent." Nocturnal coughing to clear the airway of excess secretions can be confused with paroxysmal nocturnal dyspnea.

Trepopnea, dyspnea lying on one side but not the other, occurs with cardiomegaly, unilateral parenchymal lung disease, and mediastinal or endobronchial tumors.

CLINICAL FINDINGS

Chronic obstructive pulmonary disease   Two patterns predominate: "Blue bloaters" are plethoric, cough incessantly, and have wheezes and rhonchi with a wet cough; "pink puffers" are thin, wrinkled, barrel-chested, and breathe with pursed lips (auto-PEEP). On examination, the chest is hyperresonant, with distant breath sounds and a prolonged expiratory phase. End-inspiratory retraction at the costal margin is consistent with hyperinflation and air trapping.

Congestive heart failure   Dyspnea on exertion progresses to orthopnea and paroxysmal nocturnal dyspnea. Rales, S3 gallop, jugular venous distention, and edema are diagnostic signs **(Plate 41).**

Asthma   Intermittent or persisting wheezing is the sine qua non of asthma.

Recurrent pulmonary embolism   Consider this in patients with a stepwise increase in dyspnea, pleuritic chest pain, or a predisposing factor such as cancer or oral contraceptive use.

Interstitial lung disease   It is distinguished by cyanosis on exertion, clubbing of the fingers, and fine "Velcro" rales **(Plate 52).**

Lung cancer   Suspect cancer in a smoker with unilateral wheeze or hemoptysis.

Chronic pleural effusion   Breath sounds are decreased with dullness to percussion unilaterally at the lung base.

Primary pulmonary hypertension   It occurs in women in their forties, often in those having a history of accompanying chest pain or Raynaud's phenomenon **(Plate 36).**

Cystic fibrosis   This diagnosis is usually made in childhood. The patient has pulmonary symptoms of recurrent respiratory infections and chronic, copious, thick secretions.

Kyphoscoliosis   This is evident on inspection of the thorax, but care should be taken to distinguish it from a barrel chest in emphysema.

Myasthenia gravis   Fatigable dyspnea is associated with diplopia, ptosis, or swallowing difficulty **(Plate 219).**

Tracheal stenosis   Stridor and inspiratory retraction of the supraclavicular space occurs in critical tracheal stenosis.

Mitral stenosis   Key symptoms/findings are a diastolic rumble, hemoptysis, and malar flushing, especially in a patient with a history of rheumatic fever **(Plate 28).**

Gynecomastia

PLATE 61

Chapter 37

◼ DIFFERENTIAL OVERVIEW

❑ Adolescence
❑ Drugs
❑ Cirrhosis
❑ Bilateral orchiectomy
❑ Ectopic hCG
❑ Klinefelter's syndrome

DIAGNOSTIC APPROACH

An estrogen-mediated phenomenon, gynecomastia may be produced by increased secretion of estrogens or increased peripheral conversion of testosterone and androstenedione to estradiol and estrone. It may be unilateral in one-third of cases, and it may be tender or painful.

Gynecomastia must be distinguished from breast cancer, which is an eccentric firm mass with fixation and regional adenopathy, and from a generalized increase in fatty tissue in obesity.

Gynecomastia is not a feature of central hypogonadism and does not increase the risk of developing male breast cancer.

CLINICAL FINDINGS

Adolescence Gynecomastia is a normal transient physiologic phenomenon in as many as 80% of pubertal boys, and it is often unilateral.

Drugs Exogenous estrogens, such as milk or meat from estrogen-fed cattle, may cause gynecomastia. Spironolactone, H2 antagonists, digitoxin, phenothiazines, amphetamines, reserpine, methyldopa, isoniazid, ketoconazole, imipramine, phenytoin, heroin, marijuana, antiandrogens, and anabolic steroids can all induce gynecomastia. A clue is unilateral gynecomastia or asymmetric enlargement.

Cirrhosis Look for concomitant signs such as spider angiomata, palmar erythema, ascites, and testicular atrophy **(Plate 61).**

Bilateral orchiectomy Whether traumatic or intentional in treatment of prostate cancer, gynecomastia is accompanied by decreased beard growth and muscle mass and smooth skin.

Ectopic hCG This may be produced by choriocarcinoma of the testis and tumors of the lung, liver, pancreas, colon, or stomach.

Klinefelter's syndrome Gynecomastia develops during puberty in a patient with long limbs, small firm testes, and underdeveloped secondary sexual characteristics.

Hemoptysis

◼ DIFFERENTIAL OVERVIEW

❑ Bronchitis
❑ Pneumonia
❑ Pulmonary edema
❑ Pulmonary infarction
❑ Tuberculosis
❑ Bronchogenic carcinoma
❑ Chest trauma
❑ Bronchiectasis
❑ Bronchial adenoma
❑ A-V malformation
❑ Aspergilloma
❑ Vasculitis
❑ Lung abscess
❑ Mitral stenosis
❑ Hereditary hemorrhagic telangiectasia
❑ Primary pulmonary hemosiderosis
❑ Parasitic

DIAGNOSTIC APPROACH

In primary care practice, neoplasm is the cause of less than 2% of cases of hemoptysis. A chest radiograph is nonetheless an essential component of the evaluation of every case of hemoptysis.

Differentiate hemoptysis from hematemesis. Hemoptysis is frothy, blood-tinged sputum that the patient can usually distinguish as coming from the lungs. Hematemesis is associated with nausea and vomiting, and it may be darker. Nasal or pharyngeal bleeding with posterior pharyngeal drainage could also be a source that must be considered.

Clubbing indicates a chronic disorder and may be found in association with neoplasm, bronchiectasis, and lung abscess. Massive hemoptysis is usually due to lung cancer, tuberculosis, or aortic aneurysm.

DIFFERENTIAL DIAGNOSIS

Bronchitis   Occurring in the setting of an acute vigorous productive cough, bronchitis is associated with typical upper respiratory symptoms.

Pneumonia   Fever, cough tinged with blood, pleuritic chest pain, and focal rales with consolidative findings may occur in any combination. Pneumococcus classically produces rust-colored sputum. Klebsiella may produce a tenacious "currant jelly" sputum.

Pulmonary edema   In acute left heart failure, frothy pink sputum occurs with dependent rales, S3 gallop, and dyspnea.

Pulmonary infarction   In acute pulmonary embolism, sudden onset of pleuritic chest pain and dyspnea with a pleural rub will occur. A source may be found in a unilateral swollen leg **(Plate 42).**

Tuberculosis   The classic presentation is blood-tinged sputum. Epidemiologic exposure/risk factors (e.g., being a health care worker, an Asian immigrant, or at risk for HIV) or upper lung field consolidative findings provide additional clues.

Bronchogenic carcinoma   When presenting with hemoptysis, the lung cancer is usually primary because metastatic cancer is rarely endobronchial. Environmental exposure to tobacco or asbestos or a family history of this disease increases the risk. Firm, palpable supraclavicular nodes are sometimes found.

Chest trauma   Rib fracture may cause a lung laceration. There will be exquisite tenderness over the rib segment, and the fragment will "float."

Bronchiectasis   It is recognized clinically by recurrent episodes of grossly bloody sputum (due to necrosis of bronchial mucosa) in a patient with copious amounts of purulent sputum on a chronic basis.

Hemoptysis

Bronchial adenoma   Being quite vascular, these often present with episodes of self-limited hemoptysis recurrent over years.

A-V malformation   There may be an audible bruit on auscultation of the lung.

Aspergilloma   It occurs in an immunosuppressed host with prior cavitary lung disease or bullous disease with wheezing.

Vasculitis   Goodpasture's syndrome and Wegener's are defined by hemoptysis in association with hematuria. Wegener's will be associated with a nasal septal ulcer or perforation **(Plate 111).**

Lung abscess   Unmistakably fetid sputum will be intermittently mixed with blood.

Mitral stenosis   Hemoptysis is a diagnostic pearl in a patient with a soft, low-pitched apical diastolic murmur and an opening snap. This condition is often not considered because of its rarity and the orientation toward considering pulmonary causes of hemoptysis **(Plate 28).**

Hereditary hemorrhagic telangiectasia   Telangiectasias are evident on the lips and skin, and there is usually a history of bleeding from other sites **(Plate 55).**

Primary pulmonary hemosiderosis   This occurs in young adult males with exertional dyspnea.

Parasitic   Schistosomiasis, paragonomiasis, or echinococcus should be considered as causes in international travelers or immigrants.

Hiccup

PLATE 198

▚ DIFFERENTIAL OVERVIEW

- ❏ Idiopathic
- ❏ Drugs
- ❏ Post-operative
- ❏ Pneumonia
- ❏ Liver metastasis
- ❏ Lung cancer
- ❏ Esophageal cancer
- ❏ Subdiaphragmatic abscess
- ❏ Pericarditis
- ❏ Uremia
- ❏ Central
- ❏ Hysterical
- ❏ Splenic infarction
- ❏ Thoracic aortic aneurysm

DIAGNOSTIC APPROACH

Hiccups are caused by excitation of the phrenic reflex arc or by suppression of higher centers by central lesions or metabolic abnormalities. The sound is produced by spasm of the inspiratory muscles abruptly terminated by glottis closure.

Recurrent or intractable hiccups should prompt a more thorough investigation. Hiccup with dysphagia suggests esophageal cancer, achalasia, or hiatal hernia.

CLINICAL FINDINGS

Idiopathic   Self-limited hiccups occur in an otherwise healthy patient and may be initiated by laughter or gastric distension with rapid eating/drinking.

Drugs   Alcohol, general anesthesia, barbiturates, benzodiazepines, dexamethasone, and methyldopa are causes.

Post-operative   Hiccups may be the result of general anesthesia itself or of diaphragmatic irritation with upper abdominal surgery.

Pneumonia   Hiccups are caused by diaphragmatic inflammation so there is usually pleuritic chest pain in the setting of cough, fever, and a pleural rub.

Liver metastasis   Suspect metastases if a primary cancer is known, but hiccups may be the presenting symptom. A firm mass is palpable in the right upper quadrant.

Lung cancer   Mediastinal adenopathy impinges on the phrenic nerve. Smoking history and hemoptysis are important clues.

Esophageal cancer   A tumor in the distal one-third of the esophagus is suggested by hiccups associated with dysphagia.

Subdiaphragmatic abscess   Suspect with abdominal pain, especially that which radiates to the shoulder and is associated with fever and localized upper abdominal tenderness.

Pericarditis   It is marked by chest pain relieved by leaning forward, and a 2-3 component friction rub. Consider it in the setting of myocardial infarction.

Uremia   The uremia is usually severe enough to cause a metabolic encephalopathy **(Plate 198)**.

Central   These hiccups are recognized by concomitant neurological findings. The most common central nervous system causes are sarcoidosis, encephalitis, brainstem tumor, and basilar meningitis.

Hysterical   The hiccup stops during sleep.

Splenic infarction   Hiccups accompany acute left upper quadrant abdominal pain. There is an embolic source, such as atrial fibrillation, endocarditis, or sickle cell anemia.

Thoracic aortic aneurysm   Often asymptomatic, such an aneurysm may cause a palpable pulsation in the upper chest.

Patterned Breathing

◤ DIFFERENTIAL OVERVIEW

❑ Tachypnea
❑ Paroxysmal nocturnal dyspnea
❑ Sleep apnea
❑ Kussmaul
❑ Cheyne-Stokes
❑ Kussmaul
❑ Biot's
❑ Apneustic
❑ Ataxic
❑ Stertorous

CLINICAL FINDINGS

Tachypnea   Although there are many pulmonary causes, the most important is pulmonary embolism (Se 0.92), associated with leg swelling and pleuritic chest pain. Intense tachypnea is also seen with intracranial hemorrhage **(Plate 42).**

Paroxysmal nocturnal dyspnea   A patient reports awakening from sleep with air hunger and diaphoresis, and opens a window for fresh air. Cough often occurs during an episode. This pattern is characteristic of congestive heart failure.

Sleep apnea   Roommates note loud snoring with long periods of apnea terminated by a gasping snore. Usually occurring in obese individuals, sleep apnea is associated with daytime somnolence.

Cheyne-Stokes   It is marked by periodic and sequentially increasing depth of respiration, followed by 15-60 second periods of apnea. It is seen most commonly in severe congestive heart failure, but also in meningitis, brain tumor, pneumonia, hypoxia, high-altitude sickness, and stroke. There is a delayed feedback to central respiratory centers leading to loss of fine-tuning to changes in pCO_2. The circulation time from the lung to the CNS equals one-half the cycle length. A low pontine or upper medullary lesion will produce a Cheyne-Stokes pattern unresponsive to pCO_2. These patients will be cyanotic and have CO_2 retention. Oxygen will enhance this pattern whereas in classic Cheyne-Stokes, the pattern would be suppressed.

Kussmaul   It occurs as regular, deep, fast breathing without dyspnea in acute metabolic acidosis such as ketoacidosis, salicylate or methyl alcohol toxicity, or uremia. The respirations cannot be interrupted for speech so the patient must pause to breathe. This finding is of value in the differentiation of hypotensive shock, in which tachypnea favors sepsis rather than hypovolemia.

Biot's   There are clusters of irregularly irregular breathing with abrupt starts and stops and longer periods of apnea than breathing. Seen in pontine lesions, Biot's may precede respiratory arrest.

Apneustic   Bradypnea, in which patients hold their breath at end-inspiration, is most often a sign of pontine hemorrhage, but it may also occur in basilar artery occlusion, hypoglycemia, anoxia, or severe meningitis.

Ataxic   This appears as breathing with varying tidal volumes and rates, caused by a problem with medullary chemoreceptors, but under conscious control.

Stertorous   The cheeks puff in and out with advanced increased intracranial pressure.

Chapter 41

Pneumonia Variants

◤ DIFFERENTIAL OVERVIEW

- ❏ Streptococcus pneumoniae
- ❏ Mycoplasma pneumoniae
- ❏ Haemophilus influenzae
- ❏ Chlamydia pneumoniae
- ❏ Influenza virus
- ❏ Staphylococcus aureus
- ❏ Mycobacterium tuberculosis
- ❏ Legionella pneumophila
- ❏ Klebsiella pneumoniae
- ❏ Pneumocystis carinii
- ❏ Chlamydia psittaci
- ❏ Hantavirus

DIAGNOSTIC APPROACH

Although the current trend is to use broad spectrum and multiple antibiotics without deter-mining the cause of the pneumonia, the use of clinical findings combined with low-tech bedside diagnostics, such as sputum Gram's stain, can often direct the choice of the appro-priate antibiotics. For example, in smokers with chronic bronchitis consider H. influenzae, S. pneumoniae, and B. catarrhalis.

CLINICAL FINDINGS

Streptococcus pneumoniae   Osler's triad of rigor, pleuritic chest pain, and rust-colored sputum still applies in a febrile patient with acute cough. The patient appears ill, and fever may exceed 40°. A sputum Gram's stain showing sheets of neutrophils and en-capsulated gram-positive diplococci will confirm the diagnosis.

Mycoplasma pneumoniae   The onset is subacute, with thin mucoid sputum and low-grade fever. Consider it in a young adult who has had contact with others with bronchi-tis or pneumonia within the incubation time of 2–3 weeks. Sputum Gram's stain shows sheets of neutrophils but no associated organisms (a pattern also common to atypical pneumonias caused by viruses, C. pneumoniae and Legionella). Bedside cold agglu-tinins provide a neat confirmation. Collect blood in an oxalated tube, and immerse it in wet ice for 1–2 minutes. Agglutination that occurs on the side of the tube and that dis-appears upon rewarming to body temperature indicates a positive test (at least 1:64 titer). Repeated agglutination on re-immersion helps differentiate mycoplasma from viral cold agglutinins **(Plate 232)**.

Haemophilus influenzae   Usually occurring in a smoker, H. influenzae is marked by rales without consolidative findings on examination. The sputum Gram's stain will show a background of small, pleomorphic, gram-negative coccobacilli.

Chlamydia pneumoniae   It presents like mycoplasma but with a greater degree of upper respiratory signs such as laryngitis or sinusitis.

Influenza virus   Flu-like symptoms will be prominent, with myalgias, sore throat, and malaise. The cough will produce scant sputum, and a specimen for Gram's stain will usually be unavailable.

Staphylococcus aureus   Abrupt in onset, this pneumonia makes the patient seriously ill, producing hectic fevers, chills, and productive cough. Hematogenous spread from en-docarditis may be a source, so look for a murmur, splinter hemorrhages or petechiae. The sputum Gram's stain shows large gram-positive cocci in clusters **(Plates 22, 23, 24)**.

Mycobacterium tuberculosis   The onset is subacute, associated with fatigue, anorexia, fever, and weight loss. Hemoptysis is a common presenting symptom. Look for upper lobe consolidative findings. Suspect this illness when the patient is HIV-infected, home-less, or institutionalized.

Legionella pneumophila   Cough is not prominent, but mental status changes, fever with relative bradycardia, and abdominal pain are. Sputum Gram's stain will show the "atypical pneumonia" pattern, but the patient has more toxicity than does one with mycoplasma or influenza.

Klebsiella pneumoniae   "Currant-jelly" sputum is a classic finding in this necrotizing pneumonia. Suspect it in alcoholics and other patients at risk of aspiration.

Pneumocystis carinii   Consider it when there is insidious onset of dyspnea and dry cough in an HIV-infected patient.

Chlamydia psittaci   Suspect it when there is a history of bird exposure.

Hantavirus   A prodrome of fever and myalgia leads rapidly to pulmonary edema and hypotension, in a patient with a history of rodent exposure.

◪ DIFFERENTIAL OVERVIEW

- ❏ Congestive heart failure
- ❏ Pneumonia
- ❏ Atelectasis
- ❏ Idiopathic pulmonary fibrosis
- ❏ Pulmonary sarcoidosis
- ❏ Asbestosis
- ❏ Rheumatoid lung disease
- ❏ Scleroderma

DIAGNOSTIC APPROACH

Early inspiratory rales, usually coarse and textured, are caused by bronchial obstruction. When found in emphysema or asthma, the FEV1/FVC ratio is reduced to less than 0.50. Late rales are alveolar in origin, owing to stiffening of the interstitium, causing the alveoli to pop open. Rattling secretions in the small airways (rhonchi) can sometimes be confused with rales. They are accompanied by a wet/loose cough.

CLINICAL FINDINGS

Congestive heart failure   Left ventricular failure produces dependent bibasilar rales, associated with a third heart sound.

Pneumonia   Rales caused by lobar consolidation are localized to a single area of the lung and occur in patients with fever and productive cough.

Atelectasis   A painful condition, such as recent abdominal surgery or a chest wall contusion, prevents the patient from fully expanding his lungs. The rales clear after the patient is asked to cough.

Idiopathic pulmonary fibrosis   The lung exam exhibits fixed, fine "Velcro" rales. In early fibrosis, rales occur at the lateral bases. As the disease progresses, the rales move up, in concert with the progressive worsening of dyspnea **(Plate 52).**

Pulmonary sarcoidosis   Lung involvement produces exertional dyspnea and a dry cough. Extrapulmonary signs, such as erythema nodosum, lymphadenopathy, iritis, or blue-purple shiny facial lesions of lupus pernio, suggest the diagnosis **(Plates 169, 170, 171).**

Asbestosis   Rales often precede chest radiograph findings. An occupational exposure can be elicited.

Rheumatoid lung disease   Interstitial disease with fine rales may be accompanied by a pleural rub or effusion. It occurs in the presence of active rheumatoid arthritis, with prominent synovial swelling and symmetrical polyarthritis **(Plates 88, 89).**

Scleroderma   Pulmonary fibrosis may be accompanied by pulmonary hypertension. Shiny, bound-down skin on the hands and face and dysphagia to solids are clues **(Plate 97).**

PLATES 4, 42, 52, 185, 231

◼ DIFFERENTIAL OVERVIEW

Wheezing
- ❑ Asthma
- ❑ Reactive airways disease
- ❑ Pulmonary edema
- ❑ Pulmonary embolism
- ❑ Emphysema
- ❑ Gastroesophageal reflux
- ❑ Drug/toxin reaction
- ❑ Vocal cord dysfunction
- ❑ Foreign body aspiration
- ❑ Mediastinal mass
- ❑ Carcinoid syndrome

Stridor
- ❑ Mucus plug
- ❑ Laryngeal trauma
- ❑ Angioedema
- ❑ Acute epiglottitis
- ❑ Retropharyngeal abscess

DIAGNOSTIC APPROACH

Wheezing has Se 0.14, Sp 0.99, and LR 14 for airway obstruction.

Central airway obstruction, such as that caused by aspirated foreign body or bronchogenic cancer, should be suspected when the onset of wheezing is sudden and focal, allergic markers and specific triggers are absent, and response to bronchodilator is poor. A history of aspiration or smoking and clubbing are also helpful **(Plate 52).**

Nocturnal wheezing could be the result of congestive heart failure (paroxysmal nocturnal dyspnea) or gastric aspiration with reflux.

CLINICAL FINDINGS

Asthma   Diffuse expiratory wheezing and a subjective tightness in breathing are cardinal signs. An asthma exacerbation with absence of wheeze and marked dyspnea signals severe airflow obstruction with little air movement.

Reactive airways disease   Self-limited wheezing occurs in the setting of a viral respiratory infection. The patient usually has a prior history of allergy.

Pulmonary edema   Rales are characteristic, but may be obscured by wheezes. Elevation of jugular venous pressure is usually found.

Pulmonary embolism   Diffuse or localized wheezing may be caused by the release of mediators of inflammation. Sudden-onset pleuritic chest pain, a swollen leg, and hemoptysis are important clues **(Plate 42).**

Emphysema   The course is chronic and progressive rather than episodic, and dyspnea is a hallmark. The patient is a heavy smoker with a barrel chest.

Gastroesophageal reflux   Nocturnal cough and wheeze coincide with heartburn and an acidic taste in the mouth.

Drug/toxin reaction   Beta blockers, aspirin (in a triad with nasal polyps and asthma), metabisulfate, iodinated contrast, and monosodium glutamate are common precipitants. Toluene and sulfur dioxide are inhalant precipitants.

Vocal cord dysfunction   It produces upper airway inspiratory wheeze associated with an abnormal voice.

Foreign body aspiration   It is suggested by focal wheezing and onset that occurs after loss of consciousness or dental manipulation.

Mediastinal mass   Mediastinal compression produces a superior vena cava syndrome with facial plethora, jugular venous engorgement, and prominent veins over the anterior chest.

Carcinoid syndrome   Carcinoid syndrome is recognized by brief, episodic flushing and wheezing **(Plate 4).**

Mucus plug   Acute stridor occurs in a dehydrated patient with a productive but weak cough.

Laryngeal trauma   There is a history of external neck trauma or heat/caustic inhalation.

Angioedema   Focal swelling of the tongue, lips, or periorbital region coincident with the stridor is key **(Plate 185).**

Acute epiglottitis   Severe sore throat without visible findings, thick muffled voice, and dysphagia are found in addition to the stridor.

Retropharyngeal abscess   Severe pain occurs with swallowing, leading to drooling, neck swelling, fever, and a toxic appearance **(Plate 231).**

Section IV
Abdomen

Abdominal Distension

◼ DIFFERENTIAL OVERVIEW

Ascites
- ❏ Right-sided heart failure
- ❏ Cirrhosis
- ❏ Hypoalbuminemia
- ❏ Ovarian cancer
- ❏ Portal vein thrombosis
- ❏ Hepatic vein thrombosis
- ❏ Intra-abdominal metastases
- ❏ Tuberculous peritonitis
- ❏ Chylous effusion

Gas/Bloating
- ❏ Aerophagia
- ❏ Irritable bowel syndrome
- ❏ Acquired lactase deficiency
- ❏ Carbonated beverages
- ❏ Nonabsorbable carbohydrates
- ❏ Fatty food intolerance
- ❏ Small bowel obstruction
- ❏ Gastric dilation

Other
- ❏ Obesity
- ❏ Distended bladder
- ❏ Gravid uterus

DIAGNOSTIC APPROACH

In ascites, the abdomen is globular, the skin is tense and shiny, and the umbilicus is flush. The most reliable signs of ascites are bulging flanks, transmitted fluid wave, and shifting dullness to percussion. Fluid in the bulging flanks is best appreciated by a heaviness when the examiner lifts from below **(Plate 61).**

Venous dilation on the abdominal wall can be used as a differentiating feature. Normally, as determined by stripping veins, flow below the umbilicus is downward, and above the umbilicus, upward. In portal vein obstruction, flow is normal. In inferior vena cava obstruction, flow below the umbilicus is reversed as blood is shunted to the superior vena cava **(Plate 62).**

With portal hypertension, a soft liver suggests extrahepatic obstruction, a firm liver, cirrhosis, and a very hard or nodular liver, cancer. Portal hypertension alone does not produce ascites unless there is hypoalbuminemia or increased hepatic lymphatic pressure.

Look for signs of systemic disease such as weight loss or abdominal pain. For example, gluten-induced enteropathy may present with bloating and distension, but will also manifest prominent weight loss, steatorrhea, and diarrhea **(Plate 59).**

CLINICAL FINDINGS

Right-sided heart failure   Dilated jugular veins and edema usually precede the ascites. In constrictive pericarditis, there is jugular distension, a quiet precordium, ascites, and hepatomegaly **(Plate 41).**

Cirrhosis   A history of chronic alcoholism or hepatitis is usually present. Other stigmata include dilated veins on the abdominal wall, spider angiomata, testicular atrophy, gynecomastia, hemorrhoids, and palmar erythema **(Plate 62).**

Hypoalbuminemia   Common causes include nephrotic syndrome, malabsorption, and protein-calorie malnutrition **(Plate 41).**

Ovarian cancer   Nearly two-thirds of cases presents with ascites and a palpable pelvic mass. A gastric tumor with dropped implants in the cul-de-sac could present in a similar manner **(Plate 63).**

Abdominal Distension

Portal vein thrombosis   Thrombosis produces esophageal varices, often with upper gastrointestinal bleeding and splenomegaly **(Plate 62).**

Hepatic vein thrombosis   Thrombosis is characterized by hepatomegaly and ascites. If the inferior vena cava is also obstructed, there may be massive leg edema. It most often occurs in the setting of renal cell cancer, polycythemia, or migratory thrombophlebitis **(Plates 61, 62).**

Intra-abdominal metastases   A known tumor at an intraabdominal site, palpable nodules especially in the liver or around the umbilicus, left supraclavicular adenopathy, and marked cachexia are clues **(Plate 63).**

Tuberculous peritonitis   Ascites without leg edema, loculation (no shifting dullness), night sweats, and evidence of extrapulmonary tuberculosis in other sites are important indicators of this unusual diagnosis.

Chylous effusion   Chyle is most commonly seen in association with trauma or tumor and also in filariasis (elephantiasis).

Aerophagia   Eructation (belching) is the predominant phenomenon. It is caused by drinking carbonated beverages, air swallowing with excess saliva (e.g., gum or lozenges), chronic postnasal drainage, overly dry mouth (e.g., Sjogren's or anticholinergics), or air swallowing with stress or habit, which can be observed during the interview.

Irritable bowel syndrome   A sensation of abdominal bloating is common, despite little objective increase in gas formation. These symptoms will increase after a meal and are associated with cramping abdominal pain relieved by a bowel movement, and loose stools.

Acquired lactase deficiency   Milk, cheese, and ice cream produce loose stools, flatulence, abdominal cramps, bloating, or distension. Intolerance may be acquired as an adult, especially in patients of African or Asian descent (80–90%). It may also occur transiently following a viral gastroenteritis.

Carbonated beverages   Carbonated soft drinks, beer, and effervescent medications produce belching, especially when gulped, but seldom increase flatus.

Nonabsorbable carbohydrates   Baked beans, soybeans, broccoli, and cabbage contain a nonabsorbable complex carbohydrate that may be broken down into carbon dioxide, hydrogen, and methane by colonic bacteria. Saccharin and sorbitol (in sugarless gum) and fructose, in dates, prunes, grapes and fruit juices, may also be incompletely absorbed.

Fatty food intolerance CO_2 is produced in the duodenum, eliciting a sensation of postprandial bloating.

Small bowel obstruction   Poorly localized, cramping visceral pain, bilious vomiting, and swelling with tympanitic distension are typical. High-pitched rushes are heard on auscultation. Distended coils of intestine with visible peristalsis may be seen when abdominal musculature is lax.

Gastric dilation   Upper abdominal distension, tympany, and a succussion splash are the usual signs. Delayed gastric emptying may be the result of abdominal pain, peptic ulcer, paraplegia, diabetes (ketoacidosis or autonomic neuropathy), hypocalcemia, hypercalcemia, hypokalemia, uremia, or drugs (morphine, anticholinergics).

Obesity   There is an overhanging pannus, the skin is not stretched and shiny as in ascites, and the umbilicus is a deep pit rather than protruding as in ascites.

Distended bladder   A globular mass arises from the pelvis and is dull to percussion. There is usually a strong cramping pain referred to the urethra.

Gravid uterus   Pregnancy should be evident with amenorrhea and a central pelvic mass. The uterus may enlarge rapidly with hydrops.

Abdominal/Pelvic Mass

◼ DIFFERENTIAL OVERVIEW

Abdominal Mass
- ❑ Liver enlargement
- ❑ Spleen enlargement
- ❑ Fecal mass
- ❑ Diverticulitis
- ❑ Colon cancer
- ❑ Gallbladder enlargement
- ❑ Pancreatic pseudocyst
- ❑ Crohn's disease
- ❑ Abdominal aortic aneurysm
- ❑ Renal enlargement

Pelvic Mass
- ❑ Distended Bladder
- ❑ Pregnant uterus
- ❑ Salpingitis
- ❑ Ovarian cyst
- ❑ Uterine fibromyoma
- ❑ Ovarian cancer
- ❑ Endometrial cancer
- ❑ Ectopic pregnancy
- ❑ Malignant deposit

DIAGNOSTIC APPROACH

Consider the structures in the region of the mass for clues to its origin and the presence of tenderness as an indicator of inflammation/infection. It is possible to miss initially even a relatively large mass unless a systematic four-quadrant examination is performed.

CLINICAL FINDINGS

Liver enlargement   The liver extends from under the costal margin. Liver metastases feel hard and irregular. In patients with acute hepatitis, the liver is tender and smoothly enlarged.

Spleen enlargement   A palpable spleen tip in the left upper quadrant on inspiration signifies splenic enlargement.

Fecal mass   It is commonly found in the cecum or sigmoid colon. Firm and mobile, it may disappear completely on repeat exam.

Diverticulitis   A boggy, tender, ill-defined mass may be palpable in the left lower quadrant. The patient is febrile.

Colon cancer   It presents as a vague fixed mass that is associated with a change in bowel habits and blood in the stool.

Gallbladder enlargement   An oval, movable, right upper quadrant mass develops in a patient with a history of episodic intense steady pain (biliary colic).

Pancreatic pseudocyst   It appears as a left upper quadrant, smooth, rounded, fixed mass in a patient with a history of recurrent pancreatitis.

Crohn's disease   A right lower quadrant mass arises from terminal ileum involvement, in conjunction with weight loss and recurrent diarrhea with mucus and blood.

Abdominal aortic aneurysm   This is characterized by a central pulsatile mass, often with a harsh bruit. Differentiate an aneurysm from a transmitted impulse by placing the hands parallel along the edge of the mass. If they move apart, it is expansile.

Renal enlargement   Palpated in the lateral abdomen, an irregular nodular mass associated with intermittent profuse hematuria with pyramidal clots will signify renal cancer. Renal cancer may be associated with the sudden appearance of a left scrotal varicocele.

Distended bladder   A smooth mass arises over the pelvic brim. There will usually be a prominent urge to void.

Abdominal/Pelvic Mass

Pregnant uterus   Suspect when the menstrual period is missed, and look for other signs of pregnancy, such as nausea, darkening of the areola, bluish cervix, and globular uterine enlargement.

Salpingitis   Fever, progressive abdominal pain, and an exquisitely tender, fixed adnexal swelling are found. Lateral traction of the cervix during the pelvic exam will cause pain (chandelier sign) **(Plate 77).**

Ovarian cyst   The menses are normal. The mass can be separated from the uterus on bimanual exam.

Uterine fibromyoma   Menorrhagia is common, except in subperiosteal tumors. Masses are irregular and attached to the uterus.

Ovarian cancer   Fixation of the mass in the pelvis, ascites with abdominal distension, unilateral leg edema, cachexia, and abdominal pain are clues **(Plate 63).**

Endometrial cancer   Irregular bleeding is the primary sign.

Ectopic pregnancy   Before rupture, a mildly tender adnexal mass will appear. Other signs include a missed period or irregular, spotty bleeding. With tubal rupture, there will be sudden pain, hypotension, and an ill-defined lateral mass.

Malignant deposit   It will be palpable through the rectum as a firm, shelf-like impression.

Acute Abdominal Pain

◪ DIFFERENTIAL OVERVIEW

Generalized/Periumbilical
❏ Gastroenteritis
❏ Obstipation
❏ Small bowel obstruction
❏ Large bowel obstruction
❏ Mesenteric ischemia
❏ Peritonitis
❏ Abdominal aortic dissection
❏ Sickle cell crisis

Right Upper Quadrant/Epigastrium
❏ Hepatitis
❏ Biliary colic
❏ Peptic ulcer disease
❏ Pyelonephritis
❏ Acute cholecystitis

Right Lower Quadrant
❏ Appendicitis
❏ Inflammatory bowel disease
❏ Salpingitis
❏ Rectus abdominus muscle strain
❏ Ureteral calculus
❏ Ruptured corpus luteum cyst
❏ Ruptured ectopic pregnancy
❏ Ovarian torsion

Left Upper Quadrant
❏ Pancreatitis
❏ Splenic infarction
❏ Pyelonephritis
❏ Myocardial infarction

Left Lower Quadrant
❏ Inflammatory bowel disease
❏ Diverticulitis
❏ Salpingitis
❏ Rectus abdominus muscle strain
❏ Ureteral calculus
❏ Ovarian torsion
❏ Ruptured corpus luteum cyst
❏ Ruptured ectopic pregnancy
❏ Sigmoid volvulus

DIAGNOSTIC APPROACH

History indicates the diagnosis in 85–90% of cases. Consider organs located in the region of maximal pain and the time-course of onset. The ultimate decision may require a repeated history and physical examination over several hours. Narcotic analgesics should be withheld until a diagnosis is established because they can mask the expression of diagnostic characteristics of the disease. An intrathoracic source must always be considered with upper abdominal pain. *Physical examination* can demonstrate peritoneal inflammation and rebound tenderness by eliciting pain with gentle percussion of the abdomen as opposed to sharp release of the depressed hand. Pelvic and rectal examinations are mandatory in every patient who has abdominal pain. Auscultation may reveal silence that is consistent with ileus, intermittent rushes with bowel obstruction, or hyperactivity with gastroenteritis.

Parietal pain, caused by inflammation of the parietal peritoneum, is a steadily aching pain, located directly over the inflamed area and accentuated by pressure. Tonic reflex

Acute Abdominal Pain Chapter 46

spasm of the abdominal musculature is present. *Visceral pain*, caused by obstruction of a hollow viscera, is classically intermittent and colicky, but distension may produce steady pain. The pain is poorly localized, in contrast to pain from the parietal peritoneum, which is innervated by somatic nerves. The patient with visceral colic will writhe incessantly whereas the patient with parietal pain lies still in bed. *Vascular occlusion* can be recognized by severe pain disproportionate to physical findings in a patient with vascular disease or atrial fibrillation.

If the patient is well one moment, then has excruciating pain, which is maximal at onset, consider a ruptured hollow viscera or a vascular event, such as myocardial infarction or ruptured aortic aneurysm.

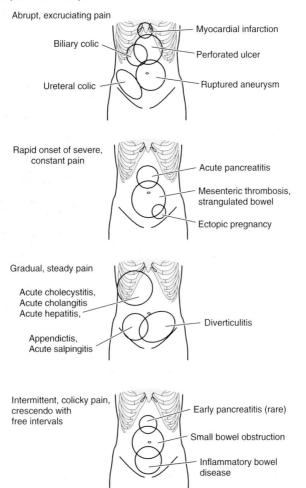

Abrupt, excruciating pain

Biliary colic

Ureteral colic

Myocardial infarction

Perforated ulcer

Ruptured aneurysm

Rapid onset of severe, constant pain

Acute pancreatitis

Mesenteric thrombosis, strangulated bowel

Ectopic pregnancy

Gradual, steady pain

Acute cholecystitis, Acute cholangitis Acute hepatitis,

Appendictis, Acute salpingitis

Diverticulitis

Intermittent, colicky pain, crescendo with free intervals

Early pancreatitis (rare)

Small bowel obstruction

Inflammatory bowel disease

Figure 8. Causes of acute abdominal pain by character and location. (Adapted from: Saunders CE, Ho MT. Current Emergency Diagnosis and Treatment. 4th ed. Norwalk, CT: Appleton & Lange, 1992, p. 111.)

Acute Abdominal Pain

CLINICAL FINDINGS

Gastroenteritis   The typical syndrome will consist of diffuse, cramping abdominal pain, fever, and nausea, with hyperactive bowel sounds and mild diffuse abdominal tenderness. Bacterial infections will cause higher fever, watery diarrhea, and foul-smelling, often bloody stools.

Obstipation   The patient is distended with stool palpable through the abdominal wall and only mild abdominal tenderness. There will usually be a history of absence of bowel movements for several days although a small amount of diarrhea may occur around the fecal obstruction.

Small bowel obstruction   The pain is colicky, severe, and poorly localized. Cramping pain occurs in short intense waves followed by complete absence of pain. Short pain-free intervals occur in proximal obstruction, and longer ones in distal. The patient is restless. Vomiting, which may become feculent, is common in proximal obstruction. The abdomen is distended in distal obstruction, and the rectum has an empty, "ballooned" feel. Tenderness to palpation is not impressive unless perforation has occurred. High-pitched hyperactive bowel sounds are characteristic, but they may be hypoactive or absent in 25%. Most patients (80%) have a history of prior abdominal surgery.

Large bowel obstruction   Constipation or change in bowel habits often precedes complete obstruction. Pain is felt below the umbilicus. Distension is prominent, but pain is less severe than with small bowel obstruction.

Mesenteric ischemia   Acute vascular occlusion usually presents with severe midabdominal pain out of proportion to the physical findings. The pain begins as colic, then progresses. In later stages, fever and hypotension occur. An embolic substrate (atrial fibrillation, or acute MI) is a key clue. The stool should be hemoccult positive. "Intestinal angina" presents with recurrent colicky abdominal pain and distension occurring 20–30 minutes after a meal and lasting 2–3 hours. This may manifest itself as food aversion or a malabsorptive diarrhea/steatorrhea with prominent weight loss. There is often a bruit in the upper abdomen.

Peritonitis   There will be early vomiting, board-like abdominal rigidity, rebound tenderness, fever, and a silent abdomen. The patient will lie absolutely still. The pain is often localized (e.g., appendicitis) before becoming generalized.

Abdominal aortic dissection   The pain is migrating, severe, tearing, and radiating to the back. The patient will often be in early shock, hypotensive and restless. There may be a pulsating, enlarged, tender aorta palpable through the abdomen. A femoral pulse may be absent. Loss of motor function and sensation in one leg suggests dissection with spinal artery compromise **(Plate 25).**

Sickle cell crisis   Diffuse abdominal pain with peritoneal signs develops in a patient with sickle cell anemia.

Hepatitis   Following a prodromal phase of anorexia and malaise, the icteric phase is dominated by right upper quadrant pain and tenderness, fever, jaundice, nausea, dark urine, and light stools.

Biliary colic   Sudden onset of steady and severe pain lasting 15 minutes to hours occurs with acute obstruction of the common bile or cystic duct. Cystic duct obstruction causes right upper quadrant pain whereas common duct obstruction causes epigastric pain, early jaundice, and prominent emesis. Pain may radiate to the scapula.

Peptic ulcer disease   Gnawing, aching, burning, or hunger pain in the epigastrium, relieved temporarily by food or antacids, suggests this diagnosis. Radiation to the back suggests perforation into the pancreas. Duodenal ulcer causes pain 1–2 hours after meals and at night.

Pyelonephritis   Typically, patients have dysuria, fever, nausea, and costovertebral angle tenderness although they may present with poorly localized abdominal pain.

Acute cholecystitis   Right upper quadrant pain radiates to the scapula and is accompanied by nausea, vomiting, and fever. Murphy's sign (inspiratory arrest on palpation over the gallbladder) is present, and a distended gallbladder is palpable in 30%. There is often a background of biliary colic. Fever and rigors herald a suppurative cholangitis.

Appendicitis   Classically, it begins as poorly localized visceral pain in the periumbilical region, moving to the right lower quadrant, where somatic pain is steadily progressive. There is localized tenderness over McBurney's point, with or without rebound tenderness. Anorexia/nausea and low-grade fever are usually present.

Inflammatory bowel disease   Pain, fever, and diarrhea with blood or mucus accompany flares. Terminal ileitis in young adults may simulate acute appendicitis. Crohn's may be recognized by systemic signs, such as arthritis.

Salpingitis   A sexually active woman presents with lower abdominal pain. Pelvic examination reveals yellow discharge from the cervix, cervical motion pain ("chandelier sign"), or tender adnexa. An exquisitely tender adnexal mass indicates a tubo-ovarian abscess **(Plate 72)**.

Rectus abdominus muscle strain   The history will suggest strain or overuse. The pain is constant and aching and is exacerbated by movement. There will be superficial tenderness over the rectus, and spasm may mimic guarding. A hematoma may simulate a localized mass.

Ureteral calculus   Severe cramping flank pain radiates to the groin. The patient is pale and unable to find a comfortable position. The urine will be dipstick positive for blood.

Ruptured corpus luteum cyst   Around the time of the menses, there occurs a sudden-onset, transient (hours), unilateral, lower abdominal and adnexal pain and tenderness. It is less severe and more diffuse than appendicitis, and it steadily improves on serial examination rather than worsening. A similar presentation during midcycle occurs with rupture of a graafian follicle (mittelschmerz).

Ruptured ectopic pregnancy   A missed or late period (85%) with an adnexal mass may be the only clue; thus, a high index of suspicion is needed. Rupture is accompanied by acute pain that may project to the shoulder, accompanied by cervical bleeding, shock, and a full, boggy cul-de-sac. There is a prior history of PID in 25%.

Ovarian torsion   The usual presentation is a young woman with acute onset of pain and a tender adnexal mass but no fever.

Pancreatitis   Left upper quadrant pain boring through to the back, prominent nausea and vomiting, and a history of heavy alcohol use or cholelithiasis are important clues. The patient sits up and leans forward, or lies on her side in a knee-chest position. Rebound will be present just above the umbilicus, and costovertebral angle tenderness occurs with inflammation of the tail of the pancreas. Hiccups are often present **(Plate 145)**.

Splenic infarction   Left upper quadrant pleuritic pain and tenderness occur in the setting of atrial fibrillation, sickle cell anemia, or neoplastic splenic enlargement. There may be a localized friction rub.

Myocardial infarction   Ischemia should be considered with upper abdominal pain although chest pain is usually present. Nausea can be seen with inferior ischemia.

Diverticulitis   It presents subacutely with low-grade fever and left lower quadrant abdominal pain. A tender mass with indistinct borders may be palpable on abdominal or rectal examination.

Sigmoid volvulus   Severe pain will suddenly occur while the patient is straining to defecate. Rapid, extreme left upper quadrant distension occurs, with vertical peristalsis.

Chapter 47

Acute Diarrhea

◼ DIFFERENTIAL OVERVIEW

- ❑ Viral gastroenteritis
- ❑ Staphylococcal enterotoxin
- ❑ E. coli
- ❑ Salmonella
- ❑ Campylobacter
- ❑ Drugs
- ❑ C. difficile colitis
- ❑ Giardia
- ❑ Shigella
- ❑ Yersinia
- ❑ Entamoeba histolytica
- ❑ Typhoid fever
- ❑ Vibrio parahaemolyticus
- ❑ Cryptosporidia
- ❑ Cholera
- ❑ Strongyloides

DIAGNOSTIC APPROACH

Most cases of acute diarrhea are self-limited, and evaluation for a specific cause is usually done only on those patients who show more toxicity or who have a prolonged course.

Secretory diarrhea is characterized by the absence of fever and prominent nausea/vomiting with watery stools that persist when fasting. It is caused by toxins (staph, E. coli, vibrio cholera), gastrin (pancreatic cancer), calcitonin (medullary carcinoma of the thyroid), or vasoactive intestinal peptide (VIP). Invasive infection with exudative diarrhea is associated with systemic symptoms, fever, chills, and blood, pus, and proteinaceous material in the stools. It most commonly occurs with infections such as Salmonella, Shigella, Campylobacter, or enterohemorrhagic E. coli.

Small bowel diarrhea is characterized by passage of large loose stools, and with periumbilical pain. Large bowel diarrhea has frequent passage of small stools, with tenesmus.

Common pathogens in HIV-associated diarrhea are cytomegalovirus, Cryptosporidia, Isospora, Salmonella, and Giardia.

Bloody diarrhea usually indicates invasive infection, but the differential also includes superior mesenteric artery thrombosis, inflammatory bowel disease, and drug-induced or ischemic colitis.

CLINICAL FINDINGS

Viral gastroenteritis   It begins abruptly, with diarrhea, nausea, vomiting, headache, low-grade fever, abdominal cramps, and malaise. The abdomen is diffusely mildly tender, and bowel sounds are hyperactive. Diarrhea is small bowel in type.

Staphylococcal enterotoxin   It causes classic food poisoning, with acute nausea, vomiting, cramps, and diarrhea 2–8 hours after eating food that has spoiled due to lack of refrigeration.

E. coli   Enterotoxic strains produce a secretory watery diarrhea, typical traveler's diarrhea. Enteroinvasive strains produce dysentery with hemorrhagic colitis and fever.

Salmonella   Invasive infection produces an enterotoxin-mediated secretory watery diarrhea, cramps, and fever, which can progress to dysentery or bacteremia. Sources include contaminated eggs or poultry, with an incubation period of 12–36 hours.

Campylobacter   Poultry and pets are sources. Prominent cramps and strongly malodorous stools are typical symptoms.

Drugs   Phenolphthalein, magnesium-containing antacids, caffeine, digoxin, quinidine, procainamide, antibiotics, NSAIDs, colchicine, lovastatin, and fluoxetine are frequent causes of diarrhea, but almost any drug is capable of causing it.

C. difficile colitis   Suspect this when diarrhea occurs following the use of broad-spectrum antibiotics. The patient becomes febrile and exhibits toxicity.

Giardia   Mild diarrhea with cramping and gas is a frequent presentation. Heavy small bowel infection may produce loose, watery or greasy, foul, yellow stools (steatorrhea) and mucus, without blood. Malabsorption with significant weight loss often occurs when symptoms persist more than 10 days.

Shigella   Because of a fecal-oral route of spread, *Shigella* is often seen in day care centers and rural areas of developing countries. Either small or large bowel presentations may occur. The patient may exhibit toxicity with fever, bloody diarrhea, nausea, vomiting, and cramps **(Plate 171).**

Yersinia   Fever, polyarthritis, and erythema nodosum may develop in 10–40%. Localized infection of the terminal ileum and cecum can cause right lower quadrant abdominal pain.

Entamoeba histolytica   The spectrum ranges from mild to fulminant with acute bloody diarrhea, usually with lower abdominal pain. Often, these patients have traveled to rural areas that have inadequate sanitation.

Typhoid fever   "Pea soup" diarrhea may develop in the third week of an illness characterized by progressive fever, relative bradycardia, rose spots (evanescent trunk rash), splenomegaly, cough, headache, and right lower quadrant abdominal pain **(Plate 60).**

Vibrio parahaemolyticus   It develops from raw seafood, especially oysters, salmon, and red snapper sushi, usually causing mild symptoms after an incubation period of hours to days.

Cryptosporidia   This prominent pathogen in HIV infection produces a profuse, watery diarrhea. It may also come from day care centers or occupational contact with dung.

Cholera   A spectrum of diarrhea up to gray, watery, mucoid "rice water" stools with fluid losses in excess of 1 liter/hour may occur.

Strongyloides   Infection is marked by epigastric abdominal pain, watery diarrhea, urticaria, perianal itching, bronchospasm, cough, and wheezing. Endemic regions include the southern United States, Central America, tropical Asia, and Africa **(Plate 183).**

Chapter 48

Anorexia

▣ DIFFERENTIAL OVERVIEW

- ❑ Depression
- ❑ Drugs
- ❑ Anorexia nervosa
- ❑ Congestive heart failure
- ❑ Hepatitis
- ❑ Cancer
- ❑ HIV infection
- ❑ Uremia
- ❑ Addison's disease
- ❑ Mesenteric ischemia
- ❑ Hypothalamic lesion

DIAGNOSTIC APPROACH

This differential refers to protracted anorexia. Acute anorexia may occur as a migraine prodrome or in early appendicitis.

Anorexia must be differentiated from early satiety or odynophagia (aversion to swallowing due to pain).

CLINICAL FINDINGS

Depression   Depressed mood, anhedonia, sleep disturbance, and inertia are key symptoms.

Drugs   Digoxin, narcotics, diuretics, amphetamines, antidepressants (SSRIs), and antihypertensives (especially ACE inhibitors) are common causes.

Anorexia nervosa   Loss of appetite is less common than an avoidance of food due to an abnormal body perception. Suspect anorexia nervosa in very thin young women. Hypothermia, constipation, and downy lanugo hair are additional findings that should raise suspicion.

Congestive heart failure   Because anorexia only occurs in advanced heart failure, signs such as edema, dependant rales, and S3 gallop are readily evident **(Plate 41).**

Hepatitis   Anorexia may precede the appearance of clinical jaundice, but right upper quadrant discomfort and tenderness are present.

Cancer   Anorexia is prominent in gastric and pancreatic cancer and in cancer with liver metastases. A humoral substance such as tumor necrosis factor may play a role. Weight loss that is out of proportion to the anorexia is common.

HIV infection   Anorexia can occur as a primary phenomenon of the wasting syndrome, due to opportunistic infection or to medication side effects.

Uremia   Waxy edema, sallow color, and oliguria are frequent findings **(Plate 198).**

Addison's disease   Associated signs include fatigue, hypotension, and hyperpigmentation, especially of the palmar creases and buccal mucosa **(Plates 12, 13).**

Mesenteric ischemia   Patients avoid eating because of resulting abdominal discomfort. Systemic vascular disease and an abdominal bruit usually coincide.

Hypothalamic lesion   Lesions such as sarcoidosis or tumor also cause visual field defects and metabolic/thermoregulatory disorders.

Chronic Diarrhea Chapter 49

PLATES 4, 52, 58, 59, 63, 86, 166, 171

◼ DIFFERENTIAL OVERVIEW

Inflammatory
- ❏ Inflammatory bowel disease
- ❏ Giardiasis
- ❏ Cryptosporidiosis

Altered Intestinal Motility
- ❏ Irritable bowel syndrome
- ❏ Diabetic enteropathy

Osmotic
- ❏ Lactase deficiency
- ❏ Drugs
- ❏ Pancreatic insufficiency
- ❏ Post-gastrectomy
- ❏ Celiac sprue
- ❏ Small bowel lymphoma

Secretory
- ❏ Villous adenoma
- ❏ Pancreatic cholera
- ❏ Carcinoid
- ❏ Zollinger-Ellison syndrome
- ❏ Medullary carcinoma of the thyroid

DIAGNOSTIC APPROACH

Symptoms of *inflammatory* diarrhea are fever, abdominal tenderness, blood in the stool, or extraintestinal manifestations such as arthritis, erythema nodosum, pyoderma gangrenosum, or iritis. *Osmotic* diarrhea is suggested by steatorrhea or carbohydrate malabsorption. It improves with fasting. *Secretory* diarrhea is evidenced by large volume and watery stools.

Increased stool bulk is an early sign of malabsorption. Stools are difficult to flush and leave oil in the bowl. Increased flatulence occurs with carbohydrate malabsorption. Protein-losing enteropathy is associated with peripheral edema and ascites. Malabsorption of fat-soluble vitamins may cause specific deficiencies, such as vitamin A (night blindness and dry eyes), vitamin D (paresthesias and cramps), or vitamin K (easy bruising) deficiencies.

CLINICAL FINDINGS

Inflammatory bowel disease   Active inflammation causes abdominal pain, fever, bloody or purulent stools, and tenesmus. Extraintestinal manifestations such as axial or monoarticular arthritis, pyoderma gangrenosum, iritis, or hepatitis provide further clues when present **(Plates 58, 86, 171).**

Giardiasis   Diarrhea is mild with prominent gas and cramps. A history of ingestion of a ground water source (e.g., from a stream) is common.

Cryptosporidiosis   Watery diarrhea in children attending day care or in adults with AIDS is the typical presentation.

Irritable bowel syndrome   Constipation and diarrhea with mucous stools wax and wane over years without worsening. Cramping abdominal pain, usually in the left lower quadrant, is relieved by defecation.

Diabetic enteropathy   Diabetes is notable for nocturnal diarrhea, which occurs with autonomic neuropathy (orthostatic hypotension, impotence) **(Plate 166).**

Lactase deficiency   Bloating, cramps, and diarrhea occur after eating milk products. Lactase deficiency may be acquired in adulthood or occur transiently as a sequela to a viral gastroenteritis.

Chapter 49

Chronic Diarrhea

Drugs   Laxative abuse may be hidden in patients with bulimia. Antibiotics, caffeine, digitalis, quinidine, sorbitol (sugar-free gums), and NSAIDs also cause diarrhea.

Pancreatic insufficiency   Stools are malodorous, bulky, and greasy. Often, two flushes are necessary to completely clear the toilet. In adults, there is usually a preceding history of recurrent acute pancreatitis, or cystic fibrosis with recurrent URIs and small size for age.

Post-gastrectomy   Patients may have diarrhea because of "dumping syndrome" or "blind loop syndrome." The former is caused by carbohydrate-rich foods, and the diarrhea is associated with orthostatic lightheadedness, sweating, and tachycardia. The latter produces fat malabsorption with the bulky, malodorous stools previously described.

Celiac sprue   Stools have an appearance similar to those from patients with pancreatic insufficiency. In addition, weight loss and symptoms of vitamin deficiency such as ecchymoses, glossitis, and peripheral neuropathy are prominent. Dermatitis herpetiformis (grouped vesicles on extensor surfaces) occur in a minority of patients with gluten-sensitive enteropathy **(Plate 59).**

Small bowel lymphoma   It presents insidiously with abdominal pain, weight loss, clubbing, peripheral edema, and abdominal mass **(Plates 52, 63).**

Villous adenoma   Watery diarrhea occurs independent of food or fluid intake and often with excessive mucous secretion. Hypokalemia results.

Pancreatic cholera   Vasoactive intestinal peptide (VIP) causes watery, massive diarrhea, which leads to electrolyte abnormalities. Myopathy, flushing, or neuropathy may also occur.

Carcinoid   Episodic diarrhea coincides with flushing. Telangiectasias, cyanosis, pellagra-like skin lesions, bronchospasm, and right-sided valvular lesions are useful clues **(Plate 4).**

Zollinger-Ellison syndrome   Although patients may present with diarrhea, refractory or unusually located gastric ulcers are the more typical manifestations.

Medullary carcinoma of the thyroid   Diarrhea is associated with metastases and a poorer prognosis.

Chronic/Recurrent Abdominal Pain

PLATES 12, 13, 58, 63, 71, 86, 134, 171

◪ DIFFERENTIAL OVERVIEW

- ❏ Irritable bowel syndrome
- ❏ Peptic ulcer disease
- ❏ Cholecystitis
- ❏ Chronic pancreatitis
- ❏ Inflammatory bowel disease
- ❏ Intermittent mesenteric ischemia
- ❏ Pancreatic cancer
- ❏ Gastric cancer
- ❏ Endometriosis
- ❏ Recurrent intestinal obstruction
- ❏ Sickle cell anemia
- ❏ Radiculopathy
- ❏ Adrenal insufficiency
- ❏ Lead poisoning
- ❏ Porphyria

DIAGNOSTIC APPROACH

Examining a patient during an episode of pain is important for diagnosis. A significant proportion of patients with chronic abdominal pain will remain undiagnosed despite extensive testing. For these patients, repeated history and examination, during which one looks for new symptoms or any change in the pattern of symptoms, may eventually yield a formulation.

CLINICAL FINDINGS

Irritable bowel syndrome Typically, pain is experienced as cramping relieved by a bowel movement. The pain often changes in location, but the hepatic and splenic flexures and the sigmoid colon are frequent sites. Bowel movements may be either loose or constipated. Gaseous abdominal distension is often reported and can be seen.

Peptic ulcer disease A typical presentation will be chronic dyspepsia with an epigastric gnawing or hunger pain, both of which are briefly relieved by food or antacids.

Cholecystitis It may occur as biliary colic with repeated episodes of steady right upper quadrant pain that lasts 15 minutes to hours and then is completely relieved, or as acute cholecystitis, with acute progressive pain with a tender gallbladder.

Chronic pancreatitis A sequela of recurrent bouts of acute pancreatitis, it is usually alcoholic in origin. At this phase, there is often a pancreatic malabsorptive syndrome with steatorrhea. A pseudocyst may be palpable.

Inflammatory bowel disease Crohn's disease in particular may be confined to the terminal ileum, producing right lower quadrant pain. There will be concomitant fever, localized tenderness, and mucous, bloody, or diarrheal stools **(Plates 58, 86, 171).**

Intermittent mesenteric ischemia Ischemia presents as episodes of cramping or dull midabdominal pain that comes 15–30 minutes after a meal and lasts as long as 2–3 hours. Considerable weight loss caused by avoidance of eating can occur. Mesenteric artery luminal compromise is usually atherosclerotic in origin and found in patients with other atherosclerotic symptoms such as claudication or angina.

Pancreatic cancer Pain occurs in 75% of patients, especially with involvement of the body or tail of the pancreas, with deep abdominal pain radiating into the back. There is a vaguely palpable, deep, fixed mass in the left upper quadrant. Wasting, jaundice, clay-colored stools, dark urine, and migratory thrombophlebitis (Trousseau's sign) are other indicators **(Plate 63).**

Gastric cancer It presents with continuous epigastric pain, anorexia, and nausea **(Plate 71).**

Chronic/Recurrent Abdominal Pain

Endometriosis   Pelvic pain, which cycles in intensity with the period, is typical.

Recurrent intestinal obstruction   There is often a history of prior abdominal surgery giving rise to adhesions. The pain is midabdominal with distension. Vomiting ensues if obstruction is severe.

Sickle cell anemia   Recurrent, episodic, acute abdominal pain (sickle crisis) occurs in a patient with known sickle cell anemia.

Radiculopathy   The underlying process may be postherpetic, diabetic mononeuritis, or osteophyte impingement on a nerve root. The pain is neuritic (burning, sharp, electric), follows a dermatomal pattern, and does not cross the midline.

Adrenal insufficiency   Vague abdominal pain—sometimes severe—is associated with the insidious onset of weakness, nausea, weight loss, orthostatic hypotension, and hyperpigmentation, especially of the mucous membranes **(Plates 12, 13)**.

Lead poisoning   A wandering, poorly localized, colicky pain is associated with encephalopathy and peripheral neuropathy. A blue-black "lead line" on the gum, due to precipitation of lead salts, is a helpful clue **(Plate 134)**.

Porphyria   It presents with recurrent symptoms of generalized, severe, colicky abdominal pain.

Constipation

Chapter 51

PLATES 16, 17, 18, 97

DIFFERENTIAL OVERVIEW

❑ Lifestyle
❑ Drugs
❑ Depression
❑ Irritable bowel syndrome
❑ Hypothyroidism
❑ Hypokalemia
❑ Colon cancer
❑ Anorectal pathology
❑ Voluntary retention
❑ Megacolon
❑ Mechanical obstruction
❑ Spinal cord pathology
❑ Hypercalcemia
❑ Scleroderma

DIAGNOSTIC APPROACH

Determine what the patient means by constipation. Reduced frequency of stools? Hard stools? Irregular intervals? No bowel movement for days? Constipation may present as ill-defined abdominal pain or bloating.

With recent-onset constipation, seek an obstructing lesion, such as colon cancer, stricture, diverticular disease, inflammatory bowel disease, or foreign body. Hard stool in the vault rules out mechanical obstruction and suggests impaired emptying of the rectal vault. A change in stool caliber is more often caused by a tight sphincter than an "apple core" lesion.

CLINICAL FINDINGS

Lifestyle Lack of exercise and low intake of fluids and dietary fiber contribute to constipation.

Drugs Laxatives (chronically used), opiates, and anticholinergic medications, such as tricyclic antidepressants, ganglionic blockers, iron, calcium or aluminum-containing antacids, and calcium-channel blockers, are common sources. Dark pigmentation of the colonic mucosa on anoscopy suggests surreptitious laxative abuse with anthraquinone laxatives such as castor oil or senna.

Depression Constipation is a common presenting somatic manifestation, associated with altered mood and cognition and other "vegetative" signs.

Irritable bowel syndrome There is a longstanding history, beginning in young age, of abdominal cramps followed by bowel movements, bloating, flatulence, and constipation. Excessive nonpropulsive contractions produce small, hard "rabbit pellet" stools. Symptoms increase with psychological stress.

Hypothyroidism Constipation is seldom the main symptom. Other symptoms such as fatigue, weight gain, and cold intolerance, and findings such as enlarged thyroid, coarse hair and facial features, loss of lateral eyebrows, and delayed relaxation of ankle reflexes suggest the diagnosis (**Plates 16, 17, 18**).

Hypokalemia It is often found in patients taking diuretics or chronically using laxatives.

Colon cancer Consider cancer in patients older than 50 years of age, especially when a family history of colon cancer exists or when a recent onset of constipation, a change in stool caliber, or rectal bleeding (including occult blood) has occurred.

Anorectal pathology Inflamed or thrombosed hemorrhoids, fissures, strictures, or proctitis may contribute.

Voluntary retention Retention of stool may down-regulate the usual physiologic feedback.

Megacolon An atonic, hugely dilated colon is indicated by abdominal distension with an empty rectal vault. A psychogenic form is associated with encopresis (soiling at night).

Mechanical obstruction Symptoms include lack of passage of stool or air, vomiting (especially with small bowel obstruction), visible peristalsis with loud borborygmi, progressive abdominal distension, and severe, colicky pain.

Spinal cord pathology Constipation is caused by colonic dilation, which is associated with multiple sclerosis, tabes, or spinal cord tumors. It may be suggested by a flaccid anal sphincter with decreased anal sensation.

Hypercalcemia Serum calcium is usually greater than 12; therefore, other manifestations such as CNS effects are present.

Scleroderma Constipation is associated with dysphagia and tight, shiny skin **(Plate 97).**

Dysphagia

PLATES 71, 97, 184, 188, 189, 206, 209, 219

◼ DIFFERENTIAL OVERVIEW

- ❏ Esophagitis
- ❏ Reflux stricture
- ❏ Zenker's diverticulum
- ❏ Transfer dysphagia
- ❏ Diffuse esophageal spasm
- ❏ Foreign body
- ❏ Esophageal cancer
- ❏ Achalasia
- ❏ External compression
- ❏ Scleroderma
- ❏ Myasthenia gravis
- ❏ Globus hystericus
- ❏ Esophageal web
- ❏ Botulism

DIAGNOSTIC APPROACH

Differentiate mechanical obstruction from motor disorders (80% accuracy on history):

History	Mechanical	Motor
Pace of onset	Rapid and progressive	Gradual
Effect of solids and liquids	Solids > liquids	Solids = liquids
Effect of cold	Unchanged	Increased dysphagia
Effect of a bolus	Regurgitation	Passage by repeated swallowing, forceful drinking, Valsalva, or throwing back head and shoulders

A sensation of sticking usually occurs at the level of the obstruction although distal esophageal obstruction may be referred to the suprasternal notch. Odynophagia (painful swallowing) is usually caused by infectious esophagitis (*Candida*, HSV, CMV), severe reflux, or pill-induced esophagitis. Phagophobia (fear of swallowing) can occur in patients with hysteria, rabies, tetanus, or pharyngeal paralysis.

Weight loss may occur with dysphagia of any cause, but a major decrease, which is disproportionate to the dysphagia, suggests cancer. Hoarseness occurring *before* dysphagia is consistent with a laryngeal lesion. Hoarseness occurring *after* the onset of dysphagia suggests recurrent laryngeal involvement with esophageal or bronchogenic cancer or laryngitis due to reflux or neuromuscular disease. Hiccups signal a problem in the terminal esophagus (cancer, achalasia, hiatal hernia). Intermittent dysphagia can be found in patients with motor disorders and esophageal stricture. Unilateral wheezing with dysphagia indicates a mediastinal mass involving both the esophagus and bronchus.

CLINICAL FINDINGS

Esophagitis   The main symptoms are heartburn and odynophagia with swallowing saliva alone. Oral thrush is a clue to *Candida* esophagitis; vesicles, to herpes simplex. Mucositis may occur with radiation or chemotherapy **(Plates 184, 206, 209).**

Reflux stricture   Schatzki ring, occurring with longstanding reflux/heartburn, causes a sensation of distal obstruction. Dysphagia is intermittent and for solid food only (the classic onset occurs with swallowing meat).

Zenker's diverticulum   Halitosis and regurgitation are clues.

Transfer dysphagia   There is difficulty initiating the act of swallowing of solids or liquids. Aspiration with cough after swallowing, fluid expectoration through the nose, nasal speech, dysphonia, and dysarthria are also present. Causes include pseudobulbar palsy, myasthenia gravis, dermatomyositis, and muscular dystrophy.

Dysphagia

Diffuse esophageal spasm   Symptoms include intermittent dysphagia associated with chest pain and triggered by cold or heat.

Foreign body   Its onset is with eating, usually caused by fish or chicken bones. There is a distinct, well-localized sensation of the foreign body.

Esophageal cancer   Marked weight loss and progressively increasing dysphagia over weeks are characteristic. Occasionally, hyperkeratotic palms and soles appear **(Plate 71)**.

Achalasia   Pain with eating or drinking rapidly is caused by vigorous tertiary contractures. Food can be consumed if eaten slowly. Regurgitation occurs with changes in position (e.g., nocturnal) or exercise. Foul breath is noted from food in the esophagus.

External compression   Compression is suggested by the symptom complex of dysphagia and unilateral wheezing, with concurrent hoarseness if the recurrent laryngeal is involved. Causes include thyromegaly, mediastinal mass, descending thoracic aortic aneurysm, paraesophageal diaphragmatic hernia, left atrial enlargement, prior radiation, and surgery.

Scleroderma   Continuous dysphagia occurs with heartburn. Bound-down skin and telangiectasias are found on the hands and face **(Plate 97)**.

Myasthenia gravis   Progressive fatigue occurs with repeated swallowing. Bilateral ptosis is common **(Plate 219)**.

Globus hystericus   There is a constant lump in the throat with a sensation of food sticking at the cricoid. Symptoms can be unrelated to or relieved by swallowing. There may be a history of hysterical aphonia.

Esophageal web   Iron deficiency anemia, with pica (clay or ice craving) and pallor, is present **(Plates 188, 189)**.

Botulism   Nausea, vomiting, and stiff tongue rapidly progress to aphonia and aphagia. Symmetrical ptosis and strabismus are present.

Gastrointestinal Bleeding Chapter 53

PLATES 58, 61, 63, 71, 86, 168, 171, 188

◪ DIFFERENTIAL OVERVIEW

Upper GI
- ❑ Peptic ulcer disease
- ❑ Gastritis
- ❑ Mallory-Weiss tear
- ❑ Esophageal varices
- ❑ Esophagitis
- ❑ Epistaxis
- ❑ Esophageal cancer
- ❑ Gastric cancer

Lower GI
- ❑ Infectious diarrhea
- ❑ Diverticular bleeding
- ❑ Hemorrhoids
- ❑ Anal fissure
- ❑ Inflammatory bowel disease
- ❑ Arteriovenous malformation of the colon
- ❑ Colon cancer
- ❑ Mesenteric ischemia
- ❑ Aortoenteric fistula

DIAGNOSTIC APPROACH

With overt bleeding, determining whether a source is proximal or distal to the ligament of Treitz is key to the further diagnostic evaluation. Upper sources usually produce melena (black, tarry stools) unless the bleeding is brisk or large volume and transit is rapid. Hematemesis confirms an upper GI source and suggests a loss of more than a quarter of intravascular volume. Melena without hematemesis usually results from a lesion distal to the pylorus (e.g., duodenal ulcer) or slow bleeding. Tarry stools may be produced by as little as 100 ml of blood. Lower sources produce maroon or bright red stools. A small amount of blood only on the toilet tissue nearly always comes from a bleeding hemorrhoid or fissure. Silver stool is said to signal the presence of an ampullary carcinoma, from acholic stools combined with luminal bleeding.

Determine the hemodynamic significance of the bleeding by looking for postural lightheadedness or changes in pulse or blood pressure. Early symptoms of thirst and lightheadedness occur with loss of more than15% of intravascular volume. An orthostatic blood pressure drop of 10 mm Hg indicates a loss greater than or equal to 20% of volume. Shock with hypotension and pallor develops with 25–40% volume loss.

Occult gastrointestinal bleeding will often be discovered by an unanticipated finding of iron deficiency anemia **(Plate 188).**

Stools may be falsely colored by ingestants such as bismuth subsalicylate, iron, licorice or charcoal, which turn it black, or beets, which turn it red. These stools are not sticky. A negative stool test for occult blood will usually resolve this.

Hemoccult screening in adults older than 45 years of age will be positive in 3–5%, with Se 0.70, Sp 0.85, and LR 4.7 for colon cancer. Cancer will be found in 10–15% and polyps in another 20–30% on further evaluation. Most will be Duke's A or B1 cancer with a 5-year survival rate greater than 80%. Anyone with a single positive stool should be evaluated.

CLINICAL FINDINGS

Peptic ulcer disease   Burning or gnawing pain in the epigastrium, relieved by food intake or antacids, often precedes the bleeding episode.

Gastritis   Epigastric tenderness, pain increased by food intake, nausea, bad breath, and a furred, tooth-indented tongue are clues. Use of alcohol or NSAIDs (including aspirin) predispose patients to gastritis.

106

Chapter 53

Gastrointestinal Bleeding

Mallory-Weiss tear Protracted vomiting with retching proceeds the bleeding, often with frank hematemesis.

Esophageal varices Presenting with abrupt, painless, often massive, bleeding, esophageal varices are accompanied by spider angiomata, ascites, prominent abdominal venous pattern, and gynecomastia. There will be a history of cirrhosis, chronic liver disease, or alcoholism **(Plate 61).**

Esophagitis Bleeding is preceded by recent-onset pain and burning with swallowing.

Epistaxis Brisk posterior epistaxis with swallowed blood can cause melena.

Esophageal cancer Suspect cancer when dysphagia (food sticking) and weight loss or right supraclavicular adenopathy is present **(Plate 71).**

Gastric cancer It simulates peptic ulcer disease, but weight loss and weakness are progressive and more prominent. A vague epigastric mass may be palpated. Left supraclavicular adenopathy, abdominal mass, and nodular liver, indicative of advanced disease, are often present at diagnosis **(Plate 63).**

Infectious diarrhea Bloody diarrhea with cramping abdominal pain occurs mostly in invasive infections, such as Salmonella, Shigella, Campylobacter, enterohemorrhagic E. coli, amebiasis, and C. difficile colitis.

Diverticular bleeding This presents with painless and brisk bleeding (maroon stools) in an older patient with known diverticular disease.

Hemorrhoids Bright red blood coats the stool and toilet tissue. If the patient is examined acutely, a hemorrhoid with an erosion can usually be seen on direct inspection or anoscopy.

Anal fissure In young adults, bright red blood on the toilet tissue but not admixed with stool and pain with passing bowel movements strongly suggest a fissure. If the fissure can be visualized, the diagnosis is certain. Care must be taken to stretch the anal skin folds in a circumferential fashion to visualize the whole surface.

Inflammatory bowel disease Diarrhea, mucous, lower abdominal cramping, urgency, tenesmus, and systemic symptoms such as fever suggest this diagnosis. Erythema nodosum and pyoderma gangrenosum are helpful cutaneous clues **(Plates 58, 86, 171).**

Arteriovenous malformation of the colon It presents with painless recurrent bleeding in an older patient. Aortic stenosis and renal failure are predisposing conditions.

Colon cancer Weight loss and recent change in bowel habits, left supraclavicular adenopathy, nodular liver, acanthosis nigricans, and a rectal shelf mass suggest this. The index of suspicion is raised with a family history of colon cancer or adenomatous polyps or with ulcerative colitis **(Plates 63, 168).**

Mesenteric ischemia Abdominal pain out of proportion to examination findings is the usual acute presentation. A substrate of intestinal angina (pain after meals with food avoidance), small bowel diarrhea, vasculopathy, or atrial fibrillation will usually be the major clues.

Aortoenteric fistula Massive bright red bleeding occurs with abdominal aortic aneurysm or graft.

Heartburn

Chapter 54

PLATES 36, 97, 206, 209

 DIFFERENTIAL OVERVIEW

❏ Reflux esophagitis
❏ Drugs
❏ Gastritis
❏ Pregnancy
❏ Aerophagia
❏ Infectious esophagitis
❏ Scleroderma

DIAGNOSTIC APPROACH

Early evaluation is indicated by complications such as dysphagia, severe nausea, vomiting, weight loss or bleeding, lack of response to empiric therapy, and increase in symptoms with exertion (suggesting angina). Heartburn can mimic angina, with chest pressure radiating to the jaw or shoulder. Pain or difficulty swallowing suggests active inflammation, malignancy, achalasia, or stricture. Nocturnal pain relieved by intake of food, milk, or antacids favors peptic ulcer disease. Pain increased by meals and not interfering with daily activities favors nonulcer dyspepsia.

Improvement with empiric therapy with H2 blockers or proton-pump inhibitors, based on symptomatic presentation, can confirm the diagnosis.

The correlation between severity of heartburn and endoscopic grade of esophagitis is poor.

CLINICAL FINDINGS

Reflux esophagitis   Reflux is experienced as a retrosternal burning sensation, radiating upward. It is often accompanied by spontaneous appearance of fluid in the mouth, tasting acidic (gastric), salty (reflex salivary hypersecretion, "water brash"), or bitter (bile). Symptoms may be exacerbated by lying in the supine position, bending forward, or consuming large meals. Accompanying symptoms may include chest pain, nocturnal cough, hoarseness, repetitive throat clearing, and appearance of frothy mucus in the throat.

Drugs   Lower esophageal sphincter tone may be decreased and symptoms exacerbated, by anticholinergics, theophylline, meperidine, calcium-channel blockers, tobacco, alcohol, chocolate, and peppermint. Tetracycline, aspirin, iron, and quinidine may cause direct esophageal injury.

Gastritis   There is constant epigastric burning, which is relieved by consuming food or antacids.

Pregnancy   Heartburn may occur because of increased intraabdominal pressure and decreased lower esophageal sphincter tone may be due to estrogens and progesterone.

Aerophagia   Recurrent eructation (burping) is due to swallowed air. Common precipitants include anxiety, carbonated beverages, gum chewing, postnasal drainage, and esophageal speech.

Infectious esophagitis   It is caused by opportunistic infection with Candida, herpes simplex, or cytomegalovirus in an immunocompromised host. Thrush is a clue to Candida esophagitis. Vesicles and ulcers are often seen on the lips of patients with herpes simplex esophagitis. Cytomegalovirus esophagitis is frequently seen in those with HIV infection as part of a systemic infection along with hepatitis and retinitis (**Plates 206, 209**).

Scleroderma   Consider scleroderma in a patient with heartburn and dysphagia to solids, especially with concomitant Raynaud's and subtle tightening/binding of the skin (**Plates 36, 97**).

Chapter 55

Hepatomegaly

◼ DIFFERENTIAL OVERVIEW

- ❑ Acute hepatitis
- ❑ Chronic hepatitis
- ❑ Cirrhosis
- ❑ Right heart failure
- ❑ Fatty liver
- ❑ Hepatocellular carcinoma
- ❑ Metastatic cancer
- ❑ Lymphoma/leukemia
- ❑ Liver cysts
- ❑ Hepatic vein obstruction (Budd-Chiari)
- ❑ Primary biliary cirrhosis
- ❑ Hemochromatosis
- ❑ Amyloidosis
- ❑ Gaucher's

DIAGNOSTIC APPROACH

The mean liver span is 10.5 cm in men and 7 cm in women. Larger span correlates with greater height. A span 2–3 cm larger or smaller than these values is considered abnormal. The liver may be palpable but not enlarged (normal span) with emphysema, right-sided pleural effusion, Riedel's lobe, and thin body habitus.

An hepatic arterial bruit is heard with alcoholic hepatitis or cancer, either primary or metastatic. A friction rub may be heard with perihepatitis, metastatic cancer, or after liver biopsy.

CLINICAL FINDINGS

Acute hepatitis The liver edge is smooth and usually quite tender. Fever, malaise, anorexia, nausea, and jaundice are usually present.

Chronic hepatitis The liver edge is firm and tender.

Cirrhosis The liver edge is firm and may have small nodules, especially as it begins to shrink in size in the later stages. The nodules are small in alcoholic or nutritional cirrhosis, and large with posthepatic causes. The spleen is usually enlarged, with ascites present. Other stigmata, such as vascular spiders, venous dilation on the abdominal surface, and palmar erythema, are helpful clues. An abdominal venous hum is virtually diagnostic of portal hypertension due to cirrhosis **(Plates 61, 62).**

Right heart failure The liver may be mildly to massively enlarged, with a firm, smooth, and tender surface. An hepatojugular reflux can often be demonstrated. A pulsating liver suggests tricuspid regurgitation **(Plate 41).**

Fatty liver The liver surface is smooth and pliant and may be tender because of capsular distension. Suspect this in alcohol binging, obesity, total parenteral nutrition, pregnancy, protein-calorie malnutrition, and jejunoileal bypass.

Hepatocellular carcinoma The liver edge is hard, irregular and nontender. The liver may be massively enlarged. Cancer is associated with chronic hepatitis B.

Metastatic cancer The liver has an irregular, nodular, nontender surface. It is unusual for hepatomegaly to be the initial manifestation except in adenocarcinoma of unknown origin. Left supraclavicular adenopathy is a key clue if present **(Plate 63).**

Lymphoma/leukemia Lymphadenopathy and splenomegaly are usually prominent, and night sweats are common. Hepatomegaly can also be found in 50% of patients with acute leukemia **(Plate 158, 159).**

Liver cysts Cysts feel spherical and fluid-filled even through the abdominal wall. They occur in 30% of patients with adult polycystic kidney disease.

Hepatic vein obstruction (Budd-Chiari) Painful liver enlargement, ascites, signs of cirrhosis, and other thromboses are often seen **(Plates 61, 62).**

Primary biliary cirrhosis Marked pruritis, jaundice, splenomegaly, and an enlarged, firm, smooth liver are seen **(Plates 48, 64, 66).**

109

Hemochromatosis   Suspect this in a patient with diabetes, congestive heart failure, and bronze skin coloration. Other signs of cirrhosis are present, including ascites and spider angiomata **(Plates 61, 62, 65).**

Amyloidosis   Clues are enlargement of other viscera, such as the tongue, spleen, and heart, and peripheral neuropathy. There is usually another disease producing chronic inflammation or myeloma **(Plates 131, 157).**

Gaucher's   It may present in Ashkenazi Jews as late as the third decade with hepatosplenomegaly.

Jaundice

DIFFERENTIAL OVERVIEW

Conjugated
- ❏ Viral hepatitis
- ❏ Gallstone obstruction
- ❏ Drugs
- ❏ Carotinemia
- ❏ Alcohol-induced hepatitis
- ❏ Cirrhosis
- ❏ Pregnancy (cholestatic)
- ❏ Postoperative
- ❏ Metastatic cancer
- ❏ Pancreatic cancer
- ❏ Ampullary carcinoma
- ❏ Hepatoma
- ❏ Sclerosing cholangitis
- ❏ Primary biliary cirrhosis
- ❏ Leptospirosis
- ❏ Hepatic vein obstruction (Budd-Chiari)
- ❏ Hemochromatosis

Unconjugated
- ❏ Hemolysis
- ❏ Gilbert's syndrome
- ❏ Sepsis

DIAGNOSTIC APPROACH

Jaundice becomes clinically apparent when the bilirubin level reaches 2–2.5 mg/dL. Scleral elastin has a high affinity for bilirubin, and with a white background, it is a sensitive indicator of jaundice. Biliary obstruction gives a greenish skin tint due to biliverdin. Hemolysis gives a lemon-yellow tint when observed in natural light. An orange-yellow color is more consistent with hepatocellular disease. Pseudojaundice may be found in black patients with pigmented sclera, with carotinemia, with uremia (produces a sallow yellowish pallor), and with quinacrine (produces a yellow-green color) **(Plate 64).**

Dark urine with green foam confirms a conjugated hyperbilirubinemia and excludes hemolysis or a conjugating defect. Unconjugated bilirubin is tightly bound to albumin, which prevents glomerular filtration.

Courvoisier's Law: "In a jaundiced patient, a palpable gallbladder indicates that the jaundice is not due to stones." Painless jaundice usually suggests a gradual process, as is found in intrahepatic cholestasis. The liver in this case is usually enlarged, smooth, and nontender. A patient with hepatocellular disease appears more ill than one with obstruction. Fluctuating jaundice occurs with gallstones, ampullary carcinoma, or toxins.

Anorexia, nausea, vomiting, or weight loss within 2 weeks of the appearance of jaundice suggests acute hepatitis or gallstones. Appearance more than 2 weeks prior suggests malignant biliary obstruction, chronic hepatitis, or toxin exposure (e.g., alcohol). Generalized pruritus suggests biliary obstruction, either extrinsic due to tumor or canalicular due to drug-induced intrahepatic cholestasis.

Ascites with jaundice is an ominous sign, signifying decompensated cirrhosis with portal hypertension or malignancy with liver metastases. In portal hypertension, veins are engorged radially away from the umbilicus. In inferior vena cava obstruction, flow occurs upward over the abdominal wall. A harsh hepatic bruit may occur with malignancy, alcoholic hepatitis, or hemangioma. Splenomegaly without hepatomegaly occurs with hemolysis or portal vein occlusion.

Jaundice

CLINICAL FINDINGS

Viral hepatitis   Prodromal symptoms are anorexia, nausea, abdominal pain, arthralgias, fever, and malaise. The liver is tender and slightly enlarged. There may be an exposure history (travel to endemic areas, transfusion, consumption of raw shellfish, or intravenous drug use or needlestick injury). The urine will be dark with acholic (light) stools.

Gallstone obstruction   A pattern of right upper quadrant pain occurring in episodes over months to years is often seen. Pain radiates to the tip of the right scapula, shoulder, or back. Sudden onset of colicky pain, nausea, and vomiting followed by fever suggests passage of a gallstone that had obstructed the common bile duct.

Drugs   Estrogens produce canalicular cholestasis. Phenothiazines produce ductular cholestasis. Methyldopa causes autoimmune hemolytic anemia. Hepatotoxins include niacin, acetaminophen, isoniazid, phenytoin, sulfonamides, ketoconazole, erythromycin estolate, chlorpromazine, propylthiouracil, anabolic steroids, valproate, amiodarone, acetaminophen, vitamin A and D (in high doses), carbon tetrachloride, and amanita mushrooms.

Carotinemia   An orange-yellow hue is observed, most prominently in the palms and cheeks. The urine and sclera are normal colored. It is usually due to consumption of excessive vitamins or yellow/green vegetables. Myxedema may also produce carotinemia due to altered metabolism.

Alcohol-induced hepatitis   A history of binge drinking and the odor of ethanol on the breath are found. The liver will be enlarged (as opposed to shrunken and firm in cirrhosis).

Cirrhosis   A history of alcohol abuse is discovered. The liver edge is nodular. Signs of estrogen effect such as palmar erythema, gynecomastia, testicular atrophy, and spider telangiectasias are often present. Ascites and a prominent venous pattern on the abdominal wall are late manifestations **(Plate 61).**

Pregnancy (cholestatic)   Jaundice rarely occurs in the third trimester with intrahepatic cholestasis along with itching, pale stools, and dark urine.

Postoperative   Jaundice occurs by several mechanisms including hemolysis of transfused blood, reabsorption of a hematoma, hematoperitoneum, sepsis, hypotension, and biliary tract injury.

Metastatic cancer   The liver is nodular and firm. There is usually right upper quadrant pain, which increases with inspiration. There may be a friction rub over the liver. A primary source is usually known.

Pancreatic cancer   Deep left upper quadrant pain, dramatic involuntary weight loss proceeding the appearance of jaundice, depression, and recurrent venous thromboses are clues. A palpable, nontender gallbladder (Courvoisier's sign) suggests malignant obstruction of the common bile duct with gradual distension of the gallbladder. Edema arising in a jaundiced patient without ascites or cardiorenal disease suggests pancreatic cancer with inferior vena cava obstruction.

Ampullary carcinoma   It may rarely produce the fabled "silver stools," clay-colored acholic stools combining with bleeding. More commonly, it is recognized when acute pancreatitis is caused by blockage of the pancreatic duct in a patient with signs of cancer (e.g., weight loss) and by fluctuating jaundice.

Hepatoma   In a patient with a history of estrogen use, a harsh arterial murmur is heard over the liver.

Sclerosing cholangitis   It occurs with active inflammatory bowel disease. Inflammatory bowel disease is also associated with cholangiocarcinoma, cirrhosis, amyloidosis, and gallstones (with ileal Crohn's), each of which could produce jaundice **(Plate 58).**

Primary biliary cirrhosis   Intense pruritus, splenomegaly, xanthelasmas, and tendon xanthomas are important clues **(Plates 48, 64, 66).**

Leptospirosis   After a person swims in contaminated water, a biphasic illness begins with fever, meningismus, prominent myalgias, and conjunctivitis. One week later, jaundice, ecchymoses, and renal insufficiency develop.

Hepatic vein obstruction (Budd-Chiari)   The presentation is acute, with severe abdominal pain, hepatomegaly, ascites, and jaundice. Oral contraceptives, paroxysmal nocturnal hemoglobinuria, and polycythemia predispose to its development **(Plates 61, 64).**

Jaundice

Hemochromatosis The patient has slate gray skin. Jaundice is a late manifestation along with diabetes and congestive heart failure **(Plate 65).**

Hemolysis A spleen tip is usually palpable. The skin will have a lemon-yellow tint in natural light. With severe anemia, there will be paleness and an absence of a flushing reaction in the palmar creases. Urine and stool appear normal **(Plate 188).**

Gilbert's syndrome Mild jaundice is associated with fasting or viral syndromes. Prior mild hyperbilirubinemia may be found upon chart review.

Sepsis Prolonged hypotension results in liver dysfunction.

◼ DIFFERENTIAL OVERVIEW

Presenting Symptom
- ❏ Pregnancy
- ❏ Psychogenic
- ❏ Rumination
- ❏ Diabetic ketoacidosis
- ❏ Digitalis toxicity
- ❏ Hepatitis
- ❏ Inferior myocardial infarction
- ❏ Uremia
- ❏ Adrenal insufficiency

With Abdominal Pain
- ❏ Viral gastroenteritis
- ❏ Food poisoning
- ❏ Peptic ulcer disease
- ❏ Renal colic
- ❏ Pancreatitis
- ❏ Pyelonephritis
- ❏ Appendicitis
- ❏ Cholecystitis
- ❏ Small bowel obstruction
- ❏ Peritonitis

With Neurologic Signs
- ❏ Migraine headache
- ❏ Vestibular disturbance
- ❏ Autonomic dysfunction
- ❏ Increased intracranial pressure
- ❏ Hypercalcemia
- ❏ Cerebellar hemorrhage

DIAGNOSTIC APPROACH

Projectile vomiting (forced emesis without prior nausea) should raise the possibility of increased intracranial pressure although it can result from other conditions. Central vomiting (chemoreceptor trigger zone stimulation, usually caused by toxins) is alleviated by antidopaminergic medications, which do not work well treating nausea caused by mechanical causes such as obstruction.

Early morning nausea suggests pregnancy or metabolic causes (e.g., uremia). Vomiting of a large amount of undigested food 4–6 hours after eating is consistent with gastric retention resulting from pyloric obstruction or gastroparesis or to esophageal disorders such as achalasia or Zencker's diverticulum.

CLINICAL FINDINGS

Pregnancy   Morning sickness occurs in more than 50% of pregnant women. It usually begins after the first missed period and ends before the fourth month. Severe symptoms are usually found in women who have a history of vomiting during psychologically stressing situations.

Psychogenic   Anxiety, when causal, is manifest. Self-induced vomiting (e.g., bulimia) is not accompanied by nausea.

Rumination   Effortless regurgitation of undigested food within minutes of a meal is caused by abdominal muscle contraction and relaxation of the lower esophageal sphincter.

Diabetic ketoacidosis   Tachypnea, disorientation, and fruity breath odor (due to exhaled ketones) are important clues.

Digitalis toxicity   Obviously, the patient is taking digoxin. Visual disturbances (a yellow halo surrounding lights) may be an additional clue.

Hepatitis   Anorexia, nausea, and vomiting dominate the prodromal phase. Mild liver tenderness might be found at this stage **(Plate 64).**

Inferior myocardial infarction   Nausea appears at the onset in 70%, due to stimulation of vagal afferents. Substernal pressure/pain is usually present along with diaphoresis.

Uremia   Sallow, gray-colored, dry skin and fatigue are found **(Plate 198).**

Adrenal insufficiency   The patient is asthenic, with poorly localized abdominal pain and orthostatic hypotension. Look for hyperpigmentation, with accentuation in the palmar creases and buccal mucosa **(Plates 12, 13).**

Viral gastroenteritis   The nausea is associated with watery diarrhea, cramping abdominal pain, fever, myalgias, and mild diffuse abdominal tenderness.

Food poisoning   Staphylococcal toxin-mediated symptoms occur 1–6 hours after eating suspect food, and such symptoms are not associated with fever.

Peptic ulcer disease   Postprandial vomiting with temporary relief of pain occurs, especially with pyloric channel ulcers. The vomitus contains undigested food.

Renal colic   Severe nausea and flank pain are the major symptoms. The pain is unrelieved by position and may radiate to the groin.

Pancreatitis   Left upper quadrant pain radiating to the back is the cardinal sign and is found in 95% of patients.

Pyelonephritis   Nausea is often prominent and is associated with fever, dysuria, and flank pain/tenderness.

Appendicitis   Anorexia, nausea, and vomiting are early symptoms, followed by periumbilical then right lower quadrant abdominal pain.

Cholecystitis   Emesis occurs more frequently when sudden obstruction of the common bile duct occurs.

Small bowel obstruction   It presents with marked nausea and vomiting. The higher in the intestinal tract the obstruction is, the earlier and more severe the vomiting. Intermittent cramping abdominal pain, distension, and tinkling bowel sounds are usually present. Vomitus may contain undigested food or clear intestinal secretions. Feculent emesis may be found in distal small bowel obstruction.

Peritonitis   Early vomiting and abdominal rigidity occur.

Migraine headache   Suggested by photophobia and throbbing unilateral headache, a migraine is unmistakable when a visual aura occurs.

Vestibular disturbance   Vertigo is prominent.

Autonomic dysfunction   It is characterized by vomiting of food eaten hours previously. A succussion splash may be found on examination. Diabetic autonomic neuropathy is a common cause, and it may be accompanied by a vasomotor neuropathy (orthostatic hypotension) or diarrhea.

Increased intracranial pressure   It presents with projectile vomiting, especially on arising from sleep, associated with bifrontal or bitemporal headache. Papilledema occurs, but absence of spontaneous retinal venous pulsations is the earliest sign **(Plate 129).**

Hypercalcemia   The most common scenario is intractable vomiting in a patient with an underlying neoplasm.

Cerebellar hemorrhage   Nausea and vomiting are severe and associated with ataxia and headache.

Palpable Spleen Chapter 58

◼ DIFFERENTIAL OVERVIEW

Infection
- ❏ Infectious mononucleosis
- ❏ Viral hepatitis
- ❏ HIV infection
- ❏ Bacterial endocarditis
- ❏ Falciparum malaria
- ❏ Typhoid fever
- ❏ Brucellosis
- ❏ Schistosomiasis

Immunologic Disorders
- ❏ Immune hemolytic anemia
- ❏ Rheumatoid arthritis

Hematologic Disorders
- ❏ Thalassemia minor
- ❏ Lymphoma
- ❏ Chronic myelogenous leukemia
- ❏ Polycythemia vera

Congestive
- ❏ Congestive heart failure
- ❏ Portal hypertension

Infiltrative
- ❏ Sarcoidosis
- ❏ Lysosome storage diseases

Other
- ❏ Splenic trauma

DIAGNOSTIC APPROACH

Palpation for splenic enlargement should be done with the patient supine, the examiner's left hand lifting the posterior rib cage and the right hand probing in the left upper quadrant for a palpable edge on inspiration. A palpable spleen is usually more than 50% enlarged (over 300 gm).

A palpable spleen may be found in 3% of young adults. If there is an otherwise normal history and physical examination and if the CBC and chest X-ray are normal, the patient is without an increased risk of having/developing a systemic disease. In older adults, an underlying condition can usually be found on investigation.

Huge spleens (down to the right iliac crest) may be found in chronic myelogenous leukemia, myelofibrosis, malignant lymphoma, hairy cell leukemia, thalassemia major, Gaucher's, and chronic malaria.

Fever, peripheral adenopathy, and splenomegaly should suggest infectious mononucleosis, Hodgkin's lymphoma, sarcoidosis, serum sickness, or systemic lupus. In acute infections, the spleen will be soft and tender on palpation. In chronic and infiltrative diseases, the spleen will be firm and nontender.

Left upper quadrant masses that can be mistaken for an enlarged spleen include perinephric abscess, feces, and tumors of the kidney, adrenal gland, splenic flexure, or pancreas. Renal masses will usually retain the medial notch and will be more posterior. Colon masses will not have a well-defined edge. Pancreatic masses will be more medial.

CLINICAL FINDINGS

Infectious mononucleosis It is characterized by acute onset of fever, sore throat with exudative tonsillitis, marked fatigue, posterior cervical adenopathy, and splenic enlargement in a young adult **(Plates 229, 230).**

Chapter 58

Palpable Spleen

Viral hepatitis   A flu-like prodrome with fever, malaise, arthralgias, and urticarial rash will be followed by jaundice with a tender liver. Splenomegaly with cervical adenopathy may occur in as many as 20% of cases **(Plates 64, 183)**.

HIV infection   Mild splenomegaly may be part of the generalized lymphadenopathy of early symptomatic disease or a result of opportunistic infection.

Bacterial endocarditis   Splenomegaly occurs in 30%, coincident with peripheral petechiae (seen as splinter hemorrhages, Roth spots, or conjunctival petechiae). The underlying infection is characterized by fever and murmur, especially a new or changed murmur **(Plates 22, 23, 24)**.

Falciparum malaria   On removal of damaged red cells, the spleen will enlarge, proportionate to the development of anemia. Other clues to the diagnosis are travel to an endemic area and high, spiking fever with rigors, with the patient relatively well between paroxysms. In endemic areas, massive splenomegaly may result from an abnormally exuberant immunologic response to malaria infection **(Plate 188)**.

Typhoid fever   The classic presentation is a stepwise increase in fever to greater than 40 degrees, with relative bradycardia. The fever can persist for weeks. Rose spots, pale red blanching macules on the trunk, can be seen during the first week. Hepatosplenomegaly is present in most patients **(Plate 60)**.

Brucellosis   Symptoms are nonspecific, with fever, malaise, and weight loss in a person who has been in contact with cattle. Splenomegaly may occur in 20% and may be the only clue to the diagnosis.

Schistosomiasis   Splenomegaly occurs as a late complication, the result of hepatic fibrosis causing portal hypertension. The patient will have a history of geographic exposure and other stigmata of chronic liver disease.

Immune hemolytic anemia   The clinical presentation is usually one of anemia, with lightheadedness, palpitations, and lemon-yellow pallor (caused by anemia combined with hyperbilirubinemia) **(Plate 188)**.

Rheumatoid arthritis   Felty's syndrome, with splenomegaly, occurs in the setting of chronic rheumatoid arthritis. This finding is associated with neutropenia **(Plates 88, 89)**.

Thalassemia minor   Mild anemia and icterus may be present. Approximately 20% have a palpable spleen.

Lymphoma   Splenomegaly is a common finding and may be prominent. One or more firm lymph nodes more than 2 cm in diameter secures the diagnosis. B symptoms of fever, weight loss, and night sweats are more common in patients with Hodgkin's disease **(Plate 159)**.

Chronic myelogenous leukemia   Presenting symptoms relate to hypermetabolism (weight loss, fever, or fatigue) or to left upper quadrant discomfort from the splenomegaly itself. The spleen may become greatly enlarged.

Polycythemia vera   Splenomegaly is present in 75% and is a key finding in differentiating primary from secondary polycythemia. Other findings include plethora or dusky cyanosis, blurred vision with retinal venous engorgement, and severe pruritus aggravated by a warm bath **(Plates 26, 30)**.

Congestive heart failure   Congestive hepatosplenomegaly occurs in patients with advanced right heart failure. Concomitant findings of jugular venous distension with positive hepatojugular reflux and peripheral edema are found **(Plate 41)**.

Portal hypertension   Cirrhosis is the most common cause, but hepatic vein thrombosis can also produce the same result. Splenomegaly is congestive, and it co-occurs with ascites and visible distension of the veins on the abdominal wall (caput medusa). As a general rule, splenic enlargement in portal hypertension occurs with an intrahepatic cause. Extrahepatic causes, such as portal vein thrombosis or compression from pancreatic cancer, do not usually produce splenomegaly **(Plates 61, 62)**.

Sarcoidosis   Constitutional symptoms such as fever, fatigue, and weight loss are common but nonspecific. Lung involvement is marked by exertional dyspnea and dry rales. Lymphadenopathy, Bell's palsy, iritis, parotitis, or skin lesions such as erythema nodosum, waxy plaques, or indurated, swollen, blue-purple facial lesions of lupus pernio can provide diagnostic clues. Splenomegaly occurs in 10% **(Plates 169, 170, 171)**.

Chapter 59

Rectal Pain

◪ DIFFERENTIAL OVERVIEW

- ❑ Hemorrhoid
- ❑ Rectal fissure
- ❑ Prostatitis
- ❑ Anal fistula
- ❑ Pruritus ani
- ❑ Fecal impaction
- ❑ Coccydynia
- ❑ Perirectal abscess
- ❑ Infected pilonidal cyst
- ❑ Ulcerative proctitis
- ❑ Infective proctitis
- ❑ Proctalgia fugax
- ❑ Anal carcinoma

DIAGNOSTIC APPROACH

Tenesmus is a painful urge to defecate with little result.

CLINICAL FINDINGS

Hemorrhoid Common presentations include bright red blood on the toilet tissue, a prolapsing rectal mass, itching, or thrombosis. The latter may be quite painful, with a firm, tender, bluish rectal swelling.

Rectal fissure There is usually pain on passing a bowel movement, and bright red blood will be seen on the toilet tissue. Fissures must be searched for carefully, stretching the skin at the anal verge around the complete circumference.

Prostatitis The principal symptoms are constant perineal ache, fever, and dysuria. A boggy tender prostate is the sine qua non of diagnosis.

Anal fistula A fistula presents with persistent and irritating drainage of pus, blood, or mucous. An external opening is seen on close inspection. There is usually a history of perirectal abscess, Crohn's, or radiation. It may not be painful if it is draining.

Pruritus ani Identifiable causes include pinworms (nocturnal itching), condyloma acuminata (filiform excrescences), contact dermatitis (mild itch worsened by use of topical agents), alkaline stools (severe diarrhea), psoriasis (intergluteal pinking and scaling patches elsewhere), and Candida (bright red lesions with satellites, in diabetics or immunocompromised hosts).

Fecal impaction Symptoms are often diffuse abdominal discomfort or paradoxic diarrhea, but efforts to pass a bolus of desiccated stool are painful. The diagnosis is usually made by rectal exam.

Coccydynia Sitting or direct pressure over the coccyx is painful. The cause is usually trauma, such falling on one's buttocks.

Perirectal abscess Symptoms begin with a throbbing rectal pain, which develops into an exquisitely tender mass, palpable either externally or internally on rectal exam.

Infected pilonidal cyst Redness and tenderness develop around a sinus tract at the upper pole of the buttocks cleft. Purulent fluid may be expressed.

Ulcerative proctitis It presents with mucopurulent discharge, bleeding, and tenesmus. Systemic symptoms are rare when proctitis is confined to the rectum.

Infective proctitis It occurs most prominently in gay males who engage in receptive anal intercourse. Gonococcal proctitis presents with a purulent rectal discharge. Herpes simplex proctitis is quite painful, accompanied by tenesmus, constipation, ulceration, and discharge.

Proctalgia fugax Fleeting (<30 minutes) rectal pain occurs with spasms and no abnormalities on examination.

Anal carcinoma Carcinoma may present with pruritus, mucoid drainage, and a change in bowel habits. A painless, hard, nodular or plaque-like mass is felt on rectal exam.

Section V
Genitourinary

Chapter 60

Anuria/Oliguria

◼ DIFFERENTIAL OVERVIEW

❑ Acute tubular necrosis
❑ Prerenal azotemia
❑ Tubular toxins
❑ Bladder outlet obstruction
❑ Bilateral renal artery occlusion
❑ Nephrosclerosis
❑ Acute glomerulonephritis
❑ Interstitial nephritis
❑ Renal artery thrombosis
❑ Renal vein thrombosis
❑ Ureteral calculus with a solitary kidney
❑ Pelvic tumor
❑ Retroperitoneal fibrosis
❑ Infiltrative renal disease
❑ Vasculitis
❑ Rhabdomyolysis

DIAGNOSTIC APPROACH

Distinguish anuria from urinary retention. Nonobstructive anuria is accompanied by symptoms of uremia with vomiting, drowsiness, muscle twitch, headache, and asterixis. Urinary retention causes suprapubic pain, constant urgency, and a palpable bladder with dullness to percussion in the suprapubic region **(Plate 198)**.

CLINICAL FINDINGS

Acute tubular necrosis   The urine is reddish-brown in color and has dipstick proteinuria. It is caused by transient hypotension due to decreased cardiac output, sepsis, or hypovolemia.

Prerenal azotemia   Signs of volume depletion, such as thirst, postural hypotension, tachycardia, or dry mucous membranes, are present.

Tubular toxins   Toxins include aminoglycosides, amphotericin B, heavy metals, endotoxin, myoglobin, Bence Jones proteins, iodinated contrast, organic solvents, ethylene glycol, and paraquat. Injury occurs especially in the presence of volume depletion or sepsis.

Bladder outlet obstruction   Acute urinary retention produces a full bladder (dullness to percussion above the symphysis pubis) and is usually preceded by obstructive signs such as decreased force of stream and hesitancy. It may occur precipitously with use of drugs having an anticholinergic effect, such as tricyclic antidepressants. The prostate is usually enlarged on exam.

Bilateral renal artery occlusion   Diffuse vascular disease (e.g., claudication with diminished pulses) and hypertension are usually present. There may be an abdominal bruit if flow is still present. Acute oliguria may occur with acute obstruction (as with embolic disease from atrial fibrillation) or with use of an angiotensin-converting enzyme inhibitor.

Nephrosclerosis   It is recognized by renal failure that occurs in the setting of diabetes or poorly controlled hypertension **(Plates 37, 166)**.

Acute glomerulonephritis   It may occur as a sequela of streptococcal infection of the skin, with systemic lupus erythematosus, cryoglobulinemia, Henoch-Schonlein purpura, or systemic vasculitis. Red blood cell casts are found on microscopic examination of the urine **(Plate 178)**.

Interstitial nephritis   Concomitant fever, rash, and arthralgias are the hallmarks, and urinary eosinophils are a key clue. Drugs are the usual cause, often semisynthetic penicillins, but other antibiotics, thiazides, NSAIDs, allopurinol, cimetidine, methyldopa, and phenytoin have also been implicated. It may also be seen with infections such as streptococci, toxoplasmosis, measles, or syphilis **(Plates 181, 182)**.

Renal artery thrombosis   A source is evident, such as atrial fibrillation, recent myocardial infarction, or aortic catheterization. Acute flank/abdominal pain is a hallmark. Peripheral livedo reticularis can be seen in atheroembolism **(Plate 35).**

Renal vein thrombosis   Suspect this in a patient with underlying nephrotic syndrome or hypercoagulable state when there is an acute or subacute worsening of renal function or proteinuria. Acute thrombosis is accompanied by fever and flank pain.

Ureteral calculus with a solitary kidney   It is accompanied by flank pain and hematuria (gross or dipstick). The solitary functional kidney may be a congenital variant or acquired through trauma or unilateral renal vascular disease.

Pelvic tumor   Obstruction from bladder cancer is usually preceded by symptoms of hematuria, sterile pyuria, or pain on voiding. Locally invasive prostate cancer may cause ureteral or bladder outlet obstruction and is readily detected as a stony, hard prostate on rectal exam. Uterine cancer spreads along the broad ligaments to block the ureters; thus, it may be detected on pelvic exam. Abnormal vaginal bleeding is an early sign.

Retroperitoneal fibrosis   Fibrosis is accompanied by edema of the scrotum or legs and dull, persistent lumbar back pain. It may be part of a more widespread fibrosing process involving the mediastinum, bile ducts, Dupuytren's contracture, and Riedel's thyroiditis. Primary or metastatic retroperitoneal tumors can cause a similar picture.

Infiltrative renal disease   Amyloidosis develops in a patient with a chronic inflammatory disease.

Vasculitis   Hematuria, severe hypertension, palpable purpura, and arthralgias are clues **(Plate 110).**

Rhabdomyolysis   The urine is brown, and there is a history of muscle trauma.

Chapter 61

Dysuria

◼ DIFFERENTIAL OVERVIEW

❑ Urinary tract infection
❑ Urethritis
❑ Vaginitis
❑ Acute prostatitis
❑ Urethral calculus
❑ Reiter's syndrome

DIAGNOSTIC APPROACH

Urine dipsticks are a useful diagnostic adjunct for determining the presence of pyuria. Leukocyte esterase and nitrate tests are complementary, increasing the overall sensitivity of the testing.

Always consider a sexually transmitted infection, especially with minimal pyuria and/or a new sexual partner.

In women, ask whether burning is internal (urinary tract infection) or external (vaginitis). Women who have had a prior urinary tract infection are more than 90% accurate in identifying recurrences.

CLINICAL FINDINGS

Urinary tract infection In women, infection is experienced as acute onset of urinary urgency, urinary frequency, and an internal burning sensation with passage of urine. There is often suprapubic tenderness. In men, frequency and urgency are more prominent than burning. Bacterial bladder or upper tract infections are uncommon in young men unless a structural urinary tract abnormality is present. In older men, an infection often accompanies a high postvoid residual in bladder outlet obstruction. Fever, chills, nausea, flank pain, and costovertebral angle percussion tenderness are indicators of upper tract infection.

Urethritis It is distinguished from cystitis as sharp burning with urination but little to no bladder-irritative symptoms. There may be a purulent (gonococcal) or clear mucoid (chlamydial) urethral discharge. Often, the patient has a new sexual partner. In women, cervicitis with mucopurulent discharge may accompany urethritis **(Plates 74, 76, 77).**

Vaginitis It is characterized by external burning with urination along with vaginal discharge and itching. A pelvic examination with a visible discharge and erythema will confirm signs of infection. Severe external burning and rawness should suggest herpes simplex **(Plates 82, 83, 84).**

Acute prostatitis Burning during urination may occur, along with frequency, deep perineal pressure or aching, and pain with ejaculation or defecation. The sine qua non is a tender prostate on rectal exam, which may also be boggy. With a prostatic abscess, the prostate will be extremely tender, hot, and fluctuant.

Urethral calculus Sharp pain in the urethra will accompany passage of the calculus. In men, the calculus may be palpated in the urethra on the underside of the penis.

Reiter's syndrome It presents with urethral burning along with conjunctivitis or iritis, acute symmetrical polyarthritis, mucosal ulcerations, and/or circinate balanitis **(Plate 86).**

■ DIFFERENTIAL OVERVIEW

❑ Psychogenic
❑ Drugs
❑ Diabetes mellitus
❑ Testosterone deficiency
❑ Aortoiliac occlusion
❑ Hypogastric-cavernous occlusion
❑ Pudendal artery occlusion
❑ Venous leak
❑ Primary gonadal failure
❑ Peyronie's disease
❑ Post-prostatectomy
❑ Prolactin excess
❑ Spinal cord lesion
❑ Post-priapism

DIAGNOSTIC APPROACH

If the patient has any full nocturnal or morning erections, it implies that the vascular supply and reflex arc are normal. Organic causes may have a gradual onset, so early in the course, the symptoms fluctuate some, but soon universal erectile dysfunction is present.

A neurologic cause is implied if there is decreased pinprick sensation in the sacral dermatomes. The bulbocavernosus reflex will be normal if rectal tone is normal.

CLINICAL FINDINGS

Psychogenic   A sudden onset, usually concurrent with life stress, situational performance anxiety, or mood disorder, is typical. The occurrence of full erections during sleep or on awakening is a helpful sign.

Drugs   Many drugs can cause erectile dysfunction, including antihypertensives (beta-blockers, thiazide diuretics, methyldopa, clonidine), H2 blockers, barbiturates, phenothiazines, tricyclics, MAO inhibitors, lithium, levodopa, opiates, alcohol, antihistamines, spironolactone, ketoconazole, cancer chemotherapeutics, metoclopramide, phenytoin, and indomethacin. The diagnosis is made by the reversibility of the symptoms when the drug is discontinued.

Diabetes mellitus   When erectile dysfunction occurs, other signs of autonomic neuropathy are usually present, including orthostatic hypotension or retrograde ejaculation.

Testosterone deficiency   Erectile dysfunction is partial and associated with decreased libido. Testicular atrophy is found with soft testes less than 3.5 cm in length.

Aortoiliac occlusion   It presents with thigh pain and quadriceps atrophy combined with a femoral bruit with a decreased pulse.

Hypogastric-cavernous occlusion   It should be considered in the setting of atherosclerosis risk factors, other vascular occlusions, prior pelvic radiation therapy, or pelvic trauma.

Pudendal artery occlusion   It occurs most commonly as a result of chronic trauma from a bicycle seat. Saddle paresthesias with riding are a sign of injury.

Venous leak   A hard erection occurs, and then is unable to be maintained. This is caused by valve incompetence.

Primary gonadal failure   Small, soft testes are present.

Peyronie's disease   A firm induration is felt in the lateral aspect of the penis. The penis bends sideways with erection.

Post-prostatectomy   Radical prostatectomy for prostate cancer frequently produces retrograde ejaculation or erectile failure caused by periprostatic nerve interruption.

Prolactin excess   Gynecomastia is the usual clue.

Erectile Dysfunction

Spinal cord lesion Decreased genital sensation in addition to the erectile dysfunction should raise suspicion of a cord lesion. Causes include spinal cord trauma, tumor, or a demyelinating lesion.

Post-priapism Variations include scarring of the tunica albuginea with lateral deviation of the erect penis or sinusoidal scarring with erectile failure. Causes of priapism include injury to the upper dorsal spinal cord, leukemia, sickle cell anemia, trauma, and urethral growths with bladder cancer.

Flank Pain

Chapter 63

■ DIFFERENTIAL OVERVIEW

❏ Ureteral calculus
❏ Acute pyelonephritis
❏ Latissimus strain
❏ Perinephric abscess
❏ Renal infarction
❏ Renal trauma
❏ Renal cancer
❏ Mononeuritis
❏ Papillary necrosis

DIAGNOSTIC APPROACH

Renal pain occurs with stretching of the capsule and distension of the collecting system. The pain is usually severe and aching, with nausea, vomiting, and ileus. There may be hyperesthesia in the T 9-10 dermatome.

Ureteral pain begins in the costovertebral angle and radiates to the lower abdomen, upper thigh, testis, or labia. The pain is excruciating, with crescendo waves of colic. The patient writhes but is unable to obtain relief. Hyperesthesia over the T 12 dermatome often occurs along with tenderness over the kidney or ureter.

CLINICAL FINDINGS

Ureteral calculus The sudden-onset pain radiates from the flank to the testicle or labia. The patient is unable to find a comfortable position. The degree of severity is related to the acuteness of the obstruction. The pain may be intermittent as the stone passes through the ureter, and the symptoms progress anteriorly and downward. Microscopic/dipstick hematuria is a key to the diagnosis, and its absence should prompt a search for other causes.

Acute pyelonephritis The classic presentation involves fever, nausea, vomiting, and exquisite costovertebral angle tenderness.

Latissimus strain Pain occurs after physical strain and is reproduced by twisting and lateral bending of the torso.

Perinephric abscess Its presence is suggested by findings consistent with pyelonephritis, but systemic toxicity does not clear rapidly with appropriate antibiotics.

Renal infarction It most often occurs acutely in the setting of atrial fibrillation or recent myocardial infarction.

Renal trauma Dull pain persists after flank or abdominal blunt trauma. Microscopic hematuria is a key clue.

Renal cancer Flank pain or fullness is a late sign. The classic triad of gross hematuria, flank pain, and a palpable flank/abdominal mass occurs in the minority. Inferior vena cava invasion may produce the abrupt appearance of left varicocele or leg edema. Fever or hormonal effects (e.g., hypertension, masculinization, Cushing's) may be prominent.

Mononeuritis Pain, which is burning or electrical in nature, is in a unilateral dermatomal distribution. It may occur as a prodrome to or consequence of zoster, as a consequence of nerve root entrapment, or as a diabetic mononeuritis multiplex.

Papillary necrosis Consider this when there is a history of analgesic abuse or when the patient has diabetes.

Chapter 64

Genital Ulcer

◪ DIFFERENTIAL OVERVIEW

❑ Herpes simplex
❑ Trauma
❑ Syphilis
❑ Fixed drug eruption
❑ Behçet's syndrome
❑ Candida balanitis
❑ Granuloma inguinale
❑ Chancroid
❑ Lymphogranuloma venereum
❑ Bowen's disease
❑ Carcinoma of the penis

DIAGNOSTIC APPROACH

A sexually transmitted infection is by far the most likely cause; therefore, a careful sexual history must be taken. Because the patient is often embarrassed or ashamed, cooperation with accurate information can best be gained by first clearly explaining the purpose of the questions.

CLINICAL FINDINGS

Herpes simplex   Typically, HSV produces a cluster of flaccid vesicles and shallow ulcers on an erythematous base. They are painful with a burning, dysesthetic quality (**Plate 73**).

Trauma   The most common causes are zipper tears and human bites.

Syphilis   A single, painless, nonpurulent ulcer with an indurated, rolled border is associated with a rubbery, nontender, regional lymph node (**Plate 79**).

Fixed drug eruption   It can present as red patches, plaques, and/or ulcers on the glans. Tetracycline is the most common cause.

Behçet's syndrome   Scrotal or penile ulcers are well-demarcated and deep and heal with scarring. Suspect Behçet's when uveitis is combined with genital ulcers (**Plates 85, 86, 87**).

Candida balanitis   Multiple painful, shallow ulcers on a bright red base rapidly coalesce. The prepuce becomes edematous and constricted (phimosis). There are often small satellite lesions. Suspect Candida in persons with diabetes.

Granuloma inguinale   It begins as a papule that erodes into a velvety, red, painless granuloma. Spreading to the perianal area, it may become secondarily infected.

Chancroid   A vesicle/pustule rapidly breaks down into a saucer-shaped ulcer with a red margin. The ulcer is painful and ragged, with undermined edges covered with a grayish exudate. Unilateral lymphadenopathy develops, becoming quite painful.

Lymphogranuloma venereum   The chancre feels like a button.

Bowen's disease   The lesion is a bright-red, sharply defined, velvety plaque. Regional lymph nodes may be firm with cancer. A history of arsenic contact may be elicited.

Carcinoma of the penis   Suspect cancer if the lesion does not heal and appears as a small, raised ulcer with irregular friable edges.

◩ DIFFERENTIAL OVERVIEW

- ❏ Urinary tract infection
- ❏ Nephrolithiasis
- ❏ Anticoagulation
- ❏ Long-distance running
- ❏ Renal trauma
- ❏ Bladder cancer
- ❏ Renal cell cancer
- ❏ Transitional cell cancer
- ❏ Glomerulonephritis
- ❏ Interstitial cystitis
- ❏ Hemorrhagic cystitis
- ❏ Hemoglobinuria
- ❏ Endocarditis
- ❏ Polycystic kidney disease
- ❏ Renal artery embolism
- ❏ Renal vein thrombosis
- ❏ Endometrial implants
- ❏ Wegener's granulomatosis
- ❏ Goodpasture's syndrome

DIAGNOSTIC APPROACH

A reasonable cutoff for discriminating benign from serious causes of hematuria is 10 RBCs/HPF. Ninety-four percent of unaffected persons have less than 2 RBCs/HPF. The urine dipstick at 1+ has an Se 0.91–1.0 and Sp 0.65–0.99 for microscopic hematuria.

Initial hematuria suggests a urethral source; terminal hematuria, the prostatic urethra, trigone, or base; and total hematuria, the kidney, ureter, or bladder. Massive hematuria is usually associated with bladder neoplasm, benign prostatic hypertrophy, or trauma. Bright red urine suggests a lower urinary source. Passage of large and bulky disc-like or fragmented clots implies the bladder as source, long shoestring clots suggest a ureteral origin, and pyramidal clots are from the renal pelvis. With a presentation of painless total hematuria, a urinary tract cancer is found in 20%.

Analysis of the urine sediment is crucial. White cells and bacteria are indicative of cystitis whereas white cell casts indicate pyelonephritis. Red cell casts indicate glomerulonephritis. Red cells with a glomerular source tend to be distorted. A positive dipstick but a negative urinalysis suggests the presence of myoglobin or free hemoglobin from intravascular hemolysis. Menstrual blood contamination needs to be considered in the differential of microscopic hematuria.

Flank pain associated with hematuria may result from the passage of stones or clots. Hypertension suggests renal disease. Rash, fever, arthralgia/arthritis, or hemoptysis suggests a connective tissue disease or vasculitis. Beets, blackberries, and rhubarb, as well as pyridium, rifampin, phenothiazines, and anthracyclines, can cause red urine without blood.

CLINICAL FINDINGS

Urinary tract infection Cystitis is the most common cause of hematuria. Symptoms are urinary urgency, frequency, and/or burning. Pyuria is the sine qua non.

Nephrolithiasis Patients present with acute flank pain that radiates to the testicle or thigh; such pain is associated with microscopic or gross hematuria. The pain is often severe, causing the patient to be restless and diaphoretic.

Anticoagulation Hematuria in a patient who takes anticoagulants, even if over-anticoagulated, should be investigated for an underlying structural cause.

Long-distance running Evident by history, it can be true hematuria or myoglobinuria with a positive dipstick for hemoglobin (peroxidase).

Renal trauma Suspect with a history of blunt flank trauma.

Bladder cancer   The typical history is one of urinary frequency, penile pain following urination, and the appearance of a few drops of blood after urination.

Renal cell cancer   Renal cancer is usually recognized by painless hematuria with an abdominal mass. The hematuria is intermittently massive. Flank pain may occur with passage of clots.

Transitional cell cancer   Hematuria is the presenting finding in 80% of cases.

Glomerulonephritis   Red cell casts on microscopic examination of the urine are the hallmark. Fever, oliguria, and edema of the legs, back, and eyelids also occur.

Interstitial cystitis   It is recognized as frequent painful urination in the absence of infection.

Hemorrhagic cystitis   Cyclophosphamide is a common cause in oncology patients.

Hemoglobinuria   Urine will be dark reddish-brown and the dipstick will be positive without red cells on microscopic examination. Hemolysis results from autoimmune hemolytic anemia, transfusion, paroxysmal nocturnal hemoglobinuria, diffuse intravascular coagulation, hemolytic-uremic syndrome, malaria, and snake or spider bites.

Endocarditis   Inspect for fever, new murmur, or splinter hemorrhages **(Plates 22, 23, 24).**

Polycystic kidney disease   Bilateral flank masses, polyuria, and a family history of renal failure or polycystic kidneys are present.

Renal artery embolism   Embolism usually occurs in the setting of a murmur or arrhythmia, particularly atrial fibrillation. Sudden in onset, embolism causes a sharp, continuous pain in the flank or upper abdomen.

Renal vein thrombosis   In young adults, acute or subacute deterioration of renal function occurs in the setting of oral contraceptive use, nephrotic syndrome, trauma, or pregnancy. In older adults, hypertension and recurrent pulmonary emboli may be the presenting manifestations.

Endometrial implants   Bleeding is timed to the menstrual cycles.

Wegener's granulomatosis   Renal involvement is marked by hematuria and rapidly progressive renal failure. Pulmonary symptoms include cough, hemoptysis, and dyspnea. Upper airway involvement produces purulent or bloody nasal drainage, which leads to septal perforation and/or saddle nose deformity. Other findings can include scleritis, palpable purpura, cranial neuritis, and systemic symptoms of weakness, weight loss, and arthralgias **(Plate 111).**

Goodpasture's syndrome   This syndrome presents more focally with hemoptysis and hematuria with rapidly progressive renal failure.

Infertility

Chapter 66

◼ DIFFERENTIAL OVERVIEW

Female Factors
- ❑ Anovulation
- ❑ Tubal obstruction
- ❑ Endometriosis
- ❑ Polycystic ovary disease
- ❑ Luteal phase dysfunction
- ❑ Cervical factors
- ❑ Uterine leiomyoma
- ❑ Testicular feminization

Male Factors
- ❑ Genitourinary infection
- ❑ Erectile dysfunction
- ❑ Drugs
- ❑ Retrograde ejaculation
- ❑ Varicocele
- ❑ Germinal compartment failure
- ❑ Partial androgen resistance
- ❑ Hypogonadotrophic hypogonadism
- ❑ Primary hypogonadism

DIAGNOSTIC APPROACH

Couples should be encouraged to attempt to conceive (unprotected intercourse) for 1 year before undergoing evaluation. Ovulation usually occurs if there have been spontaneous, regular, cyclic menses, but this can be confirmed by daily measurement of basal body temperature. The sperm count and motility can be ascertained to be adequate only by semen analysis.

Interpersonal issues such as career stress, differences in desire for children (a clue is that one partner only seeks evaluation), or unacknowledged homosexual preference may interfere with effective coitus.

CLINICAL FINDINGS

Anovulation   Absence of a cyclical rise in basal temperature suggests lack of ovulation, the cause of 30% of female infertility.

Tubal obstruction   Infertility caused by pelvic inflammatory disease may occur in 10% of patients following a single episode. Repeated episodes may increase the percentage to 75%.

Endometriosis   Typical symptoms are pelvic pain with dysmenorrhea, and multiple, tender nodules along the uterosacral ligament on rectovaginal exam, a posteriorly fixed uterus, and enlarged, cystic ovaries.

Polycystic ovary disease   Virilization, menstrual abnormalities, and large cystic ovaries are clues.

Luteal phase dysfunction   Ovulation occurs, as documented by basal temperature records, but there may be evidence of inadequate estrogen production by the dominant follicle, preventing implantation.

Cervical factors   The cervical mucous should be examined for viable sperm, following coitus, ideally just before ovulation.

Uterine leiomyoma   The uterus has knobby projections on examination.

Testicular feminization   The patient has well-developed breasts but lacks pubic and axillary hair, ovaries, and a uterus.

Genitourinary infection   Occult prostatitis with mild prostate tenderness should be sought. Qualitative sperm changes and leukocytes appear in the semen.

Erectile dysfunction   This is obvious by history.

Drugs   Alcohol or marijuana is often associated with testicular atrophy. Antihypertensive medications may produce problems via impotence.

Retrograde ejaculation   The male partner will experience orgasm without ejaculation. Look for sperm on urinalysis. Diabetes and prior urologic surgery are common underlying causes.

Varicocele   A "bag of worms" is visible and palpable in the scrotum. Testicular size may be reduced. A Valsalva maneuver with the patient standing may uncover a subtle varicocele.

Germinal compartment failure   A history of adult mumps, trauma, cryptorchidism, and irradiation will be elicited.

Partial androgen resistance   Gynecomastia is present.

Hypogonadotrophic hypogonadism   Because it is usually due to hypopituitarism, other endocrine deficiencies are present.

Primary hypogonadism   Klinefelter's syndrome is recognized by the presence of long limbs, azoospermia, and small testes.

DIFFERENTIAL OVERVIEW

Inguinal Swelling
- ❏ Direct inguinal hernia
- ❏ Indirect inguinal hernia
- ❏ Hydrocele
- ❏ Infectious inguinal lymphadenopathy
- ❏ Malignant lymphadenopathy

Femoral Swelling
- ❏ Infectious femoral lymphadenopathy
- ❏ Femoral hernia
- ❏ Ectopic testis
- ❏ Bursal swelling
- ❏ Lipoma
- ❏ Obturator hernia
- ❏ Spigelian hernia
- ❏ Saphenous varix
- ❏ Femoral aneurysm
- ❏ Psoas abscess

DIAGNOSTIC APPROACH

Using the landmarks of the anterior superior iliac spine and the pubic spine that define the inguinal (Poupart's) ligament, separate the femoral region below from the inguinal region above. Examine the patient both lying and standing.

If you are able to get your fingers above a lump, it is not a hernia. Femoral swellings that are reducible and give an impulse on coughing include femoral hernia, saphenous varix, and psoas abscess. Signs of intestinal obstruction associated with an irreducible hernia indicate ischemia.

CLINICAL FINDINGS

Direct inguinal hernia The swelling comes directly forward on standing and retreats backward with pressure. It is globular and posterior to the spermatic cord.

Indirect inguinal hernia It appears obliquely across the abdomen. The sac is tubular and anterior to the spermatic cord, and when in the scrotum, it is anterior to the testicle.

Hydrocele It is a transilluminating swelling surrounding the testicle and extending to the inguinal canal. Downward traction on the testis will pull a hydrocele (but not a hernia) with it. In women, a hydrocele of the canal of Nuck produces a smooth, fixed, translucent swelling.

Infectious inguinal lymphadenopathy Tender nodules appear subcutaneously around the inguinal ligament, draining the external genitalia, rectum, lower abdomen and back, and upper third of the thigh. Classic examples include tender, red nodes with scabies and a hard, painless node with a chancre of syphilis **(Plate 79).**

Malignant lymphadenopathy The nodes are characterized by bulkiness and firmness, progressive growth, and early fixation without inflammation. Adenopathy in other locations, splenomegaly, weight loss, or night sweats are helpful confirmatory signs.

Infectious femoral lymphadenopathy A tender swollen lump develops with a source of cutaneous infection in the lower two-thirds of the leg.

Femoral hernia Occurring more commonly in women, it is recognized by its femoral position. If reduced, it will tap the fingers when the patient coughs.

Ectopic testis There is an empty scrotum, with a lump in the inguinal canal.

Bursal swelling Located between the iliopsoas tendon and hip joint, it is tender.

Lipoma Soft in consistency with a lobulated edge, it lies completely outside the fascia.

Obturator hernia Its swelling is below the pubic ramus (compared with a femoral hernia, which is above). The hip is held in flexion.

Inguinal/Femoral Swelling

Spigelian hernia   The swelling is a few centimeters above the inguinal ligament.

Saphenous varix   It is associated with large varicosities of the legs, and a thrill is palpable. It fills gradually rather than with a pop as with a femoral hernia.

Femoral aneurysm   It presents as an expansile pulsation with a bruit.

Psoas abscess   Tender fluctuance is present both below and above Poupart's ligament. Back spasm with curvature toward the side of the lesion is a common compensatory reaction.

Pain with Intercourse

Chapter 68

PLATES 77, 82, 83, 84

◣ DIFFERENTIAL OVERVIEW

❑ Vaginitis
❑ Inadequate lubrication
❑ Pelvic inflammatory disease
❑ Herpes simplex vulvitis
❑ Endometriosis
❑ Size disparity
❑ Narrow introitus
❑ Vaginismus
❑ Ovarian cyst
❑ Meatal caruncle
❑ Bartholinitis
❑ Unruptured hymen

DIAGNOSTIC APPROACH

Pain greatest on intromission is found with inadequate lubrication and vaginal inflammation. Pain greatest with deep penetration is found with inflammation of deep structures, as in PID. The ability to insert a tampon rules out mechanical obstruction.

Did pain occur with the first effort at intercourse, or has it occurred concomitantly with a situational problem? Failure to localize the site of pain suggests a psychogenic source.

CLINICAL FINDINGS

Vaginitis Vaginal itching, irritation, and increased discharge that is often malodorous are present **(Plates 82, 83, 84).**

Inadequate lubrication Dryness occurs due to inadequate arousal in younger women (too little foreplay, anxiety, fear, conflict). Postmenopausal atrophic vaginitis with scant secretions is a common cause in older women.

Pelvic inflammatory disease Pain on cervical motion and mucopurulent discharge from the cervical os are diagnostic **(Plate 77).**

Herpes simplex vulvitis Usually very painful, this vulvitis has vesicles or shallow grouped ulcers on an inflamed base.

Endometriosis Pelvic pain cycles with the menses. The pain occurs both spontaneously and with intercourse.

Size disparity This is self-evident in a small woman who has a large partner.

Narrow introitus After healing of a perineal laceration (e.g., postpartum), the vaginal inlet is tight and has difficulty admitting a speculum.

Vaginismus This is suggested by involuntary spasm with attempted pelvic examination.

Ovarian cyst A mildly to moderately tender adnexal mass may be palpable.

Meatal caruncle A red growth is present on the urinary meatus.

Bartholinitis A tender red cyst appears at the edge of the vulva.

Unruptured hymen Pain may occur in a young woman during her first intercourse.

Chapter 69

Polyuria

◪ DIFFERENTIAL OVERVIEW

❑ Urinary tract infection
❑ Diabetes mellitus
❑ Diuretic therapy
❑ Bladder outlet obstruction
❑ Nephrogenic diabetes insipidus
❑ Central diabetes insipidus
❑ Psychogenic polydipsia

DIAGNOSTIC APPROACH

Mechanisms of polyuria include the following: loss of renal concentrating ability (parenchymal disease); decreased bladder capacity; solute diuresis of glucose (diabetes), urea (hypercatabolic states), mannitol or radiocontrast; postobstructive and post-ATN nephropathy; and decreased responsiveness of the tubule to aldosterone with sodium diuresis (cystic renal disease, Bartter's syndrome, or resolving ATN).

Nocturia without polyuria occurs with congestive heart failure, cirrhosis, nephrotic syndrome, chronic renal failure, beta-blockers, and diuretics.

CLINICAL FINDINGS

Urinary tract infection   Infection causes frequency of urination with irritative symptoms, but it does not increase urine volume.

Diabetes mellitus   Poorly controlled diabetes may cause excessive thirst and glycosuria, which is easily detected on urine dipstick. Blurred vision and weight loss are additional findings **(Plate 166).**

Diuretic therapy   The cause is evident from the medication history, but hidden sources, such as diet pills or alcohol, must be sought.

Bladder outlet obstruction   The prototypical cause is benign prostatic hypertrophy. There is a sensation of incomplete voiding and frequent passage of small amounts of urine.

Nephrogenic diabetes insipidus   The key to diagnosis is looking for the protean underlying conditions, which may include renal amyloidosis, myeloma, lithium therapy, hypercalcemia, hypokalemia, medullary cystic disease, analgesic nephropathy, obstructive nephropathy, amphotericin B, or demeclocycline **(Plates 131, 157).**

Central diabetes insipidus   The sudden onset of polyuria and excessive thirst, especially for large volumes of cold drinks, is characteristic. Look for signs of underlying hypothalamic lesions such as craniopharyngioma, metastatic cancer, head trauma, posthypophysectomy, or sarcoidosis **(Plates 169, 171).**

Psychogenic polydipsia   Urine output is consistent with the intake of large volumes of fluid, with wide fluctuation in output and lack of nocturia. The urine is dilute.

DIFFERENTIAL OVERVIEW

❏ Benign prostatic hypertrophy
❏ Acute bacterial prostatitis
❏ Chronic prostatitis
❏ Adenocarcinoma
❏ Prostatic calculus
❏ Prostatic abscess

DIAGNOSTIC APPROACH

The normal prostate is heart-shaped with a median raphe and a mass of 20–25 g. Carefully examine the posterior surfaces of the lateral lobes because this is where most prostate cancer originates.

In screening for prostate cancer, digital rectal examination looking for nodules, induration, or asymmetry has Se 0.69, Sp 0.89, and LR 6.3. Examination may help to calibrate PSA values in the "gray zone" of 4–10. For example, a large gland may offer an explanation for a mildly elevated PSA, but a small gland or one with induration or asymmetry should raise the suspicion of prostate cancer.

Examination followed by biopsy of any prostate nodule is the appropriate tactic because the clinical examination alone is not accurate enough in distinguishing benign causes from adenocarcinoma.

CLINICAL FINDINGS

Benign prostatic hypertrophy   The prostate is diffusely enlarged and firm (consistency of the tip of the nose). The gland may be slightly asymmetric, but architectural landmarks are maintained. There may be local induration from fibrous tissue. Obstructive symptoms usually begin early, characterized by decrease in caliber and force of stream and by hesitancy.

Acute bacterial prostatitis   Dysuria, urgency, frequency, fever, and a dull ache in the perineum are the main symptoms. The gland is boggy and quite tender to palpation.

Chronic prostatitis   It is characterized by mild persistent urethritis, with early morning mucoid secretions in the urethra and with a moderately tender to nontender gland.

Adenocarcinoma   A palpable stony nodule, flat induration, or obliteration of the raphe or lateral sulcus should raise suspicion. A deep adenocarcinoma may not be palpable.

Prostatic calculus   A calculus produces a palpable nodule, which is often like a grain of sand. There may be digital crepitation. A calculus may be indistinguishable from adenocarcinoma on examination.

Prostatic abscess   Infection presents as a soft, hot, and exquisitely tender mass of the anterior rectal wall.

Chapter 71

Proteinuria

◼ DIFFERENTIAL OVERVIEW

❑ Diabetes
❑ Drugs/toxins
❑ Acute tubular necrosis
❑ Glomerulonephritis
❑ Orthostatic
❑ Systemic lupus erythematosus
❑ Toxemia
❑ Polycystic kidneys
❑ Interstitial nephritis
❑ Renal vein thrombosis
❑ Multiple myeloma
❑ Amyloidosis

DIAGNOSTIC APPROACH

Proteinuria may present on routine urinalysis or as edema caused by reduced oncotic pressure from serum albumin loss. The dipstick is specific for albumin in concentrations of 30 mg/dL (Se 0.70, Sp 0.92, LR 8.8). False-positives may be seen with dehydration and hematuria, both of which can be detected with the dipstick (specific gravity and hemoglobin). False-negatives can occur when the protein is not albumin, e.g., with Bence-Jones proteins in myeloma. Nephrotic syndrome has more than 3.5 grams per day of proteinuria.

Systemic disease should be suspected in the presence of fever, rash, or arthritis.

CLINICAL FINDINGS

Diabetes Microalbuminuria is an early marker of nephropathy. Glycosuria is present. The diagnosis of diabetes is usually well established before this complication develops **(Plates 166, 167).**

Drugs/toxins Drugs such as nonsteroidal antiinflammatory agents, chronic acetaminophen, contrast media, angiotensin-converting enzyme inhibitors, heroin, mercury, bismuth, gold, and penicillamine can all cause renal injury and proteinuria.

Acute tubular necrosis Tubular proteinuria occurs with acute illness, especially with hypotension. "Dirty" casts can be seen on urinalysis.

Glomerulonephritis The urine sediment will show red cells or red cell casts. Marked proteinuria usually is caused by glomerular injury. Membranous glomerulonephritis is the most common cause.

Orthostatic Transient orthostatic or exercise-induced proteinuria is benign, and it may be demonstrated to be evanescent by changes in position (specimens on arising vs. 2 hours later) or testing before and after exertion.

Systemic lupus erythematosus Microscopic hematuria, malar-distribution rash, arthritis, and Raynaud's phenomenon are clues **(Plates 36, 91, 92).**

Toxemia Typically occurring in the third trimester in a primigravida, it is manifest as proteinuria, accelerated hypertension, and edema **(Plates 38, 41).**

Polycystic kidneys The onset is in the third or fourth decade, with hypertension, flank pain, hematuria, and a palpable lumpy kidney. There is often a history of renal stones.

Interstitial nephritis There will be hematuria, fever, and a maculopapular rash, usually associated with the use of antibiotics, especially methicillin. Urinary eosinophils are occasionally found **(Plate 182).**

Renal vein thrombosis Its appearance is suggested by acute flank pain, hematuria, and the sudden appearance of a left varicocele.

Multiple myeloma The dipstick will be negative or weakly positive. Bone pain, particularly in the back or ribs, is a common presentation.

Amyloidosis If occurring in the absence of systemic disease, an enlarged palpable kidney and a benign sediment may be the only clues. Systemic disease is most often marked by neuropathy, macroglossia, and waxy hemorrhagic periorbital plaques **(Plate 131, 157).**

◤ DIFFERENTIAL OVERVIEW

Pain Predominant
❑ Epididymitis
❑ Prostatitis
❑ Genitofemoral neuralgia
❑ Trauma
❑ Orchitis
❑ Testicular torsion
❑ Torsion of a testicular appendage
❑ Inguinal hernia/incarcerated

Swelling Predominant
❑ Varicocele
❑ Inguinal hernia
❑ Hydrocele
❑ Spermatocele
❑ Sebaceous cyst
❑ Testicular cancer

DIAGNOSTIC APPROACH

Testicular torsion, a medical emergency, should be the primary consideration in a patient with an acutely painful scrotum; however, epididymitis is a more common cause than torsion by a 10:1 margin.

Testicular cancer must be definitively ruled out whenever a firm induration or mass is found to be contiguous with the testicle.

Referred pain can be differentiated from scrotal pathology by a normal testicular examination.

CLINICAL FINDINGS

Epididymitis It presents gradually, often with dysuria and fever. The epididymis is cord-like, swollen, tender, and separate from the testicle. In men younger than age 35, it is usually caused by a sexually transmitted organism; in those older than age 35, by urinary coliforms. Tuberculous epididymitis adheres to the scrotum **(Plate 78).**

Prostatitis Perineal and testicular aching coincides with urinary urgency and frequency. The posterior scrotal nerve refers pain to the scrotum.

Genitofemoral neuralgia Pain in the inguinal region, testicle, and upper medial thigh may be caused by disease along the genitofemoral nerve in the retroperitoneum (e.g., abdominal aortic aneurysm, ureterolithiasis, or retrocecal appendicitis) or by superficial entrapment after an appendectomy or hernia repair.

Trauma History is key. The scrotum may be swollen and tender, resembling torsion. Trauma can cause a hematoma, contusion, or rupture of the testis.

Orchitis Usually caused by mumps or varicella and occurring 7–10 days after the parotitis, it is unilateral and associated with fever, swelling, pain, and tenderness.

Testicular torsion Sudden in onset, testicular torsion causes the retracted testicle to lie high in the scrotum. It is recognized by an anterior or horizontal position of the testicle, a nontender epididymis palpable anteriorly, and an absent cremasteric reflex. Usually occurring before age 30, there may be a history of recurrent attacks.

Torsion of a testicular appendage There will be a small, tender nodule at the head of the testis or upper epididymis. A "blue dot sign" seen through the skin at the tender point is pathognomonic.

Inguinal hernia/incarcerated A hernia appears as a pliant mass extending through the inguinal ring and increasing with Valsalva. The examining finger is unable to get above the hernia, but the hernia usually can be reduced through a patent inguinal ring. Bowel sounds are present over the hernia. With incarceration, the hernia will be increasingly painful, tender, and irreducible.

Scrotal Pain/Swelling

Varicocele The scrotum feels like a "bag of worms" and is bluish, nontender, and increased in size when standing. It usually occurs on the left (the left spermatic vein empties directly into the renal vein). The acute appearance of a varicocele in an elderly man suggests a retroperitoneal mass, especially a renal tumor.

Hydrocele It is appreciated as a large, pear-shaped mass anterior to and above the testicle. The skin is stretched shiny red and transilluminates. The testis is usually obscured. About 10% of testicular tumors present with a hydrocele.

Spermatocele It is a cystic structure on top of the testicle, usually smaller than 2 cm in size, which also transilluminates.

Sebaceous cyst It is spherical, marble-sized, firm, yellow, and superficial within the scrotal skin.

Testicular cancer Cancer appears as a firm, heavy, nontender mass in the testicle that does not transilluminate. It retains the testicular shape until it penetrates the tunica albuginea with soft projections, adhering to the scrotum. With metastasis, there may be an associated enlarged left supraclavicular node. If it produces hCG or estrogen, there may be gynecomastia. One-third present with pain, tenderness, and swelling, and 95% occur in men aged 20–45 years.

Secondary Amenorrhea   Chapter 73

PLATES 15, 57, 166, 168

◤ DIFFERENTIAL OVERVIEW

❑ Pregnancy
❑ Menopause
❑ Functional amenorrhea
❑ Drugs
❑ Anorexia nervosa
❑ Post-contraceptive
❑ Endometrial scarring
❑ Endocrinopathy
❑ Hyperprolactinemia
❑ Premature ovarian failure
❑ Polycystic ovaries
❑ Chromophobe adenoma
❑ Ovarian tumors
❑ Panhypopituitarism
❑ Müllerian dysgenesis

DIAGNOSTIC APPROACH

Evaluation should always begin with history and a urine hCG for pregnancy. On physical examination, attention should be paid to darkening of the areola, clitoromegaly, and evidence of estrogenization of the vagina.

Estrogen sufficiency can be assessed by observing a fern-like pattern of cervical mucous on a slide or by giving medroxyprogesterone for 5 days and looking for withdrawal bleeding. Bleeding suggests suppression of LH surge as seen in functional amenorrhea or polycystic ovaries.

CLINICAL FINDINGS

Pregnancy   A bluish cervix with enlarged uterus and darkening of the areola are clues.

Menopause   Manifestations include hot flashes, emotional lability, and decreased vaginal secretions. The average age of onset is age 50.

Functional amenorrhea   Amenorrhea may be triggered by emotional stress, concurrent illness, sudden weight loss, drug use (oral contraceptives or phenothiazines), or physical stress including athletic training. It often occurs in young professional women who work long hours, eat lightly, and engage in vigorous daily aerobic activity. Loss of cyclic LH production may cause mild hirsutism and acne because of stimulation of ovarian androgens.

Drugs   Increase prolactin: phenothiazines, tricyclic antidepressants, MAO inhibitors, calcium channel blockers, methyldopa, and reserpine. Estrogenic activity: digoxin, marijuana, and oral contraceptives. Ovarian toxicity: busulfan, chlorambucil, cisplatin, cyclophosphamide, and fluorouracil.

Anorexia nervosa   An overly thin habitus especially with a decrease in weight, yellow pallor from hypercarotenemia, lanugo (downy) hair, and hypotension are clues. The disorder frequently is hidden by the patient. Enlarged parotid glands and eroded dental enamel occur with coexisting bulimia **(Plate 57)**.

Post-contraceptive   Amenorrhea rarely lasts more than 6 months following discontinuation of contraceptives.

Endometrial scarring   A prior history of septic abortion, radiation therapy, or curettage with endometrial adhesions may be underlying causes.

Endocrinopathy   An endocrine disorder is usually evident by the time amenorrhea occurs; the exception is mild hypothyroidism. Uncontrolled diabetes can produce amenorrhea, especially in the setting of insulin resistance **(Plate 166, 168)**.

Hyperprolactinemia   Galactorrhea, when present with amenorrhea, distinguishes hyperprolactinemia. Microadenomas may enlarge with pregnancy so that prolonged postpartum amenorrhea is suspicious for prolactin-secreting adenoma. Failure to lactate in addition suggests Sheehan's syndrome (postpartum pituitary necrosis) **(Plate 15)**.

Premature ovarian failure   The presence of another autoimmune glandular disease provides a clue.

Polycystic ovaries   Characterized by amenorrhea, infertility, hirsutism, and obesity, the patient has ovaries that are bilaterally enlarged and cystic.

Chromophobe adenoma   These adenomas often enlarge to the point that headache and visual field defects (bitemporal hemianopsia) are present at the time that amenorrhea develops. Hypothyroidism, adrenal insufficiency, and diabetes insipidus may accompany the amenorrhea.

Ovarian tumors   Bilateral ovarian tumors rarely cause amenorrhea, but granulosa-cell tumors, which produce excess estrogen, and arrhenoblastomas with virilization do.

Panhypopituitarism   Panhypopituitarism is usually due to postpartum hemorrhage, heralded by failure of lactation, failure of menses to restart, loss of body hair, and asthenia.

Müllerian dysgenesis   Cyclic abdominal pain and distension, hirsutism, large and lobulated ovaries, obesity, and acanthosis nigricans are findings.

Urinary Incontinence Chapter 74

PLATES 119, 127, 128, 166

◼ DIFFERENTIAL OVERVIEW

- ❏ Cystitis
- ❏ Benign prostatic hypertrophy
- ❏ Pelvic floor relaxation
- ❏ Drugs
- ❏ Prostatitis
- ❏ Diabetes
- ❏ Cough
- ❏ Multiple sclerosis
- ❏ Spinal cord compression
- ❏ Decreased cortical inhibition
- ❏ Vesicovaginal fistula

DIAGNOSTIC APPROACH

On examination, test for stress-induced leakage with a full bladder, palpate for bladder distension after voiding, and check for post-void residual. Do a pelvic examination looking for pelvic floor laxity, atrophic vaginitis, urethritis, or pelvic mass, and do a rectal examination for tone, fecal impaction, and prostate nodule. Check neurosacral reflexes and perineal sensation. The bulbocavernosus reflex tests the integrity of the reflex arc. Squeezing the glans penis or clitoris produces reflex contraction of the rectal sphincter. An intact reflex arc but absent perineal sensation suggests a cord lesion or multiple sclerosis.

Urge incontinence: Urine loss is accompanied by a strong desire to void. Incontinence is preceded by a warning of seconds to minutes. Leakage is periodic but frequent, and nocturnal incontinence is common. Voluntary control of the anal sphincter is intact, and sacral sensation and reflexes are preserved. The post-void residual is low. It is usually a result of detrusor instability caused by stroke, Alzheimer's, brain tumor, Parkinson's, bladder outlet obstruction, spinal cord lesion, or interstitial cystitis.

Reflex incontinence: Voiding occurs without stress or warning. Sacral reflexes are preserved, but voluntary sphincter control and perineal sensations are impaired. Post-void residual is increased. Usually caused by a spinal cord lesion, incontinence may be mimicked by cortical damage with decreased awareness of signals to void.

Stress incontinence: Incontinence of small amounts of urine occurs with increased abdominal pressure (e.g., coughing, laughing, sneezing). Stress-induced detrusor instability is suggested by a 5–15 second delay between stress and leakage and by nocturnal leakage.

Overflow incontinence: There is frequent leakage of small amounts of urine, hesitancy, decreased flow, and incomplete emptying. The post-void residual is increased, and the bladder is palpable. Common mechanisms include bladder outlet obstruction, caused by benign prostatic hypertrophy or urethral stricture, decreased detrusor tone due to a herniated disc, or peripheral neuropathy caused by diabetes, pernicious anemia, tabes, or cauda equina.

CLINICAL FINDINGS

Cystitis Urinary frequency, urgency, and burning are hallmarks. Perineal sensation and reflexes are preserved. It may result from bacterial infection or interstitial cystitis.

Benign prostatic hypertrophy Hypertrophy may produce problems with urine retention or overflow of a chronically full (palpably distended) bladder. Prostate size on rectal examination correlates imperfectly with bladder outlet obstruction.

Pelvic floor relaxation It is usually due to prior childbirth, to aging in women, or to prior prostate surgery in men. Urine loss occurs with laughing, coughing, sneezing, and lifting. On pelvic examination, a cystocele is found during Valsalva. Symptoms are often exacerbated in the elderly by diuretic use.

Drugs Many drugs exacerbate incontinence, including decongestants and tricyclic antidepressants (with anticholinergic activity), diuretics, theophylline, and alcohol (which overwhelms bladder capacity), alpha-agonists (which increase sphincter tone), and calcium channel blockers (which decrease bladder smooth muscle contractility).

Prostatitis   Deep pelvic pain is accompanied by a sense of urgency, and patients cannot hold their urine long enough to get to a toilet.

Diabetes   Incontinence occurs without warning. There are usually associated signs of neuropathy, such as erectile dysfunction and peripheral or autonomic neuropathy. Glycosuria with increased urine volume also contributes **(Plate 74).**

Cough   Immediate leakage occurs with stress, and delayed leakage is caused by involuntary bladder contractions.

Multiple sclerosis   Incontinence occurs with detrusor spasticity with functional outlet obstruction or reflex incontinence. Associated findings include patchy numbness, hyperreflexia, and optic neuritis **(Plates 119, 127, 128).**

Spinal cord compression   Compression is associated with sensory and motor findings in the legs. Voluntary sphincter control and perineal sensations are reduced, but sacral reflexes remain intact.

Decreased cortical inhibition   Socially inappropriate urination may occur in patients with Alzheimer's disease, Parkinson's, stroke, or brain tumor.

Vesicovaginal fistula   Occurring most often after childbirth trauma, there is leakage of urine through the vagina.

◼ DIFFERENTIAL OVERVIEW

❑ Ovulatory bleeding
❑ Threatened abortion
❑ Uterine fibroid
❑ Dysfunctional bleeding
❑ Cervical erosion or polyp
❑ Ovarian senescence
❑ Retained products of gestation
❑ Ectopic pregnancy
❑ Oral contraceptives
❑ Anticoagulation therapy
❑ Thrombocytopenia
❑ Hypothalamic-pituitary-gonadal immaturity
❑ Cervical cancer
❑ Endometrial cancer

DIAGNOSTIC APPROACH

The differential above applies to unanticipated (noncyclic) bleeding. First establish that bleeding is uterine and not from the rectum or urethra. Any postmenopausal bleeding should be thoroughly evaluated for cervical or endometrial cancer.

Passage of clots or inability to control bleeding with tampons is consistent with heavy flow.

CLINICAL FINDINGS

Ovulatory bleeding   Minor bleeding may occur near the midpoint between cycles, and is associated with weight gain, breast tenderness, bloating, or dysmenorrhea.

Threatened abortion   Bleeding occurs when signs of pregnancy are present: morning nausea, breast swelling, darkening of the nipple and areola, bluish cervix, and an enlarged uterus.

Uterine fibroid   These occur in 30% of women older than age 35; thus, they may fortuitously coexist with another source of bleeding. They commonly cause heavy menses, which occur cyclically. Fibroids are palpable as an asymmetric, rubbery, lumpy uterus.

Dysfunctional bleeding   It occurs with stress or exercise. Prolonged bleeding occurs after amenorrhea. Bleeding may be stopped with ethinyl estradiol and induced with medroxyprogesterone. It is diagnostic if the cycle normalizes after bleeding is stopped.

Cervical erosion or polyp   They cause intermenstrual and postcoital spotting, and are visible on pelvic exam.

Ovarian senescence   Bleeding without ovulation results in irregular intermenstrual intervals, periods of amenorrhea, and heavy, prolonged bleeding.

Retained products of gestation   These are a main cause of bleeding occurring post-abortion (spontaneous or induced).

Ectopic pregnancy   A delayed period is followed by spotting to continuous bleeding and unilateral pelvic pain with an adnexal mass. Rupture is signaled by hypotension, marked tenderness, and severe pain radiating to the shoulder.

Oral contraceptives   Breakthrough bleeding may occur with a dosage change, missed doses, or psychologic stress.

Anticoagulation therapy   This is easily recognized as heavy periods occurring in a patient on anticoagulants.

Thrombocytopenia   A low platelet count may present with heavier than normal menstrual flow and petechiae observed on the lower legs (**Plate 187**).

Hypothalamic-pituitary-gonadal immaturity   This is a common cause of irregular bleeding in adolescents.

Cervical cancer   Bleeding is post-coital, intermenstrual, and spotting.

Endometrial cancer   Intermenstrual or postmenopausal bleeding is usually manifest as heavy periods and a watery discharge containing some blood.

Chapter 76

Vaginal Discharge

◼ DIFFERENTIAL OVERVIEW

❑ Physiologic discharge
❑ Candida vaginitis
❑ Bacterial vaginosis
❑ Trichomoniasis vaginitis
❑ Atrophic vaginitis
❑ Irritant dermatitis
❑ Gonorrheal cervicitis
❑ Chlamydia cervicitis
❑ Herpes simplex
❑ Cervical cancer

DIAGNOSTIC APPROACH

It is important to distinguish burning on urination due to cystitis, which is internal and accompanied by irritative signs (urinary frequency), from dysuria due to vaginitis, which feels external as the urine passes over an inflamed vulva. Similarly, it is important to distinguish vaginitis, characterized by discharge and pruritus, from cervicitis, with discharge and pelvic pain.

CLINICAL FINDINGS

Physiologic discharge   Maximal mucous production occurs in midcycle.

Candida vaginitis   Infection often occurs in the setting of recent antibiotic or steroid use or diabetes. The onset is just before the menses, when pH decreases. Intense pruritus causes vulvar erythema, edema, fissures, and excoriation. The discharge is thick, white, and adherent, resembling cottage cheese. On KOH prep, budding yeast and branching hyphae are usually abundant, but the sensitivity is only 80% **(Plate 84)**.

Bacterial vaginosis   Symptoms tend to be mild. The discharge is turbid, thin, pasty, gray to creamy yellow, and musty smelling. "Clue cells," which are epithelial cells that appear stippled due to the surface adhesion of bacilli, may be seen on microscopic examination in 45%. The background contains numerous short motile rods.

Trichomoniasis vaginitis   The discharge is copious; thin; frothy-white, gray or greenish-yellow; and fishy smelling, especially after application of KOH. Petechial hemorrhages on the cervix occasionally produce a strawberry-like appearance. Mobile, flagellated organisms are seen on a saline mount in 25% **(Plates 82, 83)**.

Atrophic vaginitis   Occurring in postmenopausal women, symptoms include vaginal and vulvar itching, burning, or soreness. The mucosa is thinned and erythematous, and there is a scant watery discharge.

Irritant dermatitis   It is most often caused by douching, using contraceptive products, or using scented tissue paper. A forgotten diaphragm or tampon may cause a malodorous discharge.

Gonorrheal cervicitis   This produces a thick, creamy, purulent, profuse, irritating discharge and involves the cervix, vagina, and urethra. Wet prep reveals many leukocytes. Gram-negative intracellular diplococci may be found in 50% **(Plate 77)**.

Chlamydia cervicitis   A yellow-white mucopurulent discharge issues from the cervical os (will appear yellowish on a white swab). Erythema, easy bleeding with swabbing, and cervical ectropion are common concomitants. Cervical motion tenderness (chandelier sign) will usually be present **(Plate 77)**.

Herpes simplex   Cervical infection produces ulceration, with a grayish exudate and a profuse watery discharge. Inguinal adenopathy may be present. The initial episode is often accompanied by a flu-like systemic illness. Multinucleated giant cells may be seen in scrapings from the lesions.

Cervical cancer   Cervical bleeding—a copious, watery, bloodstained, foul-smelling discharge—is the principal sign.

Section VI
Musculoskeletal/ Extremities

Acute Knee Pain

◼ DIFFERENTIAL OVERVIEW

❑ Degenerative joint disease
❑ Chondromalacia patellae
❑ Collateral ligament sprain
❑ Meniscal tear
❑ Cruciate tear
❑ Infrapatellar quadriceps tendinitis
❑ Acute monoarticular arthritis
❑ Anserine bursitis
❑ Hamstring injury
❑ Baker's cyst
❑ Septic joint
❑ Hemarthrosis
❑ Patellar fracture
❑ Patellar dislocation
❑ Osteochondritis desiccans
❑ Osteonecrosis

DIAGNOSTIC APPROACH

Careful questioning concerning the mechanism of injury is most important. Overuse injury or undue stress caused by unbalanced walking is a common source. A sensation of "giving away" on stepping down is a symptom of posterior horn meniscus or anterior cruciate tear.

Examine systematically stressing in each direction, looking for pain and/or laxity, comparing with the contralateral side. The range of motion may be limited by effusion, by a meniscal tear, or by a loose body acting as a doorstop. True locking occurs 10° short of full extension. A locked knee can flex but cannot extend fully.

McMurray's maneuver is performed by torquing the lower leg medially and laterally with the knee flexed at 90° and then extending the knee. A painful "clunk" with medial rotation indicates a lateral meniscus tear, and the same finding with lateral rotation suggests a medial meniscus tear. In Apley's maneuver, the patient lies face down with the knee flexed at 90°. If pain is produced by rotation of the knee while pulling up on the lower leg, a medial collateral ligament injury is suggested. If pain occurs with grinding while pressing down, a medial meniscus injury is suggested. An anterior drawer sign is elicited as pain and a laxity when the tibia is pulled forward with the knee at 90°, indicating anterior cruciate injury.

Palpable clicks are not necessarily pathologic; they may be caused by the semitendinosus tendon slipping over the medial condyle or the iliotibial band slipping over the lateral condyle. With effusion the hollows of the knee are filled, and a transmitted fluid wave can be elicited.

CLINICAL FINDINGS

Degenerative joint disease Osteoarthritis begins with mild stiffness on first arising that eventually resolves. Pain is localized to the anterior and medial aspects of the knee. Bony overgrowth of the knee (LR 3.0), bony prominences on the lateral aspects of the PIP and DIP joints (LR 1.7), and prominent crepitance on knee motion are helpful clues. Acute flares are precipitated by overuse.

Chondromalacia patellae This is a common cause of knee pain in joggers, producing retropatellar aching worse when climbing stairs. Pain can be elicited by downward pressure on the patella with the knee actively extended, and patellar crepitance can be felt on lateral movement of the patella.

Collateral ligament sprain Lateral force applied to the knee with the foot planted can cause collateral disruption. Test by stabilizing the lower leg and applying lateral (valgus or varus) force at varying angles of flexion. Pain and/or laxity are indicators.

Meniscal tear Twisting of the knee with the foot planted, flexed, and bearing weight is the usual mechanism. Pain usually appears in the joint line. The joint may lock or click.

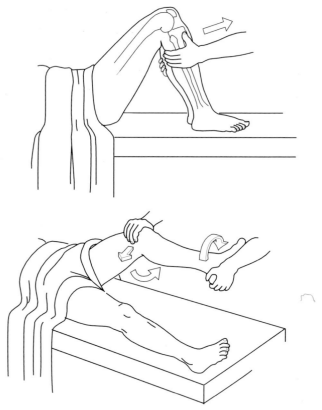

Figure 9. Anterior drawer sign in anterior cruciate injury. McMurray's maneuver in medial meniscus injury. (Adapted from: Reilly BR. Practical Strategies in Outpatient Medicine. 2nd ed. Philadelphia: W.B. Saunders, 1991, pp. 1193, 1195.)

In acute injuries, an effusion is usually found. In McMurray's maneuver, knee extension with internal rotation of the tibia stresses the medial meniscus and opens the lateral compartment, producing a painful click (palpated with a hand over the knee) as a lateral meniscal tear flips out. Extension with external rotation elicits a painful click with a medial meniscal tear. Pain without a click may also be produced by putting stress on the injured meniscus.

Cruciate tear   An anterior cruciate tear produces a sensation of "giving away" of the knee as the tibia slips forward on the femur. Pain (with acute injury) and laxity may be found with the anterior drawer sign (forward movement of the tibia when pulled at 90 ° of flexion) or the Lachman's maneuver (forward shift of the tibia at 15° flexion, more sensitive).

Infrapatellar quadriceps tendinitis   Pain and tenderness of the quadriceps tendon below the knee is accentuated by climbing stairs. A cystic/fluctuant swelling occurs with bursal inflammation. Osgood-Schlatter syndrome in adolescents produces similar pain over the anterior tibia.

Acute Knee Pain

Acute monoarticular arthritis   The knee is warm, and there may be a fever present (especially, but not exclusively, in infection). The knee is a frequent site of rheumatoid arthritis, septic arthritis (especially staphylococcal and gonococcal), gout, Lyme disease, and rheumatic fever **(Plates 75, 89, 106).**

Anserine bursitis   Medial knee pain occurs nocturnally and is exacerbated by walking in patients with osteoarthritis. There is local tenderness over the tibial ~~tuberosity~~. in sertin

Hamstring injury   A hyperextension injury produces pain and tenderness in the popliteal space.

Baker's cyst   With a synovial cyst, there is midline popliteal swelling with the knee extended, which disappears when flexed. It occurs in the setting of arthritis.

Septic joint   The knee is hot and painful, and the patient appears ill and febrile. Gonococcal sepsis is a common source in young adults, accompanied by urethritis, pustular skin lesions, and tenosynovitis **(Plate 75).**

Hemarthrosis   Suspect in hemophilia, systemic anticoagulation, and leukemia. A rapidly filling, warm, and tense knee in the setting of trauma indicates a tear of a meniscus, ligament, or fracture.

Patellar fracture   Suspect when a patient falls directly onto the knee. The patella is exquisitely tender, and discrete fragments can be felt with the thumbnail.

Patellar dislocation   There is excessive lateral patellar mobility, with a sensation of the leg "giving away."

Osteochondritis desiccans   Posttraumatic pain is located in the medial knee compartment in young adults. Locking may be caused by a loose body.

Osteonecrosis   Sudden severe pain with weight bearing occurs in an elderly patient or one on steroids.

Acute Monoarticular Arthritis

PLATES 21, 65, 75, 90, 100, 101, 102, 106

◼ DIFFERENTIAL OVERVIEW

❏ Trauma
❏ Gout
❏ Osteoarthritis
❏ Lyme disease
❏ Gonococcal arthritis
❏ Septic arthritis
❏ Pseudogout
❏ Septic bursitis
❏ Avascular necrosis

DIAGNOSTIC APPROACH

Ascertain that arthritis (joint inflammation) is present by eliciting pain on joint motion.

A monoarticular presentation of a polyarticular disease may be rarely seen in rheumatoid arthritis, Reiter's, ankylosing spondylitis, psoriatic arthritis, inflammatory bowel disease, and sarcoidosis. Erythema nodosum occurs with sarcoidosis or inflammatory bowel disease. Urethritis suggests gonorrhea or Reiter's.

CLINICAL FINDINGS

Trauma   History reveals acute torsion, deceleration, or a direct blow. Repetitive motion as the source of injury may not be recognized by the patient and may only be elicited on directed questioning.

Gout   The metatarsophalangeal joint of the great toe is a favored site (podagra), but ankles, knees, wrists, and olecranon bursa are also commonly affected. An alcoholic binge or thiazide diuretic may precipitate an attack. Recurrent attacks, rapid response to colchicine, and tophi are clues (**Plates 100, 101, 102**).

Osteoarthritis   Monoarticular arthritis occurs as an acute flare superimposed on a long-standing history of osteoarthritis. Heberden's and Bouchard's nodes will be present on the hands. The affected joint will have an increase in bony mass and will be crepitant within its range of motion (**Plate 90**).

Lyme disease   Travel to or residence in an endemic area is a prerequisite. A flu-like illness with fever and arthralgias and/or an expanding annular red rash with a clear center precedes the arthritis by days to months (**Plate 106**).

Gonococcal arthritis   Consider this in a sexually active young adult. The initial phase of fever, polyarthralgia, tenosynovitis, and pustular or necrotic skin lesions is followed in several days by a septic joint. Concurrent urethritis or cervicitis (accompanied by a purulent discharge) is helpful but not universally present (**Plate 75**).

Septic arthritis   Usually occurring in a compromised host or in a previously damaged or prosthetic joint, it involves large joints, such as the knees. It presents with abrupt onset with fever and chills and joint pain that is progressive, severe, and throbbing. The joint will be hot and very tender to touch.

Pseudogout   It occurs in older patients and in association with hyperparathyroidism or hemochromatosis (**Plates 21, 65**).

Septic bursitis   Usually appearing in the prepatellar or olecranon bursa, septic bursitis exhibits cellulitis with normal joint motion. Fever, lymphangitis, and a cutaneous portal of entry are important clues.

Avascular necrosis   Consider this when precipitating factors such as steroids or air, fat, or nitrogen embolism are present.

▨ DIFFERENTIAL OVERVIEW

Ankle Pain
❏ Ankle sprain
❏ Fibular fracture
❏ Achilles tendinitis
❏ Acute gout

Foot Pain
❏ Plantar fasciitis
❏ Acute gout
❏ Hallux valgus (bunion)
❏ Sciatica
❏ Metatarsalgia
❏ Metatarsal stress fracture
❏ Tibialis anterior tendinitis
❏ Pes planus
❏ Calcaneal fracture
❏ Interdigital neuroma
❏ Posterior tibial nerve entrapment

DIAGNOSTIC APPROACH

In acute *ankle* injury, ability to bear weight for four steps *and* absence of bone tenderness at the posterior edge or the tip of either malleolus rule out a significant fracture (presence of any has Se 1.0, Sp 0.61).

In acute *foot* injury, ability to bear weight for four steps *and* absence of bone tenderness at the navicular or the base of the fifth metatarsal rule out a significant midfoot fracture (presence of any has Se 0.98, Sp 0.30).

CLINICAL FINDINGS

Ankle sprain Inversion injury is most common, stretching the calcaneofibular or anterior talofibular ligaments, with pain, swelling, and exquisite tenderness over the anterolateral ankle. The anterior drawer sign is helpful in determining stability (and degree of injury), with an anterior shift of the foot on the tibia of greater than or equal to 4 mm being abnormal. The medial ligament is unlikely to be torn unless a fibular fracture and subluxation of the ankle joint exist. Comparison with the uninjured foot is helpful.

Fibular fracture Following trauma, the distal fibula is exquisitely tender, swollen, and ecchymotic. The patient may be able to bear weight despite the fracture.

Achilles tendinitis The patient presents with a tender Achilles tendon with a fusiform swelling. It occurs in athletic overuse but also in spondyloarthropathy, rheumatoid arthritis, and familial hypercholesterolemia. With overuse, the inflammation is maximal at 2–6 cm from the insertion; with spondyloarthropathy, maximal at the insertion. Tendon rupture will be sudden, marked by inability to rise onto the toes, with a palpable gap in the tendon. Posterior calcaneal bursitis, arising from rubbing at the heel of the shoe, can simulate this.

Acute gout Classically, it presents as podagra (acute painful swelling, dusky redness, and exquisite tenderness of the metatarsophalangeal joint of the great toe) or unilateral inflammatory ankle swelling without a history of trauma (**Plate 102.**)

Plantar fasciitis The pain is greatest with weight bearing after a period of inactivity. The medial plantar aspect of the foot (distal to the calcaneus) is tender, and pain is increased by forced dorsiflexion of the toes. It occurs more often in obese persons or those with flat feet.

Hallux valgus (bunion) A tender bursa is found over the prominence formed by lateral drift of the first metatarsal head.

Sciatica The L4 dermatome projects to the instep, the L5 to the dorsal foot, and S1 to the heel and lateral foot. The pain is usually dysesthetic (numb or burning). There will be no

155

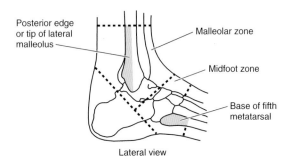

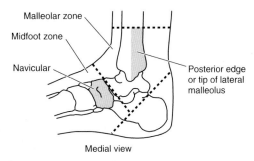

Figure 10. Surface anatomy in ankle and midfoot injuries. (Adapted from: Stiell IG, McKnight RD, Greenberg GH, et al. Implementation of the Ottawa ankle rules. JAMA 1994;271(11):828.)

palpable tenderness or swelling at the site of pain. Knee (L4) or ankle (S1) reflexes may be decreased or absent.

Metatarsalgia   Pain occurs over the mid-metatarsal heads with weight bearing. There is often a callus formed over a prominent metatarsophalangeal joint, and the plantar foot is tender to pressure. Common causes include a high arch or use of high-heeled shoes.

Metatarsal stress fracture   Pain and tenderness develop over the midshaft of the second or third metatarsal. This is a common injury in runners.

Tibialis anterior tendinitis   Pain with exquisite point tenderness occurs at the tendon insertion onto the lateral foot and is increased with foot eversion.

Pes planus   Flat feet may produce pain in the instep after prolonged standing or walking. Signs include an absent longitudinal arch, valgus heel deviation, and a prominent navicular.

Calcaneal fracture   Prominent heel pain will occur after the patient has fallen from a height.

Interdigital neuroma   Symptoms are burning pain and cramping of the third and fourth toes, which are relieved by rubbing the forefoot. Compressing the forefoot and pushing up in the third intermetatarsal space produces a palpable click with reproduction of the patient's symptoms. Tenderness is maximal between the metatarsals, and a nodule may be felt.

Posterior tibial nerve entrapment   Entrapment of the nerve in the tarsal tunnel produces burning and numbness from the medial malleolus, via the sole into the toes. Risk factors include valgus heel deviation and ankle fracture. There may be a Tinel's sign at the ankle.

Chapter 80

Arthritis/Dermatitis

DIFFERENTIAL OVERVIEW

❑ Lyme disease
❑ Erythema nodosum
❑ Rheumatoid arthritis
❑ Systemic lupus erythematosus
❑ Psoriatic arthritis
❑ Disseminated gonococcemia
❑ Sarcoidosis
❑ Scleroderma
❑ Dermatomyositis
❑ Reiter's syndrome
❑ Rheumatic fever
❑ Behçet's syndrome
❑ Still's disease
❑ Hypersensitivity vasculitis

CLINICAL FINDINGS

Lyme disease   Erythema migrans, a rapidly expanding annular rash with a clearing center, is the key early finding. The site of the Ixodid tick bite at the center of the lesion is usually intensely indurated, vesicular, or necrotic. The arthritis is an asymmetric oligoarthritis that usually occurs after the rash has resolved **(Plate 106).**

Erythema nodosum   A prodromal syndrome of fever, chills, malaise, and polyarthralgia is followed by the development of lesions that are discrete, tender, slightly raised subcutaneous nodules on the shins or ankles. They represent a hypersensitivity reaction to group A streptococcal infection, tuberculosis, sarcoidosis, inflammatory bowel disease, or drugs such as oral contraceptives and sulfonamides **(Plate 171).**

Rheumatoid arthritis   Symmetric polyarticular arthritis with synovial proliferation, especially of the wrist, and morning stiffness lasting more than 1 hour characterize the early joint involvement. Rheumatoid nodules appear over extensor surfaces. Vasculitic lesions are frequently found on the digits, appearing as small red or purpuric macules that progress to painful nodules or ulcers **(Plates 88, 89).**

Systemic lupus erythematosus   A classic butterfly rash occurs in 40% and is exacerbated by sun exposure. A diffuse maculopapular rash in sun-exposed areas heralds disease flares. Discoid lesions and scaling plaques that range in color from red to violaceous, with central atrophy and telangiectasias, occur in 20%. Vasculitis, in the form of painful ulcers on the extremities, palpable purpura, or lupus profundus (firm nodules in the subcutaneous fat on the forehead, cheeks, buttocks, and upper arms) are found. The arthritis is typically one of symmetric fusiform swelling of the proximal interphalangeal and metacarpophalangeal joints, diffuse puffiness of the hands, and tenosynovitis **(Plates 36, 91, 92, 93, 110).**

Psoriatic arthritis   Psoriatic plaques, erythematous with a silvery scale, are critical to diagnosis, but may be hidden in the scalp, umbilicus, or gluteal folds. Nail changes such as pitting or yellow discoloration of the nail plate are other clues. The arthritis typically involves the proximal interphalangeal and distal interphalangeal joints, creating sausage digits. The arthritis may become erosive, leading to telescoping of the hands. One-fourth of patients have axial skeletal arthritis **(Plates 103, 104, 105).**

Disseminated gonococcemia   Acral lesions are typically hemorrhagic pustules, but petechiae, hemorrhagic papules, or hemorrhagic bullae can occur. Fever, rigor, tenosynovitis, and polyarthritis are other findings **(Plate 75).**

Sarcoidosis   Transient maculopapular eruptions of the trunk, face, and extremities are often accompanied by uveitis, adenopathy, and parotid enlargement. Translucent reddish-brown to purple indolent plaques may develop on the face (lupus pernio), buttocks, or extremities. Joint symptoms consist of migratory transient arthralgias **(Plates 169, 171).**

157

Scleroderma   Early findings are primarily Raynaud's phenomenon and puffy fingers. Later findings include sclerodactyly (smooth, shiny tapered fingers with taut, bound-down skin); contractures with "claw hand" deformity; expressionless face (with thin lips, a beak-like nose, and sunken cheeks); microstomia; mat telangiectasias on the nail folds, face, lips, oral mucosa, or trunk; and calcinosis with leathery crepitation over the joints **(Plates 97, 98, 113).**

Dermatomyositis   The classic skin manifestation is a lilac-colored heliotrope rash on the eyelids and in a butterfly distribution. Gottron's papules are violaceous, scaly, flat lesions on the extensor aspect of the interphalangeal joints, elbows, knees, and medial malleoli; these occur as a late manifestation. Proximal muscle aching/weakness, not arthritis, is prominent. The patient is unable to reach overhead or arise from a chair. Neck flexors are more involved than extensors **(Plates 94, 95, 96).**

Reiter's syndrome   Arthritis, urethritis, conjunctivitis, and mucocutaneous ulcers are found. The arthritis is asymmetric and additive, usually involving the lower extremity joints. Solitary sausage digits may be seen. Tendinitis and fasciitis are common. The mucocutaneous lesions are eroded red vesicles or papules of the corona and glans, which when confluent are called circinate balanitis. Pustules may change into thick hyperkeratotic plaques on the palms and soles, keratoderma blennorrhagicum.

Rheumatic fever   There is an acute migratory polyarthritis with fever. Subcutaneous nodules appear over the bony prominences of the elbows, knuckles, ankles, scapulae, and occiput. They are associated with carditis. Erythema marginatum, appearing as evanescent pink lesions with serpiginous borders, is also associated with carditis **(Plate 108).**

Behçet's syndrome   The classic triad is arthritis, iritis, and oral and genital ulcerations. Recurrent aphthous ulcers are a *sine qua non.* They begin as macular erythema that develops into superficial gray ulcers. Scrotal or labial ulcerations are also found. Hypopyon uveitis, a hallmark, is a rare finding. The arthritis is primarily of the knees and ankles **(Plates 85, 86, 87).**

Still's disease   Skin lesions are red, flat, and less than 1 cm in diameter. Lesions are evanescent, occurring with fever spikes. A migratory polyarthralgia occurs **(Plate 107).**

Hypersensitivity vasculitis   After an upper respiratory infection, young adults may develop palpable purpura over the extensor surfaces and buttocks. Arthritis, edema, and colicky abdominal pain, followed by bloody stools, secures the diagnosis **(Plate 110).**

Chapter 81

Axillary Swelling

DIFFERENTIAL OVERVIEW

❑ Infectious lymphadenopathy
❑ Lipoma
❑ Pyogenic infection
❑ Malignant lymphadenopathy
❑ Tuberculous abscess
❑ Axillary artery aneurysm

DIAGNOSTIC APPROACH

Examine other node-bearing regions because axillary adenopathy may be the presenting manifestation of generalized adenopathy. Examine for fluctuance (suggesting abscess) versus discrete, rubbery nodules (suggesting lymphadenopathy).

CLINICAL FINDINGS

Infectious lymphadenopathy   The lymph nodes are tender, and a primary infected source is usually apparent in the extremity. Cat-scratch disease commonly produces prominent unilateral axillary lymphadenopathy **(Plate 174).**

Lipoma   The lesion feels soft and may be somewhat translucent. The skin wrinkles when it is raised from the lipoma. A long history of slow growth is an important clue.

Pyogenic infection   Erythema, tenderness, or fever is usually present unless the abscess is under the pectoralis muscle. It often begins as a furuncle, and it may be recurrent, hidradenitis suppurativa. The primary infection may be in the distal extremity. On occasion, a thoracic empyema will point to the axilla.

Malignant lymphadenopathy   Hodgkin's disease and local metastases from breast or lung cancer are the most common causes of isolated axillary lymphadenopathy. A primary breast lesion can usually be found (i.e., the metastasis is not larger than the primary) although it may be obscured by large breasts **(Plate 51).**

Tuberculous abscess   Tuberculosis develops as a fluctuant swelling appearing over weeks to months, with little of the usual inflammatory signs.

Axillary artery aneurysm   An aneurysm presents as a superficial pulsating mass, with a weak radial pulse and dilated arm veins. There is usually either a history of local trauma or signs of endocarditis.

Bony Prominence

Chapter 82

PLATES 14, 90

DIFFERENTIAL OVERVIEW

Age 15–25 Years
❑ Fracture
❑ Callus
❑ Subperiosteal hematoma
❑ Exostosis (osteochondroma)
❑ Osteoma
❑ Enchondroma
❑ Osteosarcoma

Age 25–40 Years
❑ Acromegaly
❑ Giant cell tumor
❑ Periosteal fibrosarcoma

Age Older Than 40 Years
❑ Osteoarthritis
❑ Paget's disease
❑ Metastatic cancer
❑ Multiple myeloma

CLINICAL FINDINGS

Fracture   It usually occurs in the setting of acute trauma, with prominent pain; however, tibial and metatarsal stress fractures may be more subacute/subtle.

Callus   Overlayering around an old fracture may present as a hard swelling over bone.

Subperiosteal hematoma   After a local injury, a permanent thickening may develop, most commonly over the anterior shin.

Exostosis (osteochondroma)   Most commonly found around the knee, these are bone-hard projections away from the joint, unilateral and arising from the epiphysis.

Osteoma   It appears as a hard nodule over membranous bone, most commonly at the vertex of the skull.

Enchondroma   It usually appears as a painless expansion of the fingers or chondrosternal junctions.

Osteosarcoma   It appears as an expansion in the upper tibia or humerus, arising from the metaphysis.

Acromegaly   Growth hormone excess is marked by a symmetrical overgrowth of the head, face, and hands. There is a decrease in the temporal visual field **(Plate 14).**

Giant cell tumor (osteoclastoma)   Commonly found around the knee or distal radius, they encompass the entire end of the bone.

Periosteal fibrosarcoma   A painful, asymmetric swelling over the lower femur is a typical presentation.

Osteoarthritis   Bony exostoses around the distal interphalangeal and proximal interphalangeal joints of the hands with stiffness and deformity and those around the knees are typical. There are irregular coarse crepitations **(Plate 90).**

Paget's disease   Frontal bossing of the skull, kyphosis, and bowing of the femurs may produce a simian appearance. Headaches and sensorineural hearing loss are common.

Metastatic cancer   The bone is not greatly enlarged, and is often warm and painful. Primary lesions in the breast, lung, prostate, kidney, thyroid, or uterus are usually known.

Multiple myeloma   Multiple painful lesions occur in the skull, ribs and vertebrae, often with pathological fractures. A bedside test for proteinuria is positive in 60% of cases. A clear urine will become cloudy when heated to 50–60° C, and then clear again when heated further, as a result of the presence of Bence-Jones proteins.

Chapter 83

Elbow Pain

DIFFERENTIAL OVERVIEW

❏ Lateral epicondylitis
❏ Olecranon bursitis
❏ Medial epicondylitis
❏ Bicipitoradialis tendinitis
❏ Cubital tunnel syndrome
❏ Radial head fracture
❏ Septic arthritis
❏ Gout
❏ Elbow dislocation
❏ Rupture distal biceps tendon
❏ Epitrochlear lymphadenitis

CLINICAL FINDINGS

Lateral epicondylitis   There is exquisite point tenderness over the lateral epicondyle. Pain is intensified by resisted extension of the wrist.

Olecranon bursitis   Marked by fluctuant swelling over the olecranon, it is most often traumatic, but if septic, it will be tender.

Medial epicondylitis   There is tenderness over the medial epicondyle. Pain is intensified with resisted flexion of the wrist. Ulnar neuritis also occurs in as many as one-half of patients with medial epicondylitis.

Bicipitoradialis tendinitis   There is pain and tenderness over distal biceps tendon. The usual source is repetitive elbow flexion, such as from throwing a ball.

Cubital tunnel syndrome   Ulnar nerve distribution pain and tingling with hypothenar wasting is prominent, and pressure in the cubital tunnel reproduces the symptoms.

Radial head fracture   Resulting from a fall onto an outstretched hand, there is impaired forearm rotation and exquisite tenderness over the radial head (immediately distal to the lateral epicondyle).

Septic arthritis   Pain is severe and aggravated by movement. The joint is warm and tender, and the paraolecranon grooves are fluid-filled. Fever is present but often low-grade. N. gonorrhea is the most common cause in patients younger than 30 years of age and S. aureus in those older than 30 **(Plate 75)**.

Gout   Acute pain, redness, and swelling occur, as in septic arthritis, but fever is usually absent **(Plate 100)**.

Elbow dislocation   Typically caused by a fall onto an outstretched arm, the olecranon protrudes abnormally. The arm is held at 130°, and neither active nor passive movement is possible.

Rupture distal biceps tendon   The tear occurs with a "pop" at maximal resisted flexion, such as lifting a heavy weight. There is antecubital pain, and the biceps tendon is no longer palpable there, instead forming a knot in the biceps mass of the upper arm.

Epitrochlear lymphadenitis   Tender nodes are palpable in the medial elbow. Causes include bacterial infection of the ulnar aspect of the hand, cat-scratch disease, and secondary syphilis **(Plates 80, 81, 174)**.

Hip Pain

◪ DIFFERENTIAL OVERVIEW

❑ Osteoarthritis
❑ Trochanteric bursitis
❑ Ischial bursitis
❑ Iliopectineal bursitis
❑ Iliopsoas bursitis
❑ Nerve root compression
❑ Meralgia paresthetica
❑ Obturator inflammation
❑ Iliac apophysitis
❑ Hip fracture
❑ Aortoiliac insufficiency
❑ Polymyalgia rheumatica
❑ Ankylosing spondylitis
❑ Septic arthritis
❑ Avascular necrosis femoral head

DIAGNOSTIC APPROACH

In disease of the hip joint, the earliest limitation is internal rotation with the hip hyperextended. The hip joint is palpated just below the inguinal ligament lateral to the femoral artery. Tenderness and/or crepitance are usually felt there with movement. Manual internal and external rotation of the hip with the knee and hip in flexion usually reproduces pain as does percussion of the heel with the examiner's palm.

CLINICAL FINDINGS

Osteoarthritis   The onset is gradual, beginning with minor aching or stiffness exacerbated by prolonged standing, walking, or stair-climbing. Stiffness present after prolonged inactivity loosens with use and then worsens with continued activity. The range of motion is limited, and there may be crepitance. With advanced disease, there may be a limp, antalgic gait, and positive Trendelenburg's sign (buttock falls when standing on the opposite foot) indicative of abductor weakness. The hip is held in flexion, external rotation, and adduction **(Plate 90).**

Trochanteric bursitis   Pain occurs in the lateral aspect of the hip, often radiating into the knee, and is exacerbated at night. Prominent tenderness over the greater trochanter is characteristic.

Ischial bursitis   It causes buttock pain, worse on sitting, usually induced by prolonged sitting on a hard surface. Pain may radiate posteriorly down the leg. The patient will be tender over the ischial spine.

Iliopectineal bursitis   It causes pain on hip flexion and tenderness localized to the lateral border of Scarpa's triangle.

Iliopsoas bursitis   The pain worsens with hyperextension of the hip. Flexion and external rotation reproduce the pain.

Nerve root compression   L1 and L2 impingement may be referred to the hip. Reversed straight leg raising will increase the pain.

Meralgia paresthetica   A characteristic burning dysesthesia over the anterolateral thigh is caused by entrapment of the lateral femoral cutaneous nerve at the anterior superior iliac spine.

Obturator inflammation   This is recognized by a positive obturator sign, and pain increases with internal rotation of the hip.

Iliac apophysitis   Pain and tenderness are located over the iliac crest at the insertion of the tensor fascia lata.

Hip fracture   Fracture should be suspected after any fall in an elderly patient. The leg will be shortened and externally rotated. The pain is usually severe although ambulation may be possible.

Aortoiliac insufficiency   Advanced atherosclerosis produces claudication (pain with walking, relieved by rest) that radiates to the hip and buttock.

Polymyalgia rheumatica   There is bilateral aching of the proximal musculature (hips and shoulders) in an elderly patient, with prominent weakness on arising from a chair. Passive range of motion is preserved.

Ankylosing spondylitis   Sacroiliac and lumbar spine involvement are concurrently present, with pain radiating to the hip.

Septic arthritis   Suspect infection when there is fever, a source for hematogenous seeding, or hardware in the hip. The hip is held in flexion, and there may be a bulging, tender joint capsule.

Avascular necrosis femoral head   There is a gradual onset of focal pain and limitation of movement. Predisposing conditions include chronic steroid use, hemoglobinopathy, and alcoholism.

Low Back Pain

PLATES 25, 58, 86, 90

◼ DIFFERENTIAL OVERVIEW

❑ Musculoligamentous strain
❑ Lumbar disc herniation
❑ Osteoarthritis
❑ Compression fracture
❑ Pyelonephritis
❑ Secondary gain
❑ Scoliosis
❑ Spondylolisthesis
❑ Metastatic cancer
❑ Spinal stenosis
❑ Transverse process fracture
❑ Pancreatic cancer
❑ Ankylosing spondylitis
❑ Sacroiliitis
❑ Aortic dissection
❑ Cauda equina syndrome
❑ Vertebral osteomyelitis
❑ Epidural abscess

DIAGNOSTIC APPROACH

Radicular pain has such a high sensitivity (>0.95) for nerve root compression that its absence makes important disc herniation unlikely.

Back pain at rest or unassociated with posture/movement should increase the suspicion of tumor, fracture, infection, or referred visceral pain. Spinal tenderness is a sensitive but not specific indicator. Clues to metastatic cancer include a history of cancer, unexplained weight loss, and signs of cord compression, such as motor weakness of the legs, urinary or fecal incontinence, and absent anal reflex. Recent bacterial infection, injection drug use, or immune suppression (from steroids, chemotherapy, or HIV) should raise suspicion for infection. Fever occurs in osteomyelitis (50%), epidural abscess (83%), and tuberculosis (27%).

A red flag for fracture in a young adult is major trauma, such as a fall from a height or a motor vehicle accident. In older adults, minor trauma or strenuous lifting can cause a compression fracture.

CLINICAL FINDINGS

Musculoligamentous strain   Strain usually occurs after episodic or repetitive lifting, bending, or twisting. Pain may radiate from the low back into the buttock or posterior thigh but not below the knee. There is often visible or palpable paraspinous spasm. Reproduction of the injury-inducing movement sharply exacerbates the pain.

Lumbar disc herniation   Pain, numbness, or paresthesia radiating in a dermatomal pattern from the back into the foot is the hallmark of this syndrome. L4, L5 and S1 roots are affected in more than 95% of cases. L4 compression (L3,4 disc) produces neuritic symptoms in the instep of the foot. Motor weakness of foot inversion and a diminished knee reflex may also occur, but these are not invariable results and are better considered indicators of severity. L5 compression produces symptoms in the dorsum of the foot, weakness of great toe extension, and no reflex changes. S1 compression causes symptoms in the lateral foot and heel, weakness of foot eversion, and a diminished ankle reflex. Straight leg raising, which stretches the nerve roots, reproduces pain or numbness radiating into the foot. Pain may be increased further by dorsiflexion of the foot with the leg elevated. Care must be taken not to overinterpret muscular spasm from stretching the low back or tight hamstrings as a positive test. Positive crossed straight leg raising (radicular pain in the leg opposite to that being raised) suggests a large disc or herniated fragment. Rarely, herniation of a higher disc (L3) will produce pain in the anterior thigh, quadriceps atrophy, and positive reverse straight leg raising (patient prone).

Low Back Pain

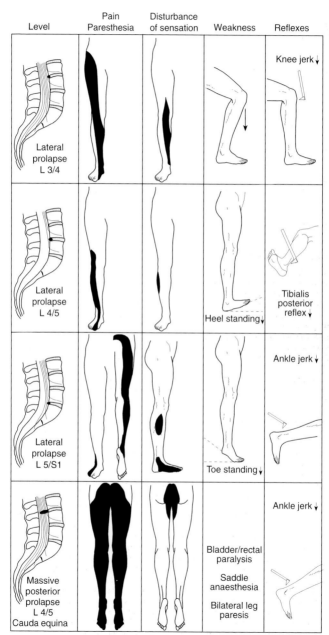

Figure 11. Lumbosacral root compression syndromes. (Adapted from: Droste C, Von Planta M. Memorix Clinical Medicine. London: Chapman & Hall 1997, p. 275.) **165**

Low Back Pain

Osteoarthritis   It is recognized as pain and stiffness with flexion and rotation in a patient with evidence elsewhere of osteoarthritis (e.g., Heberden's and Bouchard's nodes). Hypertrophied facets, osteophytes, and/or spondylolisthesis may cause root compression **(Plate 90).**

Compression fracture   Related to osteoporosis, it occurs mostly in older patients and those on steroids (Sp >0.99, LR 12). Pain suddenly brought on by flexion stress is the usual history. Pain is localized over the vertebrae or around the trunk, and there often is tenderness to palpation over the spinous processes. The upper lumbar or lower thoracic vertebrae are most commonly affected. Consider metastatic cancer, myeloma, and hyperparathyroidism as alternative causes.

Pyelonephritis   Renal infection presents with fever, prominent nausea, chills, urinary frequency, and costovertebral angle tenderness.

Secondary gain   Clues are inconsistent symptoms or physical findings (they change and lack an anatomic distribution), anger, focusing on attribution of symptoms with relatively less concern about what can be done to cure the problem, and impending litigation.

Scoliosis   Functional scoliosis disappears with flexion while structural scoliosis increases.

Spondylolisthesis   This is often asymptomatic, but when symptoms occur, flexion and extension of the low back is painful, and motion is limited. A palpable shelf is present at the level of the defect and increases with flexion.

Metastatic cancer   Back pain is of insidious onset, is not relieved by lying down (Se 0.90), often occurs at night, and is described as "boring" or "expansile." A history of cancer and unexplained weight loss are specific findings (0.98 and 0.94 respectively). Myeloma, prostate, breast, lung, and colon cancers are common sources.

Spinal stenosis   This occurs most commonly in elderly patients as chronic low back pain with evidence elsewhere (hands or knees) of osteoarthritis. The pain is worsened by standing without walking (unlike claudication) and relieved by sitting (unlike disc disease) or flexing the spine and hips. The pain may radiate into the legs and is often bilateral and poorly localized.

Transverse process fracture   Its origin is violent muscular contraction of the psoas. There is exquisite tenderness lateral to the spinous process. It may be associated with retroperitoneal bleeding leading to hypovolemic shock.

Pancreatic cancer   This cancer presents insidiously with relentless, dull upper lumbar backache with abdominal pain. Weight loss and depression are prominent.

Ankylosing spondylitis   It occurs in young men, presenting with gradual onset of back stiffness, especially in the morning. Active or old iridocyclitis (iridic adhesions or dark spots in the anterior chamber), arthritis, and a prior history of inflammatory bowel disease are clues. Schober's maneuver revealing limited flexion is sensitive but not specific **(Plates 58, 86).**

Sacroiliitis   The sacroiliac joints, marked by the sacral dimples, are deeply tender.

Aortic dissection   Acute onset, moving, tearing back pain, a restless and "shocky" patient, asymmetric femoral pulses, abdominal pulsation, and an abdominal bruit are key findings **(Plate 25).**

Cauda equina syndrome   Urinary retention or overflow incontinence, saddle anesthesia, bilateral leg weakness/numbness, and anal sphincter laxity are found. Ankle jerks are decreased, but knee jerks are increased (due to unopposed quadriceps). It is most commonly caused by a herniated disc.

Vertebral osteomyelitis   Low-grade fever, dull continuous and progressive back pain, and tenderness to percussion over the spine are found.

Epidural abscess   The characteristic presentation is radicular pain or progressive muscular weakness in a febrile patient with localized back pain and tenderness. The pain is increased with recumbency, sudden movements, or Valsalva. Spinal percussion tenderness has Se 0.86, Sp 0.60, and LR 2.2. Lhermitte sign, an electric-like sensation shooting down the back, is often present. Early signs of impending paraplegia include extensor plantar reflex (toes pointing downward), leg weakness, and urinary retention.

Chapter 86

Muscle Cramps

⬛ DIFFERENTIAL OVERVIEW

- ❏ Ordinary muscle cramp
- ❏ Overuse
- ❏ Dehydration
- ❏ Drugs/toxins
- ❏ Hypokalemia
- ❏ Hyponatremia
- ❏ Hyperventilation
- ❏ Vascular insufficiency
- ❏ Restless legs syndrome
- ❏ Hypocalcemia
- ❏ Dystonia
- ❏ Amyotrophic lateral sclerosis
- ❏ Hemifacial spasms
- ❏ Spinal cord lesion
- ❏ Muscle enzyme deficiency
- ❏ Myotonic dystrophy
- ❏ Black widow spider bite
- ❏ Tetanus

DIAGNOSTIC APPROACH

Generalized cramps suggest chronic disease of the motor neuron such as amyotrophic lateral sclerosis. Cramps recurrent and localized to one muscle group suggest nerve root disease.

An ordinary muscle cramp is a diagnosis of exclusion following a careful inspection and metabolic laboratory evaluation. Fleeting twitches or prolonged contractions are not caused by common cramps.

Myotonia is difficulty releasing a grip (handshake or doorknob) that improves with repeated contractions.

CLINICAL FINDINGS

Ordinary muscle cramp   Cramping presents as a painful involuntary cramp of a single muscle with a palpable knot. It is most often nocturnal appearing in the legs (calf and ventral foot), accompanied by local fasciculations and relieved by stretching.

Overuse   A painful cramp occurs during exercise/use. As a result of inappropriate contractions of opposing muscle groups, unusual postures often result. Swimmer's cramp is a striking example of this. "Professional cramps" also occur with the overuse of muscle groups, e.g., writer's cramp or lip and facial muscle cramping in horn players.

Dehydration   It appears with excessive sweating and loss of salt as in vigorous exertion or fever. A similar phenomenon occurs during dialysis, probably because of hyposmolarity.

Drugs/toxins   Statins can produce muscle toxicity perceived as muscle aching, pain, and cramps. Strychnine poisoning can cause spasms that are clonic rather than tetanic and that affect the whole body rather than primarily the extremities. Ergot excess, usually occurring in patients with frequent migraines, causes muscle pains and intermittent claudication.

Hypokalemia   These cramps appear like ordinary muscle cramps and occur in the setting of diuretic use.

Hyponatremia   Sodium loss is most often caused by diuretics or SIADH.

Hyperventilation   Painless carpal-pedal spasms appear along with tingling around the mouth, and in the hands and feet. The patient often does not recognize their rapid/deep breathing.

Vascular insufficiency   Intermittent claudication, not a true cramp, is predictably precipitated by exertion and relieved by rest.

Restless legs syndrome   Nocturnal creeping, aching, or writhing sensations appear in the legs. Underlying causes include iron deficiency anemia, pregnancy, rheumatoid arthritis, and uremia **(Plates 189, 198)**.

Hypocalcemia   Tetany, paroxysmal, or sustained contraction (hours to days) of the extremities and increased excitability of the nerves to mechanical stimulation, are found. Paresthesias and positive Chvostek's and Trousseau's signs will usually be present. An "accoucheur's hand" may develop, with the distal fingers extended, metacarpophalangeal joints flexed, and the thumb drawn into the palm, either spontaneously or in response to blood pressure cuff compression of the arm (Chvostek's sign).

Dystonia   Sustained postures develop as a result of simultaneous contraction of antagonist and agonist muscles, occurring with antipsychotic or antidepressant medications.

Amyotrophic lateral sclerosis   Weakness, atrophy, and fasciculations accompany the cramps **(Plate 132)**.

Hemifacial spasms   Any facial movement, such as blinking, leads to a fine twitching or prolonged facial spasm. It is caused by compression of the facial nerve in the posterior fossa.

Spinal cord lesion   Symptoms include stiffness, muscle cramps, and flexor spasms of the thigh, knee, and foot set off by cutaneous or visceral stimuli. Autonomic signs such as sweating, piloerection, and incontinence are also present.

Muscle enzyme deficiency   Phosphorylase/phosphofructokinase deficiency causes painful cramps evoked by vigorous exertion. Carnitine palmityl deficiency causes cramps to occur during prolonged exercise, especially when the patient is fasting, following a low carbohydrate diet, or spending time in a cold climate.

Myotonic dystrophy   The hallmark is delayed relaxation of voluntary contraction.

Black widow spider bite   Persistent muscle rigidity and painful cramps occur in persons who have been bitten.

Tetanus   Involuntary spasm is superimposed on continuous stiffness. Trismus ("lockjaw") occurs early in the course, along with rigid hyperextension of the neck. There will usually be a cutaneous infected source.

Chapter 87

Nail Phenomena/Clubbing

▨ DIFFERENTIAL OVERVIEW

Phenomena
- ❏ Pitting
- ❏ Transverse depression
- ❏ Transverse white line
- ❏ Nailfold telangiectasias
- ❏ Nailfold infarcts
- ❏ Splinter hemorrhages
- ❏ Onycholysis
- ❏ Spoon nails
- ❏ Blue-green nails
- ❏ White nails
- ❏ Half-and-half nails
- ❏ Yellow nails
- ❏ Blue lunulae
- ❏ Red lunulae
- ❏ Black longitudinal streak

Clubbing
- ❏ Bronchogenic cancer
- ❏ Tuberculosis
- ❏ Endocarditis
- ❏ Inflammatory bowel disease
- ❏ Familial
- ❏ Trauma
- ❏ Grave's disease
- ❏ Cirrhosis
- ❏ Cystic fibrosis
- ❏ Cyanotic congenital heart disease
- ❏ Pulmonary fibrosis
- ❏ Mediastinal Hodgkin's disease
- ❏ Mesothelioma
- ❏ Lung abscess
- ❏ Bronchiectasis
- ❏ Hypertrophic osteoarthropathy
- ❏ Pachydermoperiostosis

DIAGNOSTIC APPROACH

Nails contain an archive of information about physiologic conditions affecting growth, similar to the way tree rings reflect the weather of summers past. If examined closely, they may also contain the subtlest of clues to important systemic illness, such as endocarditis.

Clubbing is most sensitively detected by loss of the normal nail angle when seen in profile, or by putting corresponding fingers back to back and looking for loss of the diamond of light. Springiness or ballotability of the base of the nail is another early sign. The overlying skin is smooth and shiny, and the nailbeds are cyanotic. Nails of patients with chronic paronychia may be confused with clubbing (**Plate 52**).

When clubbing is present, specifically examine for findings of associated illness including peripheral stigmata of endocarditis, murmurs, splenomegaly, jaundice, wheezes, rales, pleural effusion, supraclavicular adenopathy, hepatomegaly, abdominal mass, thyromegaly and ophthalmopathy.

Unilateral clubbing may be caused by impairment of the vascular supply to the arm. Causes include aortic or subclavian artery aneurysm, anomalous aortic arch, pulmonary hypertension with patent ductus arteriosus, brachial arteriovenous fistula, superior sulcus lung tumor, and recurrent shoulder dislocation. *Unidigital clubbing* may be caused by median nerve injury or sarcoidosis. *Clubbing of toes without fingers* can be seen in coarctation of the aorta.

CLINICAL FINDINGS

Pitting   It is most commonly caused by psoriasis, but it can also seen in patients with eczema, lichen planus, and alopecia areata **(Plate 103)**.

Transverse depression   Systemic stresses (e.g., severe infection, myocardial infarction or trauma) cause transient thinning of the nail plate (Beau's lines), which gradually grows out.

Transverse white line   They are found with transient hypoalbuminemia and systemic stress (Mees' lines). They are also classically described with arsenic poisoning **(Plate 115)**.

Nailfold telangiectasias   Observe using a plus-40 diopter objective on the ophthalmoscope, enhanced using an oil droplet. Thick vessels with a glomerular appearance are consistent with dermatomyositis, scleroderma, or Raynaud's. Thin, meandering vessels are consistent with lupus **(Plate 113)**.

Nailfold infarcts   Bywater's lesions are small, painless, red-brown nailfold infarcts seen in rheumatic vasculitis.

Splinter hemorrhages   A longitudinal distal hemorrhage with the appearance of a splinter most commonly results from trauma but is also seen in persons with endocarditis, vasculitis, or scurvy. Trichinosis should be suspected when all nails are involved **(Plate 22)**.

Onycholysis   Lifting and cracking of the nail (especially the fourth finger) without cutaneous disease suggests hyperthyroidism, but it can also occur with psoriasis, dermatophyte infections, or photosensitivity owing to tetracycline **(Plate 20)**.

Spoon nails   The nails appear concave. When an acquired phenomenon, it may be associated with iron deficiency, syphilis, or thyroid disease **(Plate 189)**.

Blue-green nails   This color is the unique hallmark of Pseudomonas infections **(Plate 114)**.

White nails   Hypoalbuminemic (less than 2.2) states such as nephrotic syndrome and cirrhosis produce opaque white nails with pink tips **(Plate 112)**.

Half-and-half nails   A red-brown distal band occupying 20–50% of the nail occurs in cirrhosis, diabetes and congestive heart failure (Terry's nails). A brown distal band due to melanin deposition can be found in renal failure (Lindsay's nails).

Yellow nails   A yellow "oil droplet" lesion in the nail is typical for psoriasis. Dermatophyte infection and lymphedema may also cause yellowing of the lateral nail border. A "yellow nail syndrome," with all nails yellow without cuticles, can be seen in chronic chest infections or lymphedema **(Plate 53)**.

Blue lunulae   These are found in argyria (silver), hepatolenticular degeneration (Wilson's disease), and antimalarial therapy **(Plate 6)**.

Red lunulae   Cherry red lunulae are seen in carbon monoxide poisoning, and half moons are seen in cardiac failure **(Plate 116)**.

Black longitudinal streak   Although it may be a normal finding in darkly pigmented patients, it may also be caused by a nail bed melanoma, junctional nevus, or Peutz-Jeghers syndrome **(Plate 162)**.

Bronchogenic cancer   The key clues are a smoking history, hemoptysis, and weight loss. Clubbing is rare with cancer metastatic to the lung but occurs in 5–10% of cases of bronchogenic cancer **(Plate 52)**.

Tuberculosis   Patients present with fever, night sweats, and hemoptysis. Clubbing is uncommon in uncomplicated pulmonary tuberculosis, but it may occur in as many as one-fourth of patients with chronic cavitation **(Plate 52)**.

Endocarditis   Consider this diagnosis in a patient with predisposing factors such as an artificial or rheumatically scarred valve, mitral valve prolapse, or recent dental work. Findings include a new murmur, splenomegaly, peripheral emboli, and fever **(Plates 22, 23, 24)**.

Inflammatory bowel disease   Abdominal pain, diarrhea, fever, and blood or mucous in the stools are hallmarks **(Plate 58)**.

Familial   The appearance of the fingers has been commented on for the duration of the patient's entire life.

Trauma   Jackhammer operation is a classic cause.

Nail Phenomena/Clubbing

Grave's disease Pseudoclubbing of thyroid acropachy occurs in both the fingers and the toes. Eye findings of proptosis, stare, and lid lag are usually present as are tachycardia and fine tremor **(Plates 19, 20).**

Cirrhosis Consider this in an alcoholic or a patient with chronic hepatitis. Vascular spiders, ascites, and a nodular liver edge are clues **(Plate 61).**

Cystic fibrosis It is usually diagnosed in childhood, manifested by chronic lung infections and malabsorption, but occasionally it first becomes overt in adulthood.

Cyanotic congenital heart disease Cyanosis occurs when a right-to-left shunt is present and it is manifest by blue lips and digits since infancy. Clubbing does not occur with noncyanotic congential heart disease, such as ventricular septal defect, patent ductus arteriosus, or aortic coarctation **(Plate 29).**

Pulmonary fibrosis Velcro rales are characteristic, and clubbing occurs early.

Mediastinal Hodgkin's disease "B" symptoms such as night sweats and cervical adenopathy or splenomegaly are helpful clues.

Mesothelioma Consider this when there is occupational asbestos exposure and vague persistent chest pain.

Lung abscess Abscess is unmistakable in a febrile patient with a chronic, productive fetid cough.

Bronchiectasis Chronic profusely productive cough is the primary clue.

Hypertrophic osteoarthropathy Severe, burning, deep pain in the wrists, ankles, hands, and feet increases at night or with dependency. Warmth, redness, and brawny edema are often found over the long bones (e.g., shins). Raynaud's, peripheral cyanosis, paresthesias, and muscular weakness may also occur **(Plate 36).**

Pachydermoperiostosis Hypertrophic osteoarthropathy is combined with acromegalic features such as cylindrical thickening of the limbs, paw-like enlargement of the hands and feet, hyperhidrosis and marked oiliness, and accentuation of folds in the face causing a leonine appearance.

Neck Pain

Chapter 88

◼ DIFFERENTIAL OVERVIEW

Posterior
- ❑ Musculoligamentous strain
- ❑ Cervical spondylosis
- ❑ Cervical root compression
- ❑ Posterior cervical lymphadenopathy
- ❑ Meningeal inflammation
- ❑ Cervical fracture
- ❑ Atlantoaxial subluxation

Anterior
- ❑ Anterior cervical lymphadenopathy
- ❑ Thyroiditis
- ❑ Myocardial ischemia

DIAGNOSTIC APPROACH

With neck pain after trauma, a cervical fracture must always be ruled out and the patient's neck immobilized until this is ascertained.

Assess radicular signs of nerve compression as a marker for more serious pathology. Spurling's sign, production of radicular pain with extension and lateral neck rotation, suggests narrowing of the neural foramen. Lhermitte's sign, an electrical sensation radiating down the spine with neck flexion, is a sign of a spinal cord lesion.

With neck pain in the presence of headache or fever, actively consider meningitis.

CLINICAL FINDINGS

Musculoligamentous strain Strain will usually have a traumatic origin, e.g., whiplash. Symptoms of pain with neck motion, stiffness, and spasm gradually increase over several hours. There should be no neurological deficit. Spasm may occur, with unilateral tension causing torticollis, with the head turned to one side.

Cervical spondylosis Trauma or osteoarthritic changes in the facet joints may cause subluxation or ankylosis with decreased mobility, chronic stiffness, and recurrent mild aching. Pain may radiate to the occiput, shoulders, or arms when there is compromise of the neural foramen.

Cervical root compression Pain or numbness radiating into the distribution of C5 (anterolateral shoulder and upper arm, with decreased biceps reflex), C6 (dorsoradial forearm and thumb, with decreased brachioradialis reflex) or C7 (midhand, with decreased triceps reflex) are most common. It usually results from cervical disc herniation or osteoarthritis-associated facet hypertrophy/osteophyte formation.

Posterior cervical lymphadenopathy Discrete, tender lymph nodes occur most commonly in infectious mononucleosis **(Plates 229, 230).**

Meningeal inflammation Meningitis, with headache and fever, and subarachnoid hemorrhage, with sudden-onset severe headache, are serious causes that must be considered. There will be involuntary spasm of the neck muscles, and forward flexion will produce neck stiffness and pain (Kernig's sign).

Cervical fracture Suspect fracture in a traumatic injury, such as with diving, or with sudden deceleration, such as with a motor vehicle accident. The neck will be very tender over the midline. Radiating pain or numbness increases the likelihood of significant injury.

Atlantoaxial subluxation Occurring in rheumatoid arthritis, the neck is stiff and unable to rotate, and the head is bent forward with the chin down.

Anterior cervical lymphadenopathy Tender discrete enlarged lymph nodes in the anterior cervical chain occur with viral or streptococcal pharyngitis.

Thyroiditis The thyroid gland will be exquisitely tender, associated with tachycardia and low-grade fever.

Myocardial ischemia Exertional neck pain should raise the possibility of angina, even without concomitant chest pain. An acute myocardial infarction may on occasion present with nonexertional neck/jaw pain.

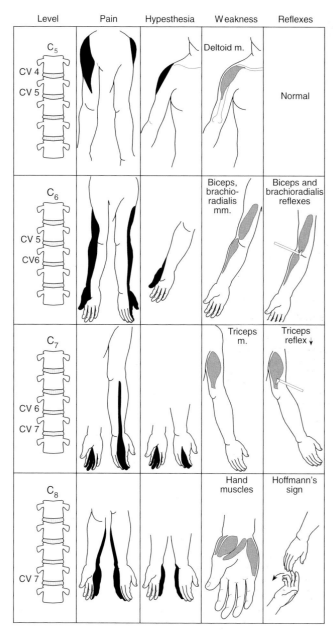

Figure 12. Cervical root compression syndromes. (Adapted from: Droste C, Von Planta M. Memorix Clinical Medicine. London: Chapman & Hall, 1997, p. 274.)

173

Periarticular Pain

◼ DIFFERENTIAL OVERVIEW

❏ Tendinitis
❏ Bursitis
❏ Tenosynovitis
❏ Myofascial pain
❏ Radicular pain
❏ Fibromyalgia
❏ Polymyalgia rheumatica
❏ Reflex sympathetic dystrophy

DIAGNOSTIC APPROACH

Periarticular pain occurs with use of a muscle group rather than movement of the joint per se. Principal symptoms are pain, stiffness, limited function, and sleep disturbance. Stiffness on awakening implies inflammation.

CLINICAL FINDINGS

Tendinitis   Tendon inflammation is usually caused by repetitive motion/overuse, as in exercising, doing assembly line work, playing musical instruments, or typing. Common syndromes include the following: *lateral epicondylitis* (tennis elbow) with pain on resisted wrist extension and supination of the forearm; *medial epicondylitis*, with pain increased by wrist flexion and pronation; *Achilles tendinitis* with posterior heel pain and tenderness; *de Quervain's tendinitis* of the thumb extensor with tenderness and swelling over the radial styloid, and pain produced by making a fist with the thumb inside then deviating it in an ulnar direction (Finkelstein's maneuver); *supraspinatus tendinitis*, with tenderness over the lateral shoulder and pain with abduction of the shoulder; and *bicipital tendinitis*, with pain in the bicipital groove and on resisted pronation of the forearm with the elbow flexed at 90°.

Bursitis   Inflammation occurs in a bursa over a bony prominence: olecranon, trochanteric, anserine (lateral knee), prepatellar, subdeltoid, and ischial. The tenderness is well-localized, and there is often palpable fluid present. The olecranon bursa is especially subject to infection, which should be suspected in the presence of fever or erythema.

Tenosynovitis   There is erythema and pain along the tendon sheath. The pain is exacerbated by movement of the tendon. Crepitance may be palpable or audible over the tendon sheath. Inflammation is usually owing to repetitive motion although disseminated gonococcemia should be considered in the presence of urethritis, fever, or pustular skin lesions **(Plate 75)**.

Myofascial pain   Pain resulting from overuse or acute injury of muscles or tendons is associated with discrete trigger points. The pain is usually poorly localized, and it may be associated with sensations of tingling, numbness, or hyperalgesia. Common sites include the following: temporomandibular joint with masseter muscle trigger points; shoulder pain with scapular trigger points; occipital headache with trapezius or neck trigger points; anterior chest pain with pectoralis or serratus anterior trigger points; low back pain with lumbar paraspinal trigger points; sciatic with gluteal muscle trigger points; and fascia lata in the lateral thigh, which produces a broad-based tenderness. Generalized myalgia may result from vigorous exercise, trauma, rhabdomyolysis, viral infections, or vasculitis.

Radicular pain   Nerve root compression may present as deep, aching pain in a limb. It may be recognized by a dermatomal distribution, absence of tenderness at the point of pain, and isolated motor weakness or hypoactive deep tendon reflexes.

Fibromyalgia   Diffuse aching pain and stiffness is widespread, associated with a disturbed sleep pattern, easy fatigability, a subjective sensation of swelling, and headache. Tender myofascial trigger points are characteristic and are found at the midpoint of the upper border of the trapezius, second costochondral joint, lumbar and lower cervical intraspinous ligaments, medial border of the scapula (at the origin of the supraspinatus),

Periarticular Pain

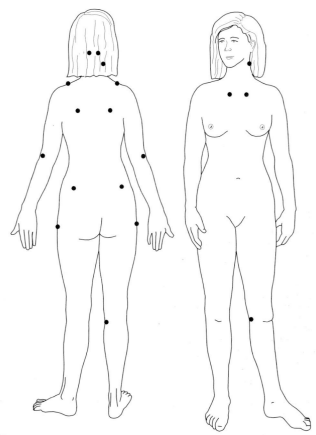

Figure 13. Fibromyalgia trigger points. (Adapted from: Rubenstein E, Federman DD. Scientific American Medicine. New York: Scientific American, 1992, p. 15:vi:7.)

distal to the lateral epicondyle over the extensor digitorum muscle, over the upper outer buttocks, and the medial collateral ligament of the knee. The American College of Rheumatology defines fibromyalgia as having widespread musculoskeletal pain, tenderness of 11 of 18 specific trigger points, and no concomitant explanatory disease.

Polymyalgia rheumatica   Diffuse severe aching in the shoulder girdle and hips occurs in association with fever, malaise, and weight loss. There is pain on arising from a squat and on resisted abduction of the shoulders. True weakness does not exclude the diagnosis but should broaden the differential. Temporal arteritis marked by headache, jaw claudication, a ropy, tender temporal artery, and visual loss is also part of the spectrum.

Reflex sympathetic dystrophy   Difficult to recognize, it is characterized by a poorly localized aching in the extremity, and vasospasm of the digits. The pain is sustained, burning, or lancinating, and nondermatomal. There is abnormal skin temperature, which is hot early in the course, and cold later. Skin color is similarly red early and cyanotic late. Perspiration is altered, dry early and moist late. There is edema of the extremity and atrophy of the hair, nails, and skin. There may be hyperpathia, overreaction to repetitive stimuli, and true weakness.

Polyarticular Arthritis
Chapter 90

PLATES 36, 58, 75, 86, 88, 89, 90, 91, 92, 97, 98, 100, 101, 102, 103, 104, 105, 106, 107, 108, 110, 113, 137, 138, 169, 171

DIFFERENTIAL OVERVIEW

❏ Osteoarthritis
❏ Rheumatoid arthritis
❏ Lyme arthritis
❏ Systemic lupus erythematosus
❏ Psoriatic arthritis
❏ Polyarticular gout
❏ Viral arthritis
❏ Scleroderma
❏ Reiter's syndrome
❏ Inflammatory bowel disease
❏ Gonococcal arthritis
❏ Ankylosing spondylitis
❏ Systemic vasculitis
❏ Sarcoidosis
❏ Pseudogout
❏ Acute rheumatic fever
❏ Still's disease

DIAGNOSTIC APPROACH

Ascertain that the pain is articular; that is, it is exacerbated by the function of the joint. Periarticular phenomena, such as bursitis or tendonitis, and neuropathic causes should be sought.

Involvement of the wrists, elbows, or metacarpophalangeal joints implies inflammatory disease rather than osteoarthritis. Morning stiffness persisting for as long as 1–2 hours, relieved by NSAIDs, is typical for inflammatory arthritis, as is a history of a red joint.

Differentiating features include the following:

Erythema nodosum: Sarcoidosis, inflammatory bowel disease-related arthritis, or Behçet's. *Rash:* Lupus, Still's, vasculitis, dermatomyositis, endocarditis, disseminated gonorrhea, or Behçet's.

Fever greater than 40° C: Still's, bacterial arthritis, or lupus. *Fever preceding arthritis:* Viral arthritis, Lyme, reactive arthritis, Still's, or bacterial endocarditis. *Spiking fever:* Bacterial infection or Still's.

Splenomegaly: Rheumatoid arthritis and lupus. *Raynaud's:* Scleroderma, mixed connective tissue disease, or lupus. *Oral ulcers:* Lupus, Behçet's, or viral arthritis. *Dry eyes and mouth:* Sjogren's, mixed connective tissue disease, or lupus. *Ocular findings:* Lupus, Behçet's, sarcoidosis, or reactive arthritis.

Migratory arthritis: Gonococcemia, rheumatic fever, meningococcemia, viral arthritis, lupus, acute leukemia, or Whipple's. *Episodic recurrences:* Lyme, crystal-induced arthritis, inflammatory bowel disease, Still's, or lupus.

Morning stiffness: Rheumatoid arthritis, polymyalgia rheumatica, Still's, or viral arthritis. *Symmetric small-joint synovitis:* Rheumatoid arthritis, lupus, or viral arthritis.

CLINICAL FINDINGS

Osteoarthritis It appears as a bland (noninflammatory) symmetric polyarthritis, especially of high stress joints, such as the thumb metacarpophalangeal joint, knees, hips, and lumbar facet joints. Heberden's (distal interphalangeal joint) and Bouchard's (proximal interphalangeal joint) nodes are usually present. The stiffness increases after rest ("gelling"), with less than 15 minutes of morning stiffness, and it progressively worsens with use. There is restricted range of movement and crepitance of the joints but often relatively little pain. There are no systemic signs **(Plate 90).**

Rheumatoid arthritis It presents with a subacute symmetrical polyarthritis with synovial swelling of the proximal interphalangeal joints, metacarpophalangeal joints, and wrists; synovial bogginess; and rheumatoid nodules on extensor surfaces. Ulnar devia-

Polyarticular Arthritis

tion of the fingers, and swan neck and boutonniere's deformities are late findings **(Plates 88, 89).**

Lyme arthritis   It typically presents as a recurrent or migratory arthritis, the second phase of a syndrome that begins with a durable expanding annular rash with a clear center (erythema migrans) and a flu-like syndrome with arthralgias. The arthritis is episodic, affecting primarily large joints **(Plate 106).**

Systemic lupus erythematosus   There are symmetrical polyarthralgias or a nondeforming arthritis of the small joints, which may be migratory. Diagnostically, it is associated with a malar rash (50%) which spares the nasolabial fold, Raynaud's (30%), alopecia (40%), oral ulcers (40%), pleuritis with a rub (50%), pericarditis with a multicomponent rub (30%), and splenomegaly (15%). Evidence of vasculitis may be found with nailfold or volar pad infarcts, palpable purpura, livedo reticularis or cutaneous ulcers. In procainamide-induced lupus, polyarthritis and fever are the main manifestations **(Plates 36, 91, 92).**

Psoriatic arthritis   It is an asymmetric oligoarthritis of the distal interphalangeal joints. It may be quite erosive, with hands becoming foreshortened ("watchglass hands"). Psoriatic plaques may be hidden in the scalp, the intergluteal folds, umbilicus, or behind the ears. Nail pitting may be another clue **(Plates 103, 104, 105).**

Polyarticular gout   Flares occur rapidly, with joints becoming exquisitely painful after a few hours. There will often be a history of monoarticular arthritis (especially podagra of the great toe). The pattern will be asymmetric and oligoarticular. Tophi, which are found on the pinnae and extensor surfaces, aid in diagnosis **(Plates 100, 101, 102).**

Viral arthritis   During the preicteric phase of hepatitis B, a migratory polyarthritis, fever, and urticarial rash often occurs. Rubella and Parvovirus B19 can cause a similar clinical syndrome, with a rash and a symmetric polyarthritis of sudden onset, particularly in the hands. HIV is associated with brief episodes of severe arthralgia, acute episodic oligoarthritis, and persistent, symmetrical polyarthritis, but fever is usually not coincident **(Plates 137, 138).**

Scleroderma   Articular symptoms are mild, and sclerodactyly and generalized skin tightening is especially pronounced over the fingers, with leathery crepitance. Raynaud's phenomenon, impaired esophageal motility with dysphagia, and cuticular telangiectasias are helpful supportive evidence. Fingertip atrophy or ulcers suggest severe Raynaud's **(Plates 36, 97, 98, 113).**

Reiter's syndrome   Patients have asymmetric lower extremity arthritis, especially heel pain, plantar fasciitis, and unilateral sacroiliitis, occurring predominantly in young men. Distinctive associated findings include urethritis, iritis or conjunctivitis, oral ulcers, circinate balanitis, and keratoderma blennorrhagicum. It may arise reactively following enteric diarrhea, acute chlamydial urethritis, or HIV with M. avium-complex. Keratoderma begins as small vesicles on the soles, toes, and glans and then progresses to opaque papules, which then become hyperkeratotic coalescing plaques. Circinate balanitis begins as vesicles on the glans, which coalesce into superficial erosions **(Plate 86).**

Inflammatory bowel disease   Bowel disease is usually symptomatically active with fever, abdominal pain, diarrhea, and blood or mucous in the stools when the arthritis develops. The arthritis occurs in the knees, ankles and wrists along with fever, oral ulcers, erythema nodosum, or pyoderma gangrenosum **(Plates 58, 171).**

Gonococcal arthritis   Characteristically, there is a migratory polyarthritis and tenosynovitis, associated with pustular skin lesions on a red base, and urethritis or cervicitis. The patient will be systemically ill with fever and marked malaise **(Plate 75).**

Ankylosing spondylitis   Arthritis of the axial spine (sacroiliac and lumbar spine) begins insidiously with low back pain that worsens with bedrest and improves with exercise. Reduced flexion is readily demonstrated. Anterior uveitis may be recurrent. Aortic insufficiency is a late finding **(Plate 86).**

Systemic vasculitis   Fever and polyarthritis are common presenting manifestations of vasculitis and are accompanied by characteristic findings such as palpable purpura or hematuria. Giant cell arthritis presents with fever and polymyalgia, but joint pain is not present on careful examination **(Plate 110).**

Sarcoidosis   Prominent ankle involvement with erythema and periarticular swelling in a young woman help to distinguish sarcoidosis from gout. Erythema nodosum, waxy red-brown skin papules, and lymphadenopathy are also clues **(Plates 169, 171).**

Pseudogout (CPPD)   Suspect when osteoarthritis-like changes are present in unusual joints (wrists, shoulders, elbows, or ankles) although the knee is the most commonly involved joint.

Acute rheumatic fever   A sore throat is followed by polyarthritis with rapid worsening so that within 24 hours the joints will be markedly swollen, red, hot, and tender. After several days the original inflammation subsides but migrates to other joints. Polyarthritis and fever are more common in adults than cardiac manifestations. The fever usually lasts a week or more **(Plate 108).**

Still's disease   A high spiking fever is associated with chills and an evanescent pink rash that blanches. The arthritis is migratory at its onset **(Plate 107).**

Chapter 91

Raynaud's Phenomenon

▚ DIFFERENTIAL OVERVIEW

❑ Idiopathic
❑ Systemic lupus erythematosus
❑ Scleroderma
❑ Drugs
❑ Thoracic outlet syndrome
❑ Subclavian atherosclerosis
❑ Cryoglobulinemia
❑ Chronic vibration exposure

DIAGNOSTIC APPROACH

Cold is the usual precipitant. A classic triphasic response, occurring in 20%, begins with blanching of the extremities, often sharply demarcated, followed by cyanotic (slate-blue) discoloration with a dull aching caused by vascular stasis. With rewarming, the digits become livid purple, then deep red. The radial pulse remains normal throughout (**Plate 36**).

"White attacks" are consistent with true digital arterial closure whereas cyanosis or mottling may be caused by arteriovenous shunt closure or small arteriole vasospasm. Pain suggests severe tissue ischemia and an underlying disease.

Fever, arthralgias, or constitutional symptoms are subtle indicators of an emerging connective tissue disease. There may be a long interval between the initial appearance of Raynaud's and the diagnosis of a connective tissue disease.

Unilateral Raynaud's results from proximal vascular disease such as thoracic outlet syndrome or subclavian atherosclerosis. Unidigital Raynaud's is due to trauma or embolism to the palmar artery.

CLINICAL FINDINGS

Idiopathic   It occurs most often in young women as part of a generalized vascular hyperreactivity, associated with phenomena such as migraine.

Systemic lupus erythematosus   Of patients with this, 30–50% have Raynaud's. Malar rash, fever, serositis, and arthritis suggest the underlying diagnosis (**Plates 91, 92**).

Scleroderma   Of persons with scleroderma, 90% have Raynaud's, and it is the initial manifestation in 70%. It is part of the classic CREST syndrome of subcutaneous Calcifications, Raynaud's, Esophageal dysmotility, Sclerodactyly, and Telangiectasias. Using immersion oil and the ophthalmoscope set at 40 diopters, abnormal cuticular capillary loops consisting of enlargement, decreased numbers, and distortion of the normal delicate thin vessel structure can be seen in 80% of patients (**Plates 97, 98, 113**).

Drugs   Ergotamine, narcotics, amphetamines, beta-blockers, and vinyl chloride can all cause Raynaud's.

Thoracic outlet syndrome   Intermittent compression of the subclavian artery can produce a cold hand, but the pulse will be absent, the symptoms will not be associated with cold exposure, and the vasospasm is not as distal and well demarcated. Adson's maneuver will be positive (absent radial pulse with the head turned toward the affected side, and breath held in inspiration).

Subclavian atherosclerosis   A unilateral diminished pulse, blood pressure asymmetry, subclavian bruit, and arm claudication are the usual clinical findings.

Cryoglobulinemia   Raynaud's is associated with acrocyanosis of the tip of the nose and ears on cold exposure (**Plates 34, 35**).

Chronic vibration exposure   Raynaud's occurs as a consequence of occupations such as jackhammer operator and miner.

Shoulder Pain

Chapter 92

▧ DIFFERENTIAL OVERVIEW

- ❏ Rotator cuff tendinitis
- ❏ Bicipital tendinitis
- ❏ Acromioclavicular joint inflammation
- ❏ Acromioclavicular joint separation
- ❏ Cervical spondylosis
- ❏ Impingement syndrome
- ❏ Rotator cuff tear
- ❏ Adhesive capsulitis
- ❏ Glenohumeral joint instability
- ❏ Referred pain
- ❏ Shoulder dislocation
- ❏ Humeral neck fracture
- ❏ Glenohumeral joint arthritis
- ❏ Reflex sympathetic dystrophy
- ❏ Aseptic necrosis of the humeral head

DIAGNOSTIC APPROACH

Beware referred pain, with which life-threatening conditions can present innocuously. The patient will often try to link the pain to musculoskeletal causes, inadvertently providing false clues leading away from the correct diagnosis. Consider this if there is no pain with movement of the shoulder.

Pain with motion usually signifies periarticular pathology. Pain with resisted range of motion at midabduction ($>60°$) is found in supraspinatus tendinitis. Pain with resisted external rotation occurs with infraspinatus and teres minor inflammation, and pain with resisted internal rotation occurs with subscapularis inflammation.

CLINICAL FINDINGS

Rotator cuff tendinitis   Most often this results from supraspinatus tendinitis with pain in the location of the greater tuberosity, radiating in a C5 distribution. There is usually no major precipitating event other than repetitive motion (e.g., painting or doing carpentry work). Pain is increased with abduction and elevation of the shoulder, demonstrated by extension of both arms with the thumbs pointed downward, finding weakness on pressing down on the involved arm.

Bicipital tendinitis   Elbow flexion and forearm supination against resistance with the elbow held at the side will reproduce the pain. Tenderness is found over the long head of the biceps in the bicipital groove in the anterior aspect of the shoulder.

Acromioclavicular joint inflammation   This is found in patients who do heavy labor or play contact sports. Pain is reproduced by reaching above and in front of the body. Pain and tenderness localize over the acromioclavicular joint in the superior shoulder at the distal end of the clavicle.

Acromioclavicular joint separation   Acute shoulder injury produces an elevation and springboarding effect of the distal clavicle. The superior acromioclavicular joint will be very tender.

Cervical spondylosis   Pain is neuritic in character (numb, burning), unaffected by shoulder position, and elicited on neck motion to the side of the pain. Pain usually projects to the shoulder and lateral arm.

Impingement syndrome   A "catch" or increase in subacromial pain occurs when the arm is elevated forward while the shoulder girdle is depressed. There is a painful arc 60–120° as the thickened supraspinatus tendon is trapped between the acromion and greater tuberosity.

Rotator cuff tear   Tearing occurs with a "snap" with a fall onto an outstretched arm or direct blunt trauma. The "drop-arm" sign is positive: the arm drops to the side when re-

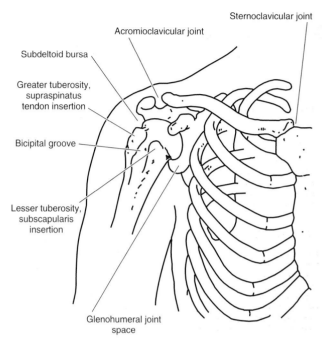

Figure 14. Surface anatomy in shoulder injury. (Adapted from: Cailliet R. Shoulder Pain. Philadelphia: FA Davis Co., 1966, p. 41.)

leased at 90° passive abduction. There will be full passive range of motion but little voluntary abduction, even after lidocaine anesthesia. On palpation, there is fine crepitance and a depression over the tendon.

Adhesive capsulitis   It occurs after a period of immobilization, causing generalized shoulder pain that is often worse at night. Active and passive range of motion is limited to a small pain-free arc. It may be associated with reflex sympathetic dystrophy.

Glenohumeral joint instability   Subsequent to a capsular tear, the shoulder "gives out" repeatedly. When the arm is gently abducted and externally rotated, a feeling of joint instability and insecurity will be elicited.

Referred pain   Myocardial ischemia radiates from the chest to the left shoulder. Aortic dissection of the ascending arch produces right neck and shoulder pain, and dissection of the transverse and descending arch produce left back and shoulder pain. Inflammation of the underside of the diaphragm produces pain in the posterosuperior shoulder, accentuated with deep breaths. A superior sulcus (Pancoast) lung cancer can produce shoulder pain in conjunction with brachial plexus findings.

Shoulder dislocation   Usually resulting from trauma while the shoulder is hyperextended, dislocation is most often anterior and characterized by loss of the shoulder's lateral rounded appearance and prominent swelling. The rounded end of the humerus can be palpated anteriorly. Assess for axillary nerve damage, radial pulse, supraspinatus tendon rupture, and humeral fracture.

Humeral neck fracture   There is a history of trauma (usually a fall onto the outstretched hand), with findings of severe pain and tenderness with ecchymosis over the proximal upper arm.

181

Glenohumeral joint arthritis   A low-grade ache increases with activity. Muscle atrophy, crepitation, and diminished motion are noted on examination.

Reflex sympathetic dystrophy   Classic findings include persistent burning pain, diffuse tenderness, immobilization of the shoulder, swelling of the arm, trophic changes (atrophy, hyperpigmentation, nail thickening, hyperhidrosis), and vasomotor instability in the hand.

Aseptic necrosis of the humeral head   The typical history is stiffness with intermittent pain of the shoulder, in the setting of predisposing medical conditions including steroids, sickle cell anemia, lupus, or dialysis.

Wrist/Hand Pain

◪ DIFFERENTIAL OVERVIEW

Phenomena
❑ Paronychia
❑ Ganglion cyst
❑ Carpal tunnel syndrome
❑ Ulnar neuropathy
❑ Trigger finger
❑ Mallet finger
❑ Digital ganglion
❑ Dupuytren's contracture
❑ De Quervain's tenosynovitis
❑ Colle's fracture
❑ Navicular fracture
❑ Metacarpal fracture
❑ Felon
❑ Bennet's fracture
❑ Smith fracture
❑ Flexor tendon rupture
❑ Reflex sympathetic dystrophy
❑ Lunate dislocation

Hands in Arthritis
❑ Osteoarthritis
❑ Rheumatoid arthritis
❑ Gout
❑ Systemic lupus erythematosus
❑ Psoriatic arthritis
❑ Scleroderma
❑ Gonococcal arthritis

DIAGNOSTIC APPROACH

With infection, swelling is most prominent in the dorsum of the hand regardless of the original location.

CLINICAL FINDINGS

Paronychia   Infection, marked by redness and swelling, is confined to the base and lateral border of the nail. When infection is chronic (e.g., resulting from Candida), the epionychium is pink and glazed, and the nail is ridged (**Plate 54**).

Ganglion cyst   It appears as a painless localized swelling over the volar or dorsal/radial aspect of the wrist. Arising from the synovial lining, it will feel compressible, and may fluctuate in size with use.

Carpal tunnel syndrome   Electrical pain and paresthesias in the thumb, index, middle, and radial aspect of the ring finger occur especially at night and may be relieved by shaking the wrist. Reproduction of the symptoms with Tinel's sign (tapping over the volar wrist) or Phalen's sign (wrist flexion for 30–60 seconds) is useful but does not rule out carpal tunnel syndrome when negative. Thenar atrophy may develop. Typical causes include keyboard use, pregnancy, and hypothyroidism (**Plate 18**).

Ulnar neuropathy   Neuropathy presents with numbness in the ulnar aspect of the hand and weakness of the intrinsics. Typically, settings include jackhammer operators and after wrist trauma.

Trigger finger   The history is one of painful snapping or locking of the finger in flexion and of a tendon sheath nodule over the palmar metacarpophalangeal joint on examination. Diabetes and rheumatoid arthritis are common precipitants (**Plates 88, 89**).

Mallet finger   Look for a flexed fingertip with inability to extend the distal interphalangeal joint, resulting from traumatic rupture of the distal extensor tendon.

183

Wrist/Hand Pain

Digital ganglion Appearing as a firm fixed nodule in a digital flexor crease, it is often confused with a sesamoid.

Dupuytren's contracture It produces painless nodular thickening of the palmar fascia with gradual development of a flexion contracture of the fingers. Diabetes and alcoholism are common triggers.

De Quervain's tenosynovitis Chronic repetitive movement of the wrist and thumb is the usual underlying cause. When the thumb is held in the palm and the wrist deviated toward the ulna (Finkelstein test), pain occurs over the anatomic snuff box. Crepitance may be felt over the radial styloid.

Colle's fracture It is produced by a fall onto an outstretched hand. Deformity is obvious, appearing as a fork profile when viewed laterally.

Navicular fracture It typically occurs after falling on an outstretched hand and should be suspected when there is tenderness over the anatomic snuff box.

Metacarpal fracture When making a fist, the knuckle prominence will be lost. There will be tenderness over the swollen area.

Felon Redness and swelling develop in the fingertip. When the pulp is indurated and has lost its resilience, pus is present.

Bennet's fracture An oblique fracture through the first metacarpal results from injury to the extended thumb, and the thumb cannot be opposed.

Smith fracture It is caused by a fall with hyperflexion of the hand. The distal fragment is displaced in a volar direction, giving a "reversed fork" appearance.

Flexor tendon rupture There is a history of sudden pain in the finger while grabbing at an object, with inability to flex in isolation. The flexor digitorum profundus may be evaluated by having the patient flex the distal interphalangeal joint while holding the proximal interphalangeal joint in extension. The sublimis function is tested by holding the other fingers in extension at the metacarpophalangeal joint and looking for flexion of the proximal interphalangeal joint.

Reflex sympathetic dystrophy Burning pain, swelling, and tenderness of the hand is associated with shoulder pain. The hand may be hot or cold and the skin moist.

Lunate dislocation The lunate occupies the hollow just distal to the radius in line with the middle finger. It becomes more hollow and tender with dislocation. Carpal tunnel symptoms may occur.

Osteoarthritis It presents with a symmetrical arthritis with bony hypertrophy of the proximal interphalangeal joint (Bouchard's) and distal interphalangeal joint (Heberden's) joints. There can be a surprising degree of deformity and crepitance without pain on motion (**Plate 90**).

Rheumatoid arthritis Characteristic findings include symmetric synovial bogginess of the metacarpophalangeal joints, intrinsic muscle wasting, ulnar deviation of the fingers, swan neck, and boutonniere's deformities of the fingers, extensor nodules, and median neuropathy (**Plates 88, 89**).

Gout It occurs less commonly in the hands than elsewhere, presenting as a single intensely inflamed joint, sometimes with a waxy yellow discoloration caused by underlying uric acid crystals (**Plates 100, 101**).

Systemic lupus erythematosus Symmetric fusiform swelling of the proximal interphalangeal and metacarpophalangeal joints, diffuse puffiness of the hands, and tenosynovitis are typical signs (**Plates 36, 91, 92**).

Psoriatic arthritis Foreshortened digits ("watchglass hand") and pitting of the nails are clues; however, the former is a late finding. Psoriatic plaques are usually present, but they may be hidden in the hair, behind the ear, or in the gluteal fold (**Plates 103, 104, 105**).

Scleroderma The earliest sign is usually Raynaud's phenomenon, followed by diffuse edema of the hands, then by bound-down skin. The digits attain a sausage configuration, and there is often atrophy of the tufts of the fingers. Cuticular telangiectasias can be observed using the ophthalmoscope (**Plates 36, 93, 97, 113**).

Gonococcal arthritis It presents acutely with asymmetric oligoarthritis, fever, and pustular/necrotic skin lesions over the hands and tenosynovitis (**Plate 75**).

Section VII
Neurologic/Psychiatric

Chapter 94

Amnesia

◤ DIFFERENTIAL OVERVIEW

- ❏ Concussion
- ❏ Alzheimer's disease
- ❏ Drugs
- ❏ Generalized seizure
- ❏ Migraine
- ❏ Korsakoff's syndrome
- ❏ Transient global amnesia
- ❏ Psychogenic
- ❏ Herpes simplex encephalitis
- ❏ Complex partial seizures

DIAGNOSTIC APPROACH

Amnesia is characterized by an inability to recall prior events and to learn new information, despite a normal level of consciousness. There must be injury to both temporal lobes in order for amnesia to occur.

CLINICAL FINDINGS

Concussion The injury will usually be recalled, witnessed or at least suspected from surface contusions. Disruption of short-term memory imprinting causes transient anterograde and retrograde amnesia, with a length proportionate to the degree of injury. Transient loss of consciousness is usual.

Alzheimer's disease Amnesia with poor short-term memory may occur before generalized dementia becomes evident.

Drugs Alcohol intoxication may cause spotty amnesia for events (alcoholic blackout). Benzodiazepines produce a similar phenomenon.

Generalized seizure The tonic-clonic motor activity is followed by a post-ictal phase of confusion and a period of time for which the patient will be amnesic.

Migraine A migraine is classically recognized by visual aura, unilateral headache, and nausea; amnesia is an infrequent but striking symptom.

Korsakoff's syndrome The patient is unable to recall new information despite a normal level of consciousness and intact immediate recall. He compensates with fantastic confabulations. Korsakoff's occurs in chronic alcoholics, especially following Wernicke's encephalopathy, marked by acute confusion, and in nonalcoholic patients with thiamine deficiency.

Transient global amnesia It appears as sudden confusion and amnesia in a previously well person. The patient appears bewildered and has intact immediate recall but is unable to imprint new information. The neurological examination is otherwise normal. Symptoms last 2–12 hours and are often followed by a headache or nausea. The attack often follows immersion in cold or hot water, emotional stimuli, physical exertion, sexual intercourse, or automobile travel.

Psychogenic Event-specific amnesia follows traumatic events such as witnessed homicide. An hysterical fugue is purposeful, arising from emotional conflict. The state may be prolonged, with the patient losing personal identity and past memories, yet new memories are readily imprinted.

Herpes simplex encephalitis Early in the course, there may be a Korsakoff-like state, due to bilateral temporal lobe infection. Fever will be present.

Complex partial seizures They may occur without any conscious awareness, with only a blank in the memory. Temporal lobe seizures are marked by auras and repetitive behaviors.

DIFFERENTIAL OVERVIEW

❑ Situational/characterologic
❑ Post-traumatic stress disorder
❑ Drugs/withdrawal
❑ Generalized anxiety disorder
❑ Phobia
❑ Agitated depression
❑ Panic disorder
❑ Hypoglycemia
❑ Hyperthyroidism

DIAGNOSTIC APPROACH

Anxiety ranges from a vague sense of uneasiness to one of imminent danger and dread. Thoughts race and concentration is difficult. There is a heightened self-awareness and startle response. Restlessness, bitten fingernails, tremor, tic, and excessive sweating are often noticeable. Sympathetic nervous system activation may cause palpitation, flushing, sweating, or diarrhea. Hyperventilation may occur, with lightheadedness and circumoral numbness.

Heightened perception and negative interpretation of normal bodily sensations is a common stimulus to visit the physician. Anxiety is commonly somatized to symptoms of chest pain, palpitations, or shortness of breath. Anxiety-related air swallowing (aerophagia) produces belching.

Repression is a defense mechanism, leading to dissociation from awareness and conversion to hysterical symptoms such as paralysis, anesthesia, aphonia, or amnesia. Blocking of one side of a conflict (a common defense mechanism) distorts the perception of reality, causing decision-making to become difficult.

CLINICAL FINDINGS

Situational/characterologic   The anxiety is usually mild, and it waxes and wanes with the precipitant stressor. This response is heightened in persons who have a character predisposed by culture or upbringing to anxious reactions to events.

Post-traumatic stress disorder   Survivors of unanticipated tragic events often experience recurrent flashbacks, nightmares, and restlessness. They become socially withdrawn and feel inadequate.

Drugs/withdrawal   Cocaine, amphetamines, hallucinogens, caffeine, ephedrine, beta-agonists, steroids, and exogenous thyroxine all cause anxiety. Withdrawal of alcohol, drugs of abuse, or nicotine can cause symptoms ranging from anxiety, irritability, and restlessness to paranoia and hallucinations.

Generalized anxiety disorder   Muscle tension, sympathetic hyperactivity, and apprehensive expectation lead to symptoms of chronic diffuse nervousness, insomnia, fatigue, irritability, and multiple somatic complaints.

Phobia   Irrational anxiety is attached to an object or situation, leading to avoidance. Common manifestations include fear of open or closed spaces, fear of heights, and fear of public speaking.

Agitated depression   It is characterized by marked restlessness and anxiety, constant worry, preoccupation with negative thoughts, and vegetative signs.

Panic disorder   Sudden, overwhelming anxiety and sense of impending doom, accompanied by dyspnea, palpitations or faintness, are classic symptoms. Episodes occur unexpectedly, resolve within 20–30 minutes, and are often recurrent.

Hypoglycemia   A diabetic develops episodic anxiety, diaphoresis, and confusion responding to glucose or food.

Hyperthyroidism   Signs might be subtle, such as fine tremor, tachycardia, lid lag, or slight thyroid enlargement **(Plates 19, 20).**

Chapter 96

Aphasia/Dysarthria

PLATES 119, 127, 128, 131, 185

◤ DIFFERENTIAL OVERVIEW

Aphasia (Central)
❏ Broca's
❏ Wernicke's
❏ Conduction
❏ Anomic
❏ Global
❏ Motor aphasia
❏ Pure word deafness
❏ Alexia without agraphia
❏ Alexia with agraphia

Dysarthria (Peripheral)
❏ Bulbar
❏ Parkinson's
❏ Multiple sclerosis
❏ Tongue infiltration

DIAGNOSTIC APPROACH

Type	Comprehension	Repetition	Naming	Fluency
Wernicke's	Impaired	Impaired	Impaired	Increased
Broca's	Grammar only impaired	Impaired	Impaired	Decreased
Global	Impaired	Impaired	Impaired	Decreased
Conduction	Normal	Impaired	Impaired	Normal
Nonfluent	Normal	Normal	Impaired	Impaired
Fluent	Impaired	Normal	Impaired	Normal
Isolation	Impaired	Echolalia	Impaired	None
Anomic	Normal	Normal	Impaired	Word-finding impaired
Word deafness	Speech only impaired	Impaired	Normal	Normal
Alexia	Reading only impaired	Normal	Normal	Normal

CLINICAL FINDINGS

Broca's   Occlusion of the superior middle cerebral artery affects the precentral gyrus, responsible for the motor part of language production. Speech is telegraphic, produced with great effort, with abnormal word order, abnormal tense use, and the omission of small words or endings, yet it is understandable. Comprehension of written or verbal speech is good. The patient is aware of the deficit and is frustrated. Hemiparesis is usually present because Broca's area is adjacent to the motor cortex.

Wernicke's   It involves the primary auditory cortex for understanding of auditory input and monitoring of speech output. Speech is fluent with normal rhythm but conveys information poorly because of circumlocutions and paraphrasic errors ("jargon aphasia"). Comprehension, repetition, and object naming are poor. The patient may be able to repeat long, complex sentences. Writing content is abnormal although penmanship may be good. Patients may not realize their deficit. There are usually no motor deficits, but a hemianopsia or quadrantanopsia may be present.

Conduction   Abnormalities result from an angular gyrus lesion, the center for integrating sensory and other associated information, often caused by "watershed" infarcts due to hypoperfusion. Speech is fluent but conveys information imperfectly, with frequent literal paraphrasic errors (fish for dish). The patient can comprehend spoken and written language but has difficulty reading aloud (although comprehension is good with silent reading). Repetition, object naming, and writing are poor. The patient may have dysgraphia (ranging from minor misspellings to agraphia), buccofacial apraxia, mild right hemiparesis, and hemisensory deficit.

Anomic   This type of aphasia arises from metabolic disorders or space-occupying lesions with pressure effects. Speech is fluent but conveys information poorly. The patient can understand both written and spoken speech and can repeat normally. There are no motor deficits.

Global   In a large middle cerebral artery infarct, hemiparesis occurs along with inability to comprehend or speak.

Motor aphasia   Frontal lobe speech is nonfluent with preserved comprehension like Broca's, but repetition of complex sentences is preserved. Upper extremity weakness (proximal greater than distal) is present.

Pure word deafness   This is caused by bilateral temporal lobe or a single, deep, left temporal lobe lesion. The patient is unable to understand spoken words, but hearing is intact, and the patient can read aloud.

Alexia without agraphia   The patient can comprehend spoken words and tracings on the palm but cannot read. He or she can write then cannot read it. The lesion is in the splenium of the corpus callosum plus the left visual cortex.

Alexia with agraphia   Lesions of the dominant angular gyrus produce Gerstmann's syndrome (finger agnosia, right-to-left disorientation, acalculia, agraphia) plus anomia and constructional apraxia.

Bulbar   Weakness of the lips, tongue, and larynx produce a decreased ability to pronounce consonants. Causes include Guillain-Barré syndrome, polio, posterior fossa meningitis (syphilis or carcinomatous), and posterior inferior cerebellar ischemia.

Parkinson's   Speech is thick and slow without normal modulations.

Multiple sclerosis   Speech is "scanning," pronouncing syllable by syllable (**Plates 119, 127, 128**).

Tongue infiltration   Thick speech may be caused by cancer of the tongue, angioedema, or amyloidosis (**Plates 131, 185**).

Chapter 97

Ataxia

◼ DIFFERENTIAL OVERVIEW

Chronic
- ❏ Vitamin B12 deficiency
- ❏ Parkinsonism
- ❏ Myopathy
- ❏ Cervical spondylosis
- ❏ Multiple sclerosis
- ❏ Multiple subcortical strokes
- ❏ Alcoholic cerebellar degeneration
- ❏ Hydrocephalus
- ❏ Frontal lobe tumor
- ❏ Cerebellar tumor
- ❏ Spinocerebellar degeneration
- ❏ Syringomyelia
- ❏ Tabes dorsalis
- ❏ Chorea

Acute
- ❏ Alcohol intoxication
- ❏ Labyrinthitis
- ❏ Cerebellar hemorrhage
- ❏ Cerebellar infarct
- ❏ Guillain-Barré syndrome
- ❏ Hysterical
- ❏ Parietal apraxia

DIAGNOSTIC APPROACH

Hemiparetic gait, a stroke residua, results from abduction/circumduction of the leg with a contralateral tilt of the body. *Paraparetic* gait, found with spinal cord disease or cerebral palsy, is marked by "scissoring," or crossing with each step. A *steppage* gait, seen with peroneal neuropathy, has a foot drop with a high step to avoid toe dragging, and the foot slaps down. In a *waddling* gait, with proximal leg weakness such as myopathy, the leg is lifted high, and the trunk leans opposite. A *Parkinsonian* gait has a forward stoop with flexion of the hips, knees, and elbows and short shuffling steps, which accelerate. An *apraxic* gait, with bilateral frontal lobe disease, is shuffling, but the gait is hesitant and not maintained. A *cerebellar/ataxic* gait is broad-based and irregular. A *sensory/ataxic* gait is broadly based with a positive Romberg. With a *vestibular* gait, the patient falls to one side whether walking or standing. With an *hysterical* gait, there is normal leg coordination while sitting but dramatic falls when standing.

A positive Romberg (unsteady with eyes closed, steady with eyes open) indicates posterior column disease. Gross lesions of the spinal cord rarely present with ataxia because of prominent weakness and spasticity. Cerebellar lesions produce dysmetria and decomposition of movement. Speech may be scanning, with each syllable pronounced separately.

With sensory ataxia, loss of touch causes little ataxia, and loss of proprioception causes severe ataxia, which increases with the eyes closed. The gait is wide-based with the feet landing with force. Both Romberg and pursuit (finger to nose or heel to shin) will be abnormal. It is caused by lesions of the peripheral nerves, posterior columns (vitamin B12 deficiency subacute combined degeneration), posterior roots (tabes), medial lemniscus, thalamus, or sensory cortex. Polyneuritis may be caused by diabetes, polyarteritis nodosa, alcohol, arsenic, Guillain-Barré, or porphyria.

Points of differentiation are as follows:

	LNM	CST	EXP	CRB
Atrophy	Yes	No	No	No
Weakness	Yes	Yes	No	No
Tone	Decr	Incr (Spast)	Incr (Rigid)	Decr
Fasciculations	Yes	No	No	No
Gait	Steppage/ waddling	Spastic/ scissoring	Shuffling/ festinating	Broad-based ataxia

NB: LMN, lower motor neuron; CST, corticospinal tract; EXP, extrapyramidal; CRB, cerebellar.

CLINICAL FINDINGS

Vitamin B12 deficiency Combined system disease with involvement of posterior and lateral columns begins with weakness and paresthesia, which is followed by leg stiffness and ataxia. Loss of vibration and position sense is associated with upgoing toes and hyporeflexia in the legs. Associated mental status changes may occur **(Plate 69).**

Parkinsonism Typical findings are a cyclic tremor, "cog-wheeling," and increased tone. The patient moves slowly with a stooped posture, shuffling gait, decreased limb movement, and slightly flexed hips and knees, turning en bloc. The pace gradually increases (festination).

Myopathy Proximal motor weakness is evident, with a waddling gait, in which the foot is lifted high and the trunk leans opposite with each step.

Cervical spondylosis It is marked by neck and arm pain with upgoing toes.

Multiple sclerosis It most commonly presents with optic neuritis or flaring and remitting patchy numbness separated in time and space. Eye findings include optic neuritis (acute with a hyperemic disc or old with a white atrophic disc), nystagmus, and internuclear ophthalmoplegia. Lhermitte's sign, an electric sensation with neck flexion, may be present. Autonomic findings of urgency, incontinence, or impotence and reflex findings of spasticity, weakness, or clonus may be found **(Plates 119, 127, 128).**

Multiple subcortical strokes They are recognized by a stepwise pattern and the associated emotional lability, brisk reflexes, increased jaw jerk, and dysarthria.

Alcoholic cerebellar degeneration It is characterized by ataxia of the legs with less prominent involvement of the arms, speech, or ocular motility. Polyneuropathy is usually present.

Hydrocephalus Ataxia is combined with memory loss and incontinence.

Frontal lobe tumor "Frontal ataxia" with a tendency to fall backward, signs of cerebellar disease, grasp and snout reflexes, incontinence, and slow mentation are features.

Cerebellar tumor Cerebellar disease produces ataxia and decomposition of movement. Involvement of the lateral lobe elicits limb ataxia (especially upper) and hypotonia. Involvement of the flocculonodular lobe causes truncal ataxia, drunken gait, and titubation of the head and trunk. If the anterior lobe is affected, there will be gait ataxia, with inability to tandem walk. Lesions of the midline cerebellum or vermis make the patient unable to stand or walk due to ataxia and dysequilibrium, but use of limbs is normal and without nystagmus when sitting or lying. Tumors are usually metastatic in adults.

Spinocerebellar degeneration A family history is prominent, and there are widespread deficits including hyporeflexia and upgoing toes. Pes cavus is often found.

Syringomyelia Prominent features include sensory disassociation with loss of pain and temperature sensation but preservation of touch and position, anterior horn cell involvement with muscle wasting, fasciculations, absent reflexes in the upper extremities, and corticospinal tract involvement with spasticity.

Tabes dorsalis The gait is a wide-based ataxia with foot slapping. Associated findings include loss of position, deep pain and temperature sensation, areflexia, and Argyll Robertson pupils, which accommodate but do not react to light **(Plate 118).**

Chorea There is decreased tone with marked hyperextensibility or joints. The gait is wide-based and lurching with excessive abnormal movements and posturing.

Alcohol intoxication There is a wide-based cerebellar gait in a patient who appears inebriated and has an alcohol odor to the breath.

Labyrinthitis   Vertigo is a prominent feature, which is exacerbated by head position. The patient will fall to one side.

Cerebellar hemorrhage   It presents with sudden onset of occipital headache, vertigo, and ocular gaze palsies, with preserved limb strength and sensation.

Cerebellar infarct   The presentation is similar to cerebellar hemorrhage, but with prominent limb, trunk, gait and speech ataxia, nystagmus, and hypotonia.

Guillain-Barré syndrome   Ataxia often develops in the early stages. Reflexes will be absent.

Hysterical   The ataxia is inconsistent, varying from moment to moment, requiring more coordination than usual.

Parietal apraxia   The patient "forgets" how to walk, but results of formal testing are normal.

Coma

DIFFERENTIAL OVERVIEW

- ❏ Alcohol intoxication
- ❏ Drug overdose
- ❏ Hypoglycemia
- ❏ Metabolic acidosis
- ❏ Subdural hematoma
- ❏ Hypothermia
- ❏ Heat stroke
- ❏ Meningitis
- ❏ Subarachnoid hemorrhage
- ❏ Head trauma
- ❏ Ischemic encephalopathy
- ❏ Epidural hematoma
- ❏ Pontine hemorrhage
- ❏ Cerebellar hemorrhage
- ❏ Psychogenic

DIAGNOSTIC APPROACH

Glasgow Coma Scale:

Eye Opening: Spontaneous (4), to voice (3), to pain (2), without (1).

Best Motor Response: Obeys commands (6), localizes pain (5), withdraws to pain (4), abnormal flexor response (decorticate) (3), abnormal extensor response (decerebrate) (2), no movement (1).

Best Verbal Response: Appropriate/oriented (5), confused (4), inappropriate words (3), incomprehensible sounds (2), no sounds (1).

Pupils: Pupillary responses are more sensitive than papilledema in detecting increased intracranial pressure. Normal pupils imply an intact midbrain and CNIII. Preserved pupillary light reflex with other signs of brainstem impairment suggests a toxic/metabolic cause. Asymmetric reactivity is consistent with an acute structural process. A unilaterally dilated pupil suggests ipsilateral uncal herniation. Hypothermia, barbiturates, and midbrain lesions produce midposition unreactive pupils. Pinpoint pupils occur with pontine lesions, opiates, and anticholinesterases. Bilateral dilated unresponsive pupils occur with anoxia, severe midbrain damage caused by transtentorial herniation, or anticholinergic drugs. Large pupils that dilate and contract automatically (hippus) but do not react to light suggest a tectal lesion.

Eye deviation: Cortical mass lesions produce ipsilateral conjugate deviation that can be overcome with calorics. Brainstem and pontine lesions produce contralateral deviation that cannot be overcome with calorics. In metabolic coma or drug overdose coma, eyes move loosely side-to-side opposite the turning of the head. A pontine or cerebellar lesion causes skew deviation (separation of horizontal axes). Ocular bobbing (briskly down, slowly up) is a result of bilateral pontine lesions. Ocular dipping (slow arrhythmic downstroke, followed by a faster upstroke) with normal calorics is consistent with anoxic encephalopathy.

Posturing: Decorticate posturing (arm flexion and leg extension) is found with hemispheric lesions or metabolic derangement. Decerebrate posturing (extension of the legs and arms) implies dysfunction of the midbrain or upper pons on a structural or metabolic basis. In response to noxious stimuli, flexion, extension, and adduction reflexes are found. Shoulder and hip abduction involve cortical activity whereas withdrawal implies voluntary behavior.

Respiratory pattern: If the patient is yawning or swallowing, coma is not very deep and brainstem function is intact. Cheyne-Stokes respiration (crescendo-decrescendo pattern with apneic pauses) is seen with herniation, metabolic encephalopathy, and congestive heart failure. Central neurogenic hyperventilation (rapid deep breathing) indicates damage to the brainstem between the midbrain and pons. Ataxic respiration occurs with midbrain lesions. Apneustic respiration with inspiratory pauses occurs with pontine lesions and precedes respiratory arrest.

Coma

Asymmetric resting muscle tone, deep tendon reflexes, or Babinski response suggests a structural lesion. A toxic/metabolic cause is suggested by preceding confusion, disorientation, and somnolence. Myoclonic jerks or clonus provide further support.

CLINICAL FINDINGS

Alcohol intoxication   The odor of alcohol will be apparent on the breath. Be wary when diagnosing the intoxicated patient. Could there be another (obscured) cause of coma such as head trauma?

Drug overdose   Narcotic overdose produces pinpoint pupils and hypoventilation. Response to naloxone is rapid and diagnostic. Barbiturate overdose will produce absent doll's eyes and corneal reflexes, but the pupillary light response will be preserved.

Hypoglycemia   The patient is taking insulin or oral hypoglycemics and responds readily to an injection of 50% dextrose.

Metabolic acidosis   The underlying disease process is usually evident (sepsis, uremia, diabetic ketoacidosis, shock). A clue is hyperventilation with Kussmaul breathing. With diabetic ketoacidosis, there will be a fruity, sweet, acetone odor to the breath.

Subdural hematoma   There will usually be a history of head trauma, headache, and fluctuating level of consciousness.

Hypothermia   Suspect with environmental exposure and a patient who is cold to the touch. Determination of the core temperature with a special thermometer is essential.

Heat stroke   Consider this in the presence of fever without perspiration.

Meningitis   Subacute onset of prominent headache, fever, and nuchal rigidity with Kernig's and Brudzinski's signs present.

Subarachnoid hemorrhage   A severe headache of instantaneous onset followed by meningeal signs, pupillary asymmetry, strabismus (third or sixth nerve palsy), and extensor posturing is the typical evolution.

Head trauma   Suspect with mastoid ecchymoses, subconjunctival hemorrhage, raccoon eyes, or hemotympanum. Clear rhinorrhea suggests basilar skull fracture. The most common cause of coma in the setting of head trauma is subdural hematoma, with gradually evolving cortical signs. Preceding headache in the setting of a head injury (however minor), especially with asymmetric motor or sensory findings suggests supratentorial bleeding. Occipital headache—especially with vertigo, ataxia, diplopia, and vomiting—suggests subtentorial bleeding **(Plate 220).**

Ischemic encephalopathy   This usually occurs after an episode of profound hypotension (cardiopulmonary arrest) or anoxia (near drowning) and is characterized by repetitive multifocal myoclonic jerks. Hypoxia, as in COPD, is accompanied by central cyanosis. Carbon monoxide poisoning produces a flushed ("cherry red") face.

Epidural hematoma   Suspect this when there is a history of head trauma, especially a temporal blow/fracture. A gradual middle meningeal bleed produces the classic signs of initial concussion with confusion, followed by a lucid interval, then deepening coma. A unilateral "blown" (fixed and dilated) pupil is an early sign of uncal herniation. Cheyne-Stokes (crescendo-decrescendo pattern with apneic pauses) implies bilateral hemisphere dysfunction with an intact brainstem and may be the first sign of transtentorial herniation.

Pontine hemorrhage   Absent corneal reflexes and doll's eyes are present, with pinpoint pupils that react to strong light on observation with a magnifying glass. The breathing pattern is apneustic (prolonged inspiratory cramp followed by an expiratory pause).

Cerebellar hemorrhage   Occipital headache, vomiting, gaze paresis, and inability to stand is followed by coma.

Psychogenic   There is usually a prior psychiatric history. Pupils are responsive and calorics produce nystagmus. The patient is flaccid or has an avoidance response.

Deep Tendon Reflex Abnormalities

PLATES 16, 17, 18, 69, 90, 119, 127, 128, 131, 132, 133, 134, 157, 166, 198

◼ DIFFERENTIAL OVERVIEW

Hyporeflexia
- ❏ Nerve root compression
- ❏ Hypothyroidism
- ❏ Acute stroke
- ❏ Diabetes
- ❏ Alcoholism
- ❏ Vitamin B12 deficiency
- ❏ Uremia
- ❏ Myopathy
- ❏ Occult cancer
- ❏ Toxins
- ❏ Guillain-Barré syndrome
- ❏ Amyloidosis
- ❏ Spinal shock
- ❏ Adie's syndrome
- ❏ Botulism
- ❏ Charcot-Marie-Tooth

Hyperreflexia
- ❏ Cervical spondylosis
- ❏ Spinal cord compression
- ❏ Multiple small strokes
- ❏ Multiple sclerosis
- ❏ Metabolic encephalopathy
- ❏ Amyotrophic lateral sclerosis

DIAGNOSTIC APPROACH

Symmetrically hyperactive or hypoactive reflexes in the presence of downgoing toes are usually normal. A positive Babinski sign (upgoing toe) is always abnormal, signifying an upper motor neuron lesion, and is usually associated with spastic weakness and hyperreflexia. Lower motor neuron lesions are marked by hyporeflexia, flaccid weakness, atrophy, and twitching.

Reflex	Level
Jaw jerk	Trigeminal
Biceps	C5-6
Brachioradialis	C5-6
Triceps	C6-7
Finger Jerk	C8-T1
Knee Jerk	L3-4
Ankle Jerk	S1

CLINICAL FINDINGS

Nerve root compression   Common presentations include asymmetric hyporeflexia affecting the ankle jerk with S1 compression, knee jerk with L3 or 4 compression, biceps and brachioradialis with C5 or 6 compression, and triceps with C7 or 8 compression.

Hypothyroidism   Generalized hyporeflexia with a delayed relaxation phase is found; it is best seen at the ankle jerk **(Plates 16, 17, 18)**.

Acute stroke   Hyporeflexia is present on the side of the hemiparesis.

Diabetes   Ankle jerks are bilaterally absent, and there is decreased vibratory sense but little motor weakness **(Plate 166)**.

Deep Tendon Reflex Abnormalities

Alcoholism   Sensory neuropathy, including decreased vibratory sense and tender feet, is typical.

Vitamin B12 deficiency   Findings include early stocking/glove neuropathy, hypoactive or hyperactive reflexes, ataxia, and mental status abnormalities ranging from irritability to frank dementia **(Plate 69).**

Uremia   Restless legs, profound distal sensory loss, muscle atrophy with areflexia, and burning sensations occur **(Plate 198).**

Myopathy   Findings include hyporeflexia (not areflexia) and weakness that is more prominent proximally than distally.

Occult cancer   Lung cancer especially may present with a neuropathy.

Toxins   Lead, arsenic, isoniazid, vincristine, and phenytoin produce hyporeflexia in the setting of a peripheral neuropathy **(Plates 133, 134).**

Guillain-Barré syndrome   Areflexia is prominent, with acute or subacute weakness and little sensory loss. Tingling occurs in the feet and hands, and the patient has difficulty with gait and use of the hands. The occurrence of bilateral facial weakness is an important clue. Autonomic dysfunction may also be present.

Amyloidosis   Presenting with a sensory neuropathy with autonomic features, it occurs in the setting of chronic inflammatory disease, such as cancer or deep tissue infection **(Plates 131, 157).**

Spinal shock   Hyporeflexia occurs in the acute stages and is associated with a sensory level and motor weakness. It can be caused by traumatic, vascular, or neoplastic processes.

Adie's syndrome   There is generalized areflexia with a large pupil that dilates slowly with near-to-far fixation to accomodation but does not respond to direct light.

Botulism   Reflexes may be decreased or normal. Key findings are a symmetric descending paralysis, early marked cranial nerve abnormalities with diplopia, dysarthria, dysphagia, and abnormal pupillary reflexes.

Charcot-Marie-Tooth   This is a familial neuropathy characterized by sensory loss, "champagne-bottle" legs, wide-spread areflexia, and pes cavus.

Cervical spondylosis   Neck pain and decreased range of motion is accompanied by muscle wasting in the hands or arms. It occurs in older patients, mostly resulting from osteoarthritis. There are often peripheral signs of osteoarthritis, such as Heberden's or Bouchard's nodes **(Plate 90).**

Spinal cord compression   There should be a high index of suspicion in the setting of known cancer. Early symptoms include back pain, paresthesias in the legs, weakness climbing stairs, constipation, or change in urinary function. Early findings include decreased pinprick, vibration or temperature sensation in the legs, slight hyperreflexia in the legs compared with the arms, and concussion tenderness over the spine. Later findings include upgoing toes, decreased sphincter tone, and a decreased sensation at a specific spinal cord level.

Multiple small strokes   These occur in hypertensive or diabetic patients. Associated signs include emotional lability, increased jaw jerk, dementia, and ataxia.

Multiple sclerosis   Suggestive symptoms include heaviness or numbness in a limb, unilateral transient visual loss, urinary incontinence, diplopia, and gait disorder. Findings include asymmetric hyperreflexia, pallor of the optic disc, internuclear ophthalmoplegia, cerebellar ataxia, dysarthria, and spasticity and weakness of the legs **(Plates 119, 127, 128).**

Metabolic encephalopathy   This is seen in uremic and hepatic encephalopathy, and myoclonic jerks are common.

Amyotrophic lateral sclerosis   A combination of upper and lower motor neuron signs in the brainstem and spinal cord without sensory loss is diagnostic. Look for increased jaw jerk, upgoing toes, and fasciculations with muscle wasting of small muscles (e.g., of the tongue) **(Plate 132).**

◼ DIFFERENTIAL OVERVIEW

Systemic
- ❑ Drugs/toxins
- ❑ Sepsis
- ❑ Hypoglycemia
- ❑ Hypercalcemia
- ❑ Hyponatremia
- ❑ Shock
- ❑ Delirium tremens
- ❑ Vitamin B12 deficiency
- ❑ Hypoxia
- ❑ Hypercapnia
- ❑ Thyrotoxicosis
- ❑ Uremia
- ❑ Hepatic encephalopathy
- ❑ Thiamine deficiency
- ❑ Heat stroke
- ❑ Hypothermia
- ❑ Lead intoxication
- ❑ Carbon monoxide poisoning

Neurologic
- ❑ Concussion
- ❑ Hypertensive encephalopathy
- ❑ Subdural hematoma
- ❑ Postictal
- ❑ Transient global amnesia
- ❑ Meningitis
- ❑ Right parietal stroke
- ❑ Encephalitis
- ❑ Vasculitis
- ❑ Carcinomatous meningitis

Hallucinations
- ❑ Drugs
- ❑ Schizophrenia
- ❑ Temporal lobe epilepsy

DIAGNOSTIC APPROACH

Delirium is characterized by gross disorientation in the presence of alertness and vigilance, disorders of perception with vivid illusions, and psychomotor and autonomic hyperactivity. It usually develops over a short time and is associated with fluctuating mental status, decreased attention, disorganized thinking as indicated by rambling irrelevant or incoherent speech, and a decreased level of consciousness. The most sensitive findings are variability in level of arousal, impaired short-term memory (e.g., digit span), and disorientation to time. Relatives or friends are helpful sources of information about the tempo and degree of impairment.

Fever, tachycardia, or hypertension should prompt a careful evaluation for a medical cause. Infection is a common cause in the elderly, especially pneumonia or urinary tract infection. Visual hallucinations have an organic cause, such as drugs, rather than schizophrenia.

Predictors of a positive CT scan in acute head injury include coma (Se 0.50), focal neurological signs (Se 0.33), skull fracture, seizure following a minor injury, and confusion.

Delirium/Hallucinations

CLINICAL FINDINGS

Drugs/toxins Delirium may be caused by drugs such as alcohol, opiates, barbiturates, salicylates, ergot, amphetamines, cocaine, or scopolamine. Toxins such as gasoline, glue, ether, liquid paper, or heavy metals can also cause delirium. Hallucinations may be precipitated by alcohol (especially during withdrawal), propranolol, bromocriptine, or cimetidine (in the elderly).

Sepsis Rigors, hypotension, and spiking fever are the major clues in a delirious patient.

Hypoglycemia Suspect this in a known diabetic patient who takes insulin or oral hypoglycemics, or in an alcoholic patient who has marginal glycogen stores. The patient will present with confusion, diaphoresis, tremor, giddiness, and tachycardia. Rapid response to oral or intravenous glucose is diagnostic.

Hypercalcemia Suspect calcium excess in those patients who have a known cancer. Causes are legion, however, and serum calcium measurement should be considered part of a "metabolic workup."

Hyponatremia Precipitating factors include polydipsia; use of lithium, diuretics or antipsychotics; or thoracic zoster.

Shock Confusion and restlessness are early and sensitive indicators. Also present are hypotension, tachycardia, and cutaneous vasoconstriction with mottling/livedo **(Plate 31).**

Delirium tremens During alcohol withdrawal, confusion is followed by autonomic arousal with tachycardia, diaphoresis, and anxiety. This may occur several days into hospitalization, and the altered mental status may make it difficult to then obtain an alcohol history.

Vitamin B12 deficiency Peripheral neuropathy and family history of pernicious anemia are helpful clues **(Plate 69).**

Hypoxia Delirium occurs with an increased A-a gradient in acute pulmonary embolism or in pulmonary edema. Cyanosis is a helpful clue.

Hypercapnia Carbon dioxide retention from alveolar hypoventilation occurs subacutely in a patient who has chronic obstructive pulmonary disease, especially during an episode of acute bronchoconstriction.

Thyrotoxicosis Fine tremor, silky skin, tachycardia, heat intolerance, lid lag, and exophthalmos are all clues, variably present **(Plate 19).**

Uremia Delirium may rarely be a presenting sign of uremia, and it is accompanied by peripheral and periorbital edema **(Plates 41, 198).**

Hepatic encephalopathy There is usually a prominent history of alcoholism. Concurrent findings of metabolic encephalopathy, such as asterixis or myoclonus, are present. Findings of chronic liver disease include spider angiomata, ascites, hemorrhoids, and distended superficial abdominal veins **(Plates 61, 62).**

Thiamine deficiency Wernicke's encephalopathy should be suspected in a delirious patient with alcoholism or malnutrition. Concurrent findings include horizontal nystagmus, ophthalmoplegia, and ataxia.

Heat stroke Outdoor exposure, especially with exercise, and a high core temperature with a paucity of sweating are found.

Hypothermia Environmental cold exposure, low core temperature, and intense vasoconstriction are found.

Lead intoxication Symptoms include fatigue, depression, confusion, episodic vague abdominal pain, and peripheral neuropathy. A gray lead line may appear on the gums **(Plate 134).**

Carbon monoxide poisoning Suspect this with exposure to engine exhaust or a kerosene space heater in a patient with a severe headache and flushed face.

Concussion Confusion immediately follows head trauma (or appears in a situation suggestive of head trauma) **(Plate 220).**

Hypertensive encephalopathy The blood pressure will be markedly elevated. There will usually be retinal hemorrhages and exudates reflective of intracranial vasculopathy as well as papilledema **(Plate 38).**

Subdural hematoma A history of head trauma or a recent fall in an elderly patient is the common scenario. A lucid interval is a classic sign of extradural middle meningeal hematoma. These patients are often intoxicated, which makes diagnosis more difficult. Suspect this when there is temporal trauma, gradual onset of contralateral hemiparesis, and a dilated reactive pupil. A plantar extensor (Babinski) reflex is consistent with a contralateral hematoma.

Postictal   If the seizure was not witnessed, clues such as tongue biting or incontinence are often present.

Transient global amnesia   Sudden, complete, anterograde loss of memory and learning develops in the presence of strong emotion or physical exertion.

Meningitis   Fever, prominent headache, photophobia, and neck stiffness/rigidity make a lumbar puncture mandatory.

Right parietal stroke   Symptoms result from impaired attention found in a nondominant hemispheric stroke. It should be suspected when atrial fibrillation is present.

Encephalitis   Fever and confusion are prominent. Temporal lobe symptoms such as hallucinations are often manifest, especially with herpes simplex encephalitis.

Vasculitis   It usually occurs in the context of active systemic connective tissue disease (fever, arthralgias, serositis) **(Plate 110).**

Carcinomatous meningitis   It is recognized by multiple cranial nerve palsies in a patient with a known primary cancer.

Schizophrenia   Auditory hallucinations, especially with a paranoid quality, are a common manifestation.

Temporal lobe epilepsy   Complex illusions with altered consciousness, automatisms, and deja vu or jamais vu phenomena occur.

Dementia

PLATES 2, 6, 69, 118, 201, 204, 220, 238

◤ DIFFERENTIAL OVERVIEW

- ❏ Alzheimer's disease
- ❏ Multi-infarct dementia
- ❏ Depression
- ❏ Drugs
- ❏ Vitamin B12 deficiency
- ❏ HIV encephalopathy
- ❏ Korsakoff's syndrome
- ❏ Brain tumor
- ❏ Normal pressure hydrocephalus
- ❏ Chronic subdural hematoma
- ❏ Neurosyphilis
- ❏ Creutzfeldt-Jakob
- ❏ Wilson's disease

DIAGNOSTIC APPROACH

Many patients are concerned about "normal forgetting" of details. This usually results from decreased attention. The fact that they recognize and worry about this distinguishes them from patients with early dementia. Normal forgetting preserves vocabulary and spelling and improves with cues. For example, patients with Alzheimer's disease cannot recall a list of related words any better than random words.

Subtle impairments in memory, attention, and concentration are often easily compensated for and therefore hard to pinpoint. Impaired judgment and abstraction on increasingly simple matters and personality changes (notably irritability) are usually noted first. The time course of onset is helpful in distinguishing dementia from delirium, but acute exacerbations of an underlying dementia that mimic delirium are common with drugs and acute physical illness

The Folstein Mini-Mental State Exam is widely used in screening for depression and following the pace of cognitive dysfunction. Orientation scores 10 points (time 5 points, place 5 points). Registration scores 3 points (immediate recall of 3 objects). Attention 3 points (spell *world* backward). Recall 3 points (repeat earlier 3 objects). Language and praxis score 9 points (name a pencil and a watch—2, "No ifs ands or buts"—1, 3-stage verbal command—3, "Close your eyes" written command—1, write a sentence—1, copy intersecting pentagrams—1). A total score of less than 24/30 suggests dementia or delirium (sensitivity 0.50–0.80, specificity 0.80–0.95). Scores of 20–24 suggest mild impairment; 16–19, moderate; and less than or equal to 15, severe.

CLINICAL FINDINGS

Alzheimer's disease   There is a progressive, smooth decline, with aphasia, apraxia, and agnosia. "Frontal release signs" including palmomental reflex and snout are usually found. Early dysphasia predicts a rapid cognitive decline. Patients with advanced disease will exhibit increased muscle tone and clonus.

Multi-infarct dementia   Cognitive impairment will occur in a stepwise fashion, usually associated with focal neurological deficits. An underlying cause such as atrial fibrillation, poorly controlled hypertension, diabetes, or carotid vascular disease with bruit will usually be evident. The Hachinski Ischemia Score helps differentiate: abrupt onset—2, stepwise deterioration—1, fluctuating mental status—2, nocturnal confusion—1, personality preserved—1, depression—1, somatic complaints—1, emotional lability—1, hypertension—1, history of stroke—2 focal signs—2, angina—1. A score of 7 or more suggests a high probability of multi-infarct dementia **(Plate 238).**

Depression   Altered mood, self-blaming, anhedonia, disordered sleep, and initiation fatigue are clues. Usually, the patient will recognize the depression.

Drugs   Dementia may be caused or worsened by anticholinergics, antiparkinson agents, antidepressants, nonsteroidal antiinflammatory drugs, antihistamines, narcotics, steroids, H2 blockers, and substances of abuse.

Dementia

Vitamin B12 deficiency Dementia is associated with peripheral neuropathy (distal "pins and needles") and pallor (macrocytic anemia). There will often be a family history of pernicious anemia or other autoimmune disease. Affected posterior columns will produce a decrease in position and vibration sense, and affected lateral columns increase deep tendon reflexes with upgoing toes. Motor weakness and spasticity may develop, with a stiff to ataxic gait **(Plate 69).**

HIV encephalopathy The patient is usually known to be HIV-infected or has risk factors. Impaired memory, poor concentration, decreased reaction time, lack of spontaneity, weakness, and ataxia are often present. Cryptococcal or toxoplasmal meningitis and CNS lymphoma can produce cognitive dysfunction in AIDS and thus confuse the differential **(Plates 201, 204).**

Korsakoff's syndrome There will be a history of advanced alcohol abuse. The patient is suggestible, confabulates, and has an inability to remember new information despite normal recall, attention span, and level of consciousness.

Brain tumor Papilledema and focal neurological signs are usually present. Frontal tumors can be relatively silent but are recognized by abulia, bradykinesia, shuffling gait, anosmia, and frontal release signs. Rapid progression of cognitive dysfunction can be found with cerebral edema.

Normal pressure hydrocephalus The classic triad includes dementia, gait disorder (slow, shuffling, wide-based, ataxic), and incontinence, in the absence of a history of subarachnoid hemorrhage, meningitis, or head injury.

Chronic subdural hematoma Early features are headache, drowsiness, and strange behavior in an elderly patient. Focal signs come later. A history of head trauma may not be obtained; thus, a high index of suspicion is needed **(Plate 220).**

Neurosyphilis An Argyll Robertson pupil (accommodates but does not react), optic atrophy, tabes dorsalis, and a remote history of a chancre are clues. General paresis produces a spastic quadriparesis **(Plate 118).**

Creutzfeldt-Jakob Myoclonus is always present, and cerebellar signs are often found.

Wilson's disease Extrapyramidal signs, a golden (Kayser-Fleischer) ring in the iris, and hepatic dysfunction are important clues **(Plates 2, 6).**

Chapter 102

Depression

◼ DIFFERENTIAL OVERVIEW

- ❑ Dysthymia
- ❑ Major depression
- ❑ Adjustment disorder with depressed mood
- ❑ Seasonal affective disorder
- ❑ Bipolar disorder
- ❑ Drug-induced
- ❑ Thyroid disease
- ❑ Dementia
- ❑ Stroke
- ❑ Paraneoplastic

DIAGNOSTIC APPROACH

Depression often presents in primary care settings masked in the form of somatic symptoms, such as anorexia, weight loss, fatigue, insomnia (especially early morning awakening), or difficulty concentrating. It is also common for the perception of symptoms produced by another organic cause to be heightened.

Anhedonia (loss of interest in favorite activities) is a key symptom to differentiate primary from secondary depression.

Once depression is identified, it is critical to assess suicide risk. The best way to do this is to straightforwardly ask such patients if they have thought of harming themselves, and if so, do they have plans. Risk factors for suicide include living alone, prior suicide attempt, family history of suicide attempt or substance abuse, general medical illness, extreme hopelessness, psychosis, and substance abuse.

CLINICAL FINDINGS

Dysthymia   Characterized by lifelong low-grade feelings of depression, negative thinking, and anhedonia with minor or no neurovegetative symptoms.

Major depression   Episodic depression/dysphoria of mood is accompanied by neurovegetative signs of appetite or sleep disturbance, psychomotor retardation or agitation, anhedonia, decreased energy, feelings of worthlessness or guilt, decreased cognition, or suicidal ideation. There may be disordered thought processes, such as paranoid ideation. There is often a family history of depression or alcoholism.

Adjustment disorder with depressed mood   This depression is triggered by a significant life stress. Thoughts are preoccupied with the precipitating event. Depressed mood is associated with anxiety, hopelessness, helplessness, and worthlessness.

Seasonal affective disorder   Recurrent winter depression appears with atypical neurovegetative signs such as hypersomnia, overeating, and carbohydrate craving.

Bipolar disorder   It usually presents as a major depression but with a history of transitory manic symptoms such as elation or expansive mood, increased energy, decreased need for sleep, inflated self-esteem, and inappropriately low concern for the consequences of actions.

Drug-induced   Alcohol, sedative, or cocaine abuse and withdrawal are commonly associated with depression. Reserpine, beta-blockers, methyldopa, estrogens, levodopa, and corticosteroids can also produce depression.

Thyroid disease   Apathetic hyperthyroidism in the elderly or hypothyroidism at any age can produce depression. Other findings such as lethargy, cold intolerance, edema, and delayed reflex relaxation phase must be sought **(Plates 16, 17, 18).**

Dementia   Subcortical dementias are often heralded by depression.

Stroke   Depression commonly accompanies limbic or frontal strokes, usually manifest as inappropriate crying **(Plate 238).**

Paraneoplastic   Depression is especially prominent in the presentation of pancreatic cancer, accompanied by unexplained weight loss and chronic vague abdominal/back pain.

Dizziness

Chapter 103

PLATES 119, 127, 128, 235

◼ DIFFERENTIAL OVERVIEW

Vertigo
❏ Benign paroxysmal positional vertigo
❏ Toxic labyrinthitis
❏ Vertebrobasilar insufficiency
❏ Ménière's disease
❏ Multiple sclerosis
❏ Acoustic neuroma
❏ Herpes zoster oticus (Ramsey-Hunt)

Disequilibrium
❏ Multifactorial disequilibrium
❏ Stroke
❏ Cerebellar disease
❏ Frontal lobe apraxia

Lightheadedness
❏ Orthostatic hypotension
❏ Common fainting (presyncope)
❏ Hyperventilation
❏ Panic attack

DIAGNOSTIC APPROACH

Differentiate between vertigo, disequilibrium, and lightheadedness. Each has its own non-overlapping differential:

• *Vertigo* is the illusory sensation of rotatory motion, either of the patient or the environment.
• *Disequilibrium* is a sensation of imbalance when standing and walking.
• *Lightheadedness* is a sensation of impending loss of consciousness.

Provide the patient with experiential examples to refine the history (e.g., vertigo after spinning around as a child).

Attempt to provoke dizziness with maneuvers to confirm a provisional diagnosis, such as observation of gait, ambulation, and turning; orthostatic vital signs; Hallpike maneuver; Romberg; and/or 3-minute hyperventilation. The *Hallpike maneuver* provokes vertigo and nystagmus by stimulation of the posterior semicircular canal with the head tilted toward the affected side at 30° below the horizontal. Have the patient look straight ahead to observe nystagmus. The *Romberg maneuver* is performed by observing the patient standing. Swaying with eyes closed suggests disordered proprioception and/or vestibular function. Swaying with eyes open or closed is cerebellar in origin.

Vertigo usually implies a vestibular lesion (rarely brainstem). Suspect a central lesion if symptoms are preceded by a headache and vomiting without tinnitus. Central dizziness is very sensitive to movement of the head and is usually constant. Other cranial nerve findings or long track signs are usually present. *Tinnitus*, pressure, or decreased hearing localizes the problem to the inner ear and indicates the involved side. *Nystagmus* may persist after vertigo clears. Spontaneous vertical nystagmus suggests a lesion at the vestibular nucleus or cerebellum. Exertional lightheadedness occurs in severe anemia, aortic stenosis, pulmonary hypertension, pericardial disease, and hypertrophic cardiomyopathy.

Feature	Peripheral (Labyrinth)	Central (Brainstem/Cerebellum)
Severity	Marked	Mild
Nystagmus	One direction only, rotatory, horizontal	Bidirectional, vertical
Tinnitus	Often present	Absent
Hallpike	Severe, 2-10-second latency, fatigues quickly	Mild, no latency or fatigue
CNS signs	None	Often present

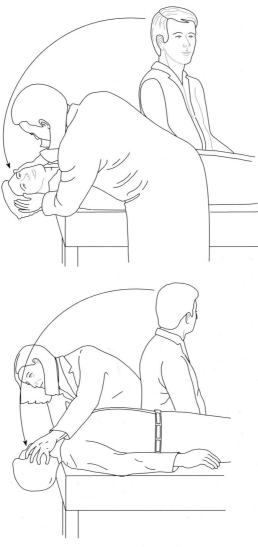

Figure 15. Eliciting positional nystagmus by Hallpike maneuver. (Adapted from: Reilly BR. Practical Strategies in Outpatient Medicine. 2nd ed. Philadelphia: W.B. Saunders, 1991, p. 204.).

CLINICAL FINDINGS

Benign paroxysmal positional vertigo   It presents as episodic vertigo of short duration, precipitated by position of the head, especially when recumbent turned toward the affected side. The Hallpike maneuver will be positive. There is no hearing deficit. A prior (remote) history of head trauma is common.

Toxic labyrinthitis   Prototypical causes include alcohol and aminoglycosides, with the latter associated with hearing loss. Salicylate intoxication produces vertigo, hyperventilation, and deafness. The history of salicylate use may be obscured by mental confusion.

Vertebrobasilar insufficiency   Occurs with the full spectrum of episodic vertigo, blurred or double vision, tingling in the face, weak legs, or dysarthria in an elderly patient. When these symptoms occur with arm usage and a subclavian bruit and asymmetric blood pressures are present, subclavian steal should be suspected.

Ménière's disease   Appears as episodic (1–3 hours), recurrent vertigo with tinnitus, unilateral decrement in hearing, distortion of sounds (diplacusis), or hypersensitivity to loud sounds. The patient is prostrated, with pallor, sweating, and spontaneous nystagmus. Fluctuation and recruitment favor Ménière's over acoustic neuroma.

Multiple sclerosis   Optic neuritis (new or old) and an afferent pupillary defect may be present. Internuclear ophthalmoplegia (when conjugate gaze is attempted, one eye will not adduct medially, and the abducting eye on lateral gaze will have nystagmus) indicates involvement of the medial longitudinal fasciculus. Transient facial numbness or diplopia is also common **(Plates 119, 127, 128).**

Acoustic neuroma   Usually presenting with slowly progressive tinnitus and hearing loss, it may also present with vertigo. Central nystagmus, diminished corneal reflexes, and facial dysesthesias may be present.

Herpes zoster oticus (Ramsey-Hunt)   Vertigo is associated with vesicles in the external auditory canal, hearing loss or tinnitus, and facial palsy **(Plate 235).**

Multifactorial disequilibrium   Ambulation requires visual, vestibular, and proprioceptive input and may be impaired when any of these are affected or with a critical mass of multiple minor impairments. Romberg and tandem gait are usually abnormal.

Stroke   Vertigo may arise when there is thrombosis of posterior inferior cerebellar artery or pontine branches. Consider this in older patients, as well as when vascular disease or atrial fibrillation is present.

Cerebellar disease   The Romberg will be positive with the eyes closed or open, and finger-to-nose pursuit will be abnormal.

Frontal lobe apraxia   The patient will appear to be walking on ice. There is difficulty initiating the gait, and turns are accomplished by pivoting around on one foot.

Orthostatic hypotension   Symptoms are only present when changing to the upright position. An orthostatic increase in pulse of 30 per minute or enough lightheadedness to cause fainting or needing to lie down is associated with a volume loss greater than 1 liter.

Common fainting (presyncope)   There is often a prodromal sensation of "graying out," nausea, clamminess, blurred vision, and pallor.

Hyperventilation   A key clue is perioral and acral tingling. Anxiety is present.

Panic attack   Dizziness is associated with severe apprehension, chest pressure, palpitations, and fear of losing control. The differential diagnosis for this includes paroxysmal tachycardia, autonomic phenomena with pheochromocytoma, hypoglycemia, and complex partial seizures.

Headache

◼ DIFFERENTIAL OVERVIEW

- ❏ Migraine
- ❏ Tension
- ❏ Acute sinusitis
- ❏ Acute glaucoma
- ❏ Postconcussive
- ❏ Cluster
- ❏ Meningitis
- ❏ Drugs
- ❏ Hypoglycemia
- ❏ Benign exertional headache
- ❏ Temporomandibular joint inflammation
- ❏ Subdural hematoma
- ❏ Subarachnoid hemorrhage
- ❏ Acute epidural hematoma
- ❏ Lumbar puncture
- ❏ Brain tumor
- ❏ Headache in HIV
- ❏ Pseudotumor cerebri
- ❏ Hypertensive encephalopathy
- ❏ Carbon monoxide intoxication
- ❏ Giant cell arteritis
- ❏ Psychogenic
- ❏ Brain abscess
- ❏ Encephalitis
- ❏ Arteriovenous malformations
- ❏ Cavernous sinus thrombosis
- ❏ Pituitary apoplexy
- ❏ Carotid artery dissection

DIAGNOSTIC APPROACH

Red flags to serious causes include the following: Sudden onset of "the worst headache of my life," especially in a non–headache-prone person; headache different from previous headaches; headache precipitated by position change, cough, or exertion; a history of trauma or fever; abnormal mental status or other neurological findings; a headache that disturbs sleep or is present immediately on awakening; immune deficiency such as HIV.

The time course helps in diagnosing headache. A "thunderclap" headache of a ruptured aneurysm peaks instantly. Cluster headache peaks over 3–5 minutes, remains at maximum for 45 minutes, and then gradually recedes. Migraine builds over hours, lasts hours to days, and is improved with sleep.

In evaluating patients with recurrent migraine, it is critical to ascertain whether the present headache differs from prior migraines and whether fever is present or spontaneous retinal venous pulsations are abnormally absent. These should prompt a search for alternative causes. If fever is present with headache, rule out meningitis.

Pain originating above the tentorium is referred to the frontal, temporal, or parietal region. Pain from the posterior fossa and below is referred to the occiput. Pain from the posterior sagittal and transverse sinuses may be referred to the eye or forehead.

Lumbar puncture, subdural hematoma, or benign intracranial hypertension can cause orthostatic headache. Occipital headache radiating to the vertex and forehead is usually a result of cervical spondylosis but can also be caused by basal subarachnoid hemorrhage, posterior fossa tumor, or meningitis.

CLINICAL FINDINGS

Migraine   A prodrome virtually always indicates migraine and is the sine qua non of migraine with aura (classic migraine). Neurological phenomena include visual scotoma (an expanding jagged bright border with a dark center, like a wildfire) or mood changes (usually depression or irritability). More unusually, a prodrome may consist of aphasia or hemiplegia. A unilateral headache follows, usually with vegetative symptoms of nausea, anorexia, or sensitivity to light and sound. The fundi may show arterial or venous dilation. Common migraine has no neurological prodrome although patients can often sense it coming on. Migraine can be recognized by vegetative symptoms, activators (e.g., red wine, stress, sleep or food deprivation, or strong odors) or deactivators (e.g., sleep, pregnancy, exhilaration, or sumatriptan). These headaches have their onset in adolescence or young adult age; new onset in older patients can occur but should prompt a search for structural causes.

Tension These are experienced as pressure, a vice or band-like sensation around the head (vertex, frontal, or temporal). Dull and steady, they worsen as the day progresses. They may last days, weeks, or months, but tension headaches are not relentlessly progressive. Anxiety, depression, and emotional conflicts are frequent precipitants.

Acute sinusitis The epicenter may be frontal (frontal sinuses), over cheeks (maxillary sinuses), between the eyes (ethmoid sinuses), or in the frontotemporal and occipital region (sphenoid sinus). Headache is a continuous or throbbing pressure sensation that is worsened by bending forward. Fever, nasal obstruction, and purulent drainage are usually present.

Acute glaucoma Orbital headache begins with aching around the rim and spreads through the trigeminal ophthalmic division. A tender hard globe, red eye with limbic flush, dull cornea, and impaired transmission of tangential light through the anterior chamber may be present **(Plates 217, 218).**

Postconcussive Contusion produces scalp tenderness at the impact site or tension-type headache. Especially after the patient's vehicle has been rear-ended in an accident, there is headache, dizziness, vertigo, memory impairment, reduced concentration, and anxiety. These symptoms may last months to years **(Plate 220).**

Cluster Cluster occurs in middle-aged men as nocturnal episodes of high intensity, steady, boring, burning, unilateral orbital pain accompanied by ipsilateral red and tearing eyes, nasal congestion, facial flushing, and diaphoresis. There also may be ipsilateral ptosis and miosis (20–40%). The headache begins a few hours after going to bed and lasts 1–2 hours. It recurs nightly for weeks to months and then disappears for years.

Meningitis Fever is the key sign. The headache is severe, generalized and constant, most intense at the base of the skull, and aggravated by forward flexion of the neck. The neck and back will be reflexively stiff to flexion (Kernig's and Brudzinski's sign). Nausea, photophobia, and altered mental status ranging from delirium to coma often accompany the headache. Clues regarding the cause include the following: petechial rash (meningococcus, enterovirus, S. aureus, leptospira); parotitis (coxsackie, LCM, EBV); vesicles (HSV); HIV (listeria, pneumococcus); diabetes (pneumococcus, gram-negative, S. aureus, cryptococcus, mucormycosis); fresh-water swimming (ameba); steroids (cryptococcus, mycobacteria); summer or fall onset (enterovirus, Borrelia, leptospira). Acute otitis, sinusitis or pneumonia, basilar skull fracture, or splenectomy suggests pneumococcal meningitis. Meningococcal meningitis is suggested by fulminant onset with vascular collapse and angular purpura with a gunmetal gray color. Tuberculous meningitis is suggested by a gradual onset and multiple cranial nerve abnormalities **(Plates 32, 233).**

Drugs Sulfamethoxazole, ibuprofen, sulindac, ketorolac, isoniazid, azathioprine, and penicillin may cause aseptic meningitis, especially in patients with systemic lupus or mixed connective tissue disease. Concurrent facial swelling, urticaria, and conjunctivitis are helpful clues. Nitrates, ergots, amphetamines, phenothiazines, alcohol, and withdrawal from caffeine may also cause headache **(Plate 182).**

Hypoglycemia Suspect this in a diabetic exhibiting diffuse sweating, throbbing frontal or generalized headache, weakness, confusion, and irritability.

Benign exertional headache It occurs more commonly in patients who have migraines. Coital headache occurs abruptly with orgasm and subsides within minutes. It is usually benign, but if it lasts for hours or is accompanied by vomiting, subarachnoid hemorrhage should be considered.

Temporomandibular joint inflammation Chewing aggravates the symptoms, and involuntary nocturnal bruxism and jaw clenching are common. Tenderness and a click over the TMJ are sensitive but not specific findings.

Headache

Subdural hematoma   Head trauma with concussion is followed by a lucid interval, then the development of mental status changes and/or focal neurological deficits such as hemiparesis, dilated pupil, and papilledema. Subdural hematoma presents with mild persistent headache, drowsiness, and confusion, and progresses to loss of consciousness **(Plate 220).**

Subarachnoid hemorrhage   Hemorrhage is sudden in onset and very severe. Headache, photophobia, nausea, meningismus, and loss of consciousness develop rapidly. A major hemorrhage has often been preceded by a similar, less severe, self-limited "herald bleed."

Acute epidural hematoma   This is usually caused by a temporal skull fracture. A progressive decrease in the level of consciousness is the rule although a brief lucid interval may follow recovery from a concussion before blood has accumulated.

Lumbar puncture   An intense occipitofrontal headache develops when the patient is upright and is relieved when supine. The onset may be as many as 12 days after the procedure. The original CNS indications for the lumbar puncture may make this difficult to recognize.

Brain tumor   The "classic" tumor headache that is worse in morning, accompanied by nausea and vomiting, occurs in less than 20%. It is relieved by lying down and worsened by straining at defecating, by coughing, or by bending over. Characteristically, it remains in the same location but is progressive, increasing in duration and severity over months. Being awakened at night with the headache is common but not diagnostic. Usually there are subtle neurological changes by the time the headache develops. Fundoscopy often shows increased intracranial pressure, manifest as absence of spontaneous venous pulsations to overt papilledema. Cerebral vomiting, without food, may occur. An occipital lobe tumor may be mistaken for migraine because of the production of scotoma **(Plate 129).**

Headache in HIV   Acute HIV causes aseptic meningitis accompanied by sore throat, diffuse maculopapular rash, and generalized lymphadenopathy. Cryptococcosis causes headache, fever, and nausea. Toxoplasmosis usually presents with encephalopathy or seizures. CNS lymphoma has headache or seizures. HIV encephalitis presents with seizures, memory loss, or decreased attention span **(Plates 201, 204).**

Pseudotumor cerebri   It presents like tumor in an obese young woman, with chronic retroorbital headache increased by eye movement. Transient blurred vision, diplopia, and vague symptoms of dizziness or facial numbness are experienced. Papilledema will often be present on examination.

Hypertensive encephalopathy   An occipital headache usually occurs with accelerated hypertension (BP>230/130), but may be seen with diastolic pressures as low as 110. The headache is worse in the morning. Hypertensive encephalopathy presents with headache, nausea, vomiting, visual disturbances, confusion, seizures, or coma. Focal neurological deficits, retinal hemorrhages, and papilledema are clues. Suspect pheochromocytoma if the headache and hypertension are paroxysmal and associated with sweating, palpitations, and weight loss **(Plate 38).**

Carbon monoxide intoxication   A prominent pounding headache develops with exposure to engine exhaust or a kerosene heater in a closed space.

Giant cell arteritis   Temporal arteritis should be considered in an elderly patient with a unilateral, dull, aching, continuous headache. It will be most intense over the temporal artery, which may be exquisitely tender and ropy or nodular. Systemic symptoms of fever and anorexia, jaw claudication (weakness, fatigue, or pain precipitated by chewing), or scalp tenderness (painful to comb the hair) often accompany the headache.

Psychogenic   Headaches are described in flamboyant terms but have no clear pattern. Terms such as lightning-like or explosive are used, but the patient experiences no visible discomfort.

Brain abscess   Parenteral drug use, lung abscess, immunodeficiency, and a parameningeal focus are clues. Fever and focal neurologic signs should be sought, but these are not universally present.

Encephalitis   Encephalitis begins acutely or subacutely with headache, fever, and signs of parenchymal involvement, such as coma, seizures, change in mental status, or focal neurological findings. Herpesvirus presents with frontal or temporal lobe neurological findings, or focal seizures, in 85%.

Arteriovenous malformations   Unilateral (always on the same side) throbbing chronic headache without aura occurs. A bruit may be heard with the stethoscope over the eye or temporal region.

Cavernous sinus thrombosis   It begins with retro-orbital headache, which is worse on sitting. Chemosis, proptosis, and painful ophthalmoplegia (deficits of cranial nerves III, IV, V) are found. Seizures or unilateral numbness or weakness may be seen. Predisposing causes include acute sinusitis, otitis, or coagulopathy.

Pituitary apoplexy   Severe bifrontal headache, drowsiness, diplopia, and visual loss (especially bitemporal hemianopia) are found.

Carotid artery dissection   Dissection occurs with neck trauma. Ipsilateral frontal, orbital, or temporal pain with Horner's syndrome and focal neurological signs are clues. A carotid bruit is often found **(Plates 120, 238).**

Chapter 105

Insomnia/Hypersomnia

◼ DIFFERENTIAL OVERVIEW

Insomnia
- ❏ Stress
- ❏ Drugs
- ❏ Medical disorders
- ❏ Phase shift
- ❏ Sleep apnea
- ❏ Conditioned insomnia
- ❏ Depression
- ❏ Restless leg syndrome
- ❏ Nocturnal myoclonus
- ❏ Nightmares

Hypersomnia
- ❏ Drugs
- ❏ Medical disorders
- ❏ Adolescence
- ❏ Narcolepsy

DIAGNOSTIC APPROACH

Insomnia may occur as difficulty falling asleep, multiple awakenings from sleep, or awakening early and being unable to fall back to sleep. If the presenting symptom is excessive daytime somnolence or fatigue, the problem may have to be reframed as one of insomnia.

CLINICAL FINDINGS

Stress   Transient insomnia is common with major life stress. Rumination occurs during the sleeplessness.

Drugs   *Insomnia:* Stimulant drugs such as caffeine, amphetamines, xanthines, nicotine, and phenylpropanolamine may cause insomnia. Benzodiazepines produce rebound anxiety and insomnia. *Hypersomnia:* Alcohol sedates, but the sleep is shallow and not restive. Tricyclic antidepressants, benzodiazepines, narcotics, and antihistamines are among the more common causes.

Medical disorders   *Insomnia:* Hyperthyroidism, congestive heart failure, COPD, nocturia, and pain are common causes. *Hypersomnia:* Those conditions producing fatigue, such as infectious mononucleosis, low cardiac output, renal failure, and hypothyroidism, cause hypersomnia **(Plates 16, 18, 19, 41, 229, 230).**

Phase shift   When the sleep–wake cycle is reset, as in alternating shift work or international travel, insomnia results. Day–night reversal is a common problem in dementia.

Sleep apnea   The roommate reports heavy snoring and interruption of breathing, which is followed by an inspiratory gasp. Patients fall asleep at inappropriate times during the day, and they may manifest behavioral abnormalities. Alcohol and sedatives worsen this condition by depressing respiratory function and REM sleep.

Conditioned insomnia   A learned behavior may result in bedtime being associated with frustration and anxiety. Patients will often sleep well in a bed other than their own.

Depression   Insomnia may be the chief complaint, manifesting as difficulty falling asleep or early awakening with inability to fall back to sleep. The manic phase of bipolar disorder will exhibit hyperactivity, racing thoughts, and speech with grandiosity.

Restless leg syndrome   It is experienced as a crawling sensation deep within the muscles, relieved by movement.

Nocturnal myoclonus   The patient may be awakened by repetitive twitching or jerking of the legs.

Nightmares   These are dream anxiety attacks, from which the patient will awaken perspiring with a rapid pulse.

211

Adolescence   Changes in the biological time clock and need for sleep are physiologic for adolescents.

Narcolepsy   This is recognized by the distinctive features of cataplexy (sudden loss of muscle tone with strong emotion, surprise, or laugh), hypnagogic hallucinations (visual or auditory waking dreams), and sleep paralysis (brief inability to move upon awakening).

Motor Weakness

PLATES 19, 25, 119, 127, 128, 130, 132, 219

DIFFERENTIAL OVERVIEW

Generalized
- ❏ Steroid myopathy
- ❏ Diabetic amyotrophy
- ❏ Polymyalgia rheumatica
- ❏ Polymyositis
- ❏ Myasthenia gravis
- ❏ Guillain-Barré syndrome
- ❏ Hyperthyroidism
- ❏ Muscular dystrophy
- ❏ Eaton-Lambert syndrome
- ❏ Metabolic myopathy

Paraparesis
- ❏ Trauma
- ❏ Multiple sclerosis
- ❏ Amyotrophic lateral sclerosis
- ❏ Guillain-Barré syndrome
- ❏ Epidural abscess
- ❏ Subacute combined degeneration
- ❏ Syringomyelia
- ❏ Aortic dissection
- ❏ Hysterical

DIAGNOSTIC APPROACH

Myopathy can be distinguished by proximal weakness (climbing stairs or combing hair), symmetrical distribution, absence of paresthesias, and pain or disturbance of bowel or bladder function. Proximal muscle weakness is more prominent in myopathy, distal weakness in peripheral nerve, or anterior horn cell disease. Bulbar weakness, manifest as difficulty speaking and swallowing, is consistent with anterior horn cell disease or neuromuscular junction disorders. Ocular weakness occurs with myasthenia gravis and myotonic or oculopharyngeal dystrophy.

Acute generalized weakness with an onset over hours can be caused by low levels of potassium, calcium, sodium, magnesium, or phosphate; by botulism; or by viral inflammatory myopathy. Spasticity, manifest as increased tone and sudden release ("clasp-knife"), occurs with any CNS lesions that cause weakness. Rigidity occurs with extrapyramidal disorders. Functional overlay should be suspected in the presence of ratcheting "give-away" weakness.

Finding	UMN	LMN	Myopathy
Atrophy	None	Severe	Mild
Fasciculations	None	Common	None
Tone	Spastic	Decreased	Nl-Decreased
Distribution	Regional	Distal/Segmental	Proximal
DTR	Increased	Decreased/Absent	Nl-Decreased
Babinski	Upgoing	Downgoing	Downgoing

NB: UMN, upper motor neuron disease; LMN, lower motor neuron disease.

CLINICAL FINDINGS

Steroid myopathy   Proximal muscle weakness develops in a patient taking chronic steroids.

Diabetic amyotrophy   Proximal weakness and atrophy of the legs, usually accompanied by anorexia, weight loss, and depression, occur in a patient with poorly controlled diabetes.

Motor Weakness

Polymyalgia rheumatica Proximal muscle aches and arthralgias are often perceived as weakness. Fever, weight loss, and temporal arteritis are also part of the spectrum.

Polymyositis Symmetrical proximal muscle weakness, with difficulty arising from a chair or climbing stairs, is the most striking finding. Difficulty swallowing may occur in 25%. Deep tendon reflexes are preserved.

Myasthenia gravis The hallmark is rapid fatigability of the muscles with progressive weakness on repetitive use, and partial recovery after rest. Fatigability is especially seen in ocular muscles with resultant ptosis or diplopia. Dysphonia with a nasal voice, decreased volume with prolonged talking, and choking with nasal regurgitation may occur **(Plates 130, 219)**.

Guillain-Barré syndrome It is characterized by an ascending motor paralysis, areflexia, and mild sensory symptoms.

Hyperthyroidism Weakness may be proximal or generalized. Fasciculations, bulbar weakness, and eye muscle involvement are present. Other signs of hyperthyroidism are usually evident, such as fine tremor, tachycardia, lid lag, and exophthalmos **(Plate 19)**.

Muscular dystrophy Early symptoms are difficulty climbing stairs and difficulty arising from a recumbent position (requiring use of the hands). Swayback, with a waddling gait due to gluteal weakness, and pseudohypertrophy of the calves may be seen. Types include: Duchenne (affects young boys); fascioscapulohumeral (onset 10–20 years); limb-girdle (affects shoulder and pelvic muscles); and myotonic dystrophy (onset is in early adulthood, with peripheral muscle wasting, frontal balding, and cataracts).

Eaton-Lambert syndrome A paraneoplastic syndrome seen most often with small cell cancer of the lung; weakness affects limbs more than cranial nerves. Reflexes are disproportionately reduced.

Metabolic myopathy Phosphofructokinase, lactate dehydrogenase, and muscle phosphorylase deficiency produce painful muscle cramps, weakness with exercise, and myoglobinuria (dipstick proteinuria). Acid maltase deficiency produces progressive weakness without myoglobinuria. Carnitine deficiency produces progressive weakness, increased by exercise.

Trauma The history is obvious. There is a flaccid paralysis, and reflexes are absent.

Multiple sclerosis Classic findings include diplopia and optic neuritis/atrophy, limb paresthesias, and internuclear ophthalmoplegia. Patchy, nondermatomal sensory symptoms separated in time and (neurological) space are also a common presentation **(Plates 119, 127, 128)**.

Amyotrophic lateral sclerosis With lower motor neuron involvement, there is a slowly progressive asymmetric weakness, muscle cramping with movement, atrophy, and fasciculations. With corticospinal involvement, stiffness is the principal symptom, with hyperactive reflexes and spasticity **(Plate 132)**.

Epidural abscess Gradual onset of motor weakness occurs with back pain and fever.

Subacute combined degeneration It is characterized by paresthesias in the hands and feet, dorsal column loss in the legs, tender muscles, weak legs, and spasticity with increased deep tendon reflexes and an upgoing plantar response.

Syringomyelia It presents with spasticity of the legs, decreased deep tendon reflexes in the arms, decreased pain and temperature sense in the arms and thorax, and weakness or wasting in the arms.

Aortic dissection Dissection of the spinal arteries will lead to sudden onset of inability to move a leg, but arm strength will be unaffected. There will be deep back pain, restlessness (so that a patient might seem to be fabricating symptoms), and a pulseless leg **(Plate 25)**.

Hysterical Normal deep tendon reflexes and *la belle indifference* are the main clues.

Peripheral Neuropathy

DIFFERENTIAL OVERVIEW

- ❑ Diabetes
- ❑ Alcohol
- ❑ Vitamin B12 deficiency
- ❑ Drugs
- ❑ Carcinomatous
- ❑ Lead
- ❑ Guillain-Barré
- ❑ Tabes dorsalis
- ❑ Syringomyelia
- ❑ Polyarteritis nodosa
- ❑ Amyloidosis
- ❑ Polymyositis
- ❑ Pellagra
- ❑ Arsenic
- ❑ Porphyria

DIAGNOSTIC APPROACH

Sensory neuropathy symptoms include positive phenomena such as tingling; pins/needles; and burning, cold, or lancinating pain. Physical findings include weakness, fasciculations, atrophy, ataxia, wide-based gait, abnormal sweating, decreased or absent deep tendon reflexes, orthostatic hypotension, hypesthesia surrounded by a zone of hyperesthesia, and vibration or position sense affected before pinprick or temperature sense.

Autonomic neuropathy symptoms include impotence, retrograde ejaculation, diaphoresis, incontinence, urinary retention, constipation, diarrhea, orthostatic dizziness, and flushing. Physical findings include delayed pupillary light response, resting tachycardia, sinus arrhythmia, and orthostatic hypotension.

Mononeuropathy affects a single peripheral nerve, caused by injury resulting from trauma, entrapment, or vascular insufficiency. Mononeuropathy multiplex affects multiple nerves over time (due to diabetes, vasculitis, or leprosy). Polyneuropathy occurs in a stocking-glove distribution and is toxic or metabolic in origin.

Injury to large myelinated nerves produces decreased light touch and proprioception with a sensation of "walking on a thick carpet" or imbalance. Injury to medium fibers causes decreased light touch and vibration sense. Injury to small unmyelinated fibers, as occurs in diabetes or amyloidosis, decreases pain and temperature sensation and produces dysesthesias.

Transverse cord lesions produce loss of all modalities below the level of the lesion and a band of hyperalgesia at the level of the lesion. Lateral cord compression is heralded by early sensory changes. Dorsal cord compression affects proprioception and tactile discrimination without pain or temperature loss. Pernicious anemia and tabes dorsalis preferentially affect the dorsal columns. Thalamic lesions produce sensory symptoms in the opposite side of the body, causing paresthesias, hyperesthesias, and hyperpathia (unpleasant burning pain with stimulation).

CLINICAL FINDINGS

Diabetes A symmetrical stocking-glove distribution is typical. Vibration and position sense is most prominently impaired initially, followed by decreased reflexes and periods of painful paresthesias and vasomotor disturbance **(Plates 123, 166).**

Alcohol A symmetrical stocking-glove neuropathy in an alcoholic patient may result from thiamine deficiency or the direct toxic effect of alcohol.

Vitamin B12 deficiency It presents as paresthesias and dysesthesias of the lower extremities, which are progressive. Combined system disease (pyramidal, posterior column, and peripheral neuropathy) is present **(Plate 69).**

Drugs Peripheral neuropathy is a common side effect of chemotherapeutic agents such as vincristine.

215

Carcinomatous   This neuropathy combines findings of a sensory polyneuropathy, muscle weakness and wasting—often with a myasthenic pattern—and subacute combined degeneration with tremor, ataxia, and dysequilibrium.

Lead   Abdominal pain, headache, ataxia, and memory loss are concurrent with the neuropathy **(Plate 134)**.

Guillain-Barré   Paresthesias are rapidly followed by the development of areflexia, weakness, and paralysis. The symptoms begin distally in the hands and feet and ascend proximally.

Tabes dorsalis   Syphilis is suggested by paroxysmal onset, absent deep tendon reflexes, absent dorsal column function, and an Argyll Robertson pupil (accommodates but does not react to light) **(Plates 118, 123)**.

Syringomyelia   It presents with a cape-like loss of pain and temperature sensation while sparing other modalities.

Polyarteritis nodosa   Consider vasculitis when polyneuritis is associated with fever, weight loss, or arterial lesions **(Plate 110)**.

Amyloidosis   It may present as a symmetrical or asymmetrical sensory–motor neuropathy. The key to diagnosis is recognition of concomitant macroglossia, waxy purpuric periorbital lesions, hepatomegaly, or congestive heart failure **(Plates 130, 131, 157)**.

Polymyositis   It presents as pain in the extremity with proximal weakness, loss of reflexes, and decrease in position and vibration sense.

Pellagra   It presents not only with subacute combined degeneration, but also with a symmetrical photodermatitis, which is brownish with a curious varnished surface appearance **(Plate 67)**.

Arsenic   Burning paresthesias in a glove or stocking distribution combined with palmar hyperkeratosis suggests arsenic intoxication **(Plate 133)**.

Porphyria   Neuropathic pain, which is associated with acute weakness, and abdominal pain (colic) are prominent features. The urine will turn a burgundy color if left exposed to light.

Radicular Pain/ Dysesthesias

PLATES 106, 119, 120, 127, 128, 132, 169, 171

◪ DIAGNOSTIC OVERVIEW

Upper Extremity
❑ Median
❑ Ulnar
❑ Radial
❑ Axillary
❑ Brachial plexus
❑ Serratus anterior
❑ Thoracic outlet syndrome
❑ Reflex sympathetic dystrophy
❑ Syringomyelia

Lower Extremity
❑ Sciatic
❑ Lateral femoral cutaneous
❑ Common peroneal
❑ Femoral
❑ Obturator

Cranial
❑ Facial
❑ Trigeminal

DIAGNOSTIC APPROACH

Paresthesias (numbness, pins and needles, hyperesthesia) are nerve-impingement symptoms. The patient usually requires prompting to be specific about distribution.

Motor function of nerve roots includes the following: C5—shoulder abduction; C6—wrist extension; C7—forearm extension at the elbow; C8,T1—digital abduction and adduction; L2,3,4—knee extension; L5—ankle and large toe dorsiflexion; and S1—plantar flexion. *Reflex* function of nerve roots includes the following: C5,6—biceps; C7,8—triceps; L2,3,4—knee jerk; and S1—ankle jerk.

Atrophic weakness of the arms and spastic weakness of the legs suggests cervical spondylosis or amyotrophic lateral sclerosis. Cervical spondylosis has pain from the neck to the back of the shoulders to the wrist, which is aggravated by arm movement. ALS has paresthesias and sensory impairment.

Beware compartment syndrome, which may be a limb-threatening emergency. There will be an injury to a compartment-bound muscle, which develops into progressive, severe, local pain. Distal paresthesias are a common early symptom—even when the distal pulse is bounding and perfusion seems good.

CLINICAL FINDINGS

Median (C6-T1) It is most often due to compression at the wrist causing carpal tunnel syndrome. Symptoms are numbness and tingling in the palmar aspect of the thumb and first two fingers. Tinel's sign (electrical pain when tapping on the volar wrist) and Phalen's sign (radicular symptoms in the hand increased by prolonged wrist flexion) are often present. Muscle wasting and loss of power in the thenar eminence occur later. When bilateral, it is associated with systemic processes such as rheumatoid arthritis, myxedema, diabetes, pregnancy, acromegaly, and amyloidosis. A complete lesion involving both forearm (pronation and radial flexion) and hand ("LOAF": lumbricales, opposition, abduction, and flexion) muscles is usually a result of trauma at the axilla or elbow.

Ulnar (C8-T1) It is usually a result of elbow trauma at the cubital fossa or Guyton's canal between the pisiform and the hook of the hamate. Typical symptoms are sensory loss in the ulnar aspect of the hand (fourth and little fingers) and motor weakness of ulnar flex-

Radicular Pain/ Dysesthesias

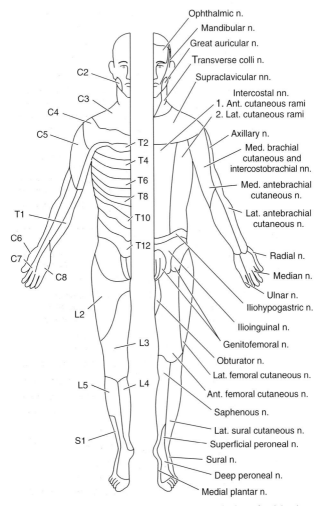

Figure 16. Anterior view of dermatomes and cutaneous projections of peripheral nerves. (Adapted from: Carpenter MB, Sutin J. Human Neuroanatomy. 8th ed. Baltimore: Williams & Wilkins, 1983.)

ion at the wrist and flexion and opposition of the ulnar digits. Longstanding injury (usually at the wrist) leads to a claw hand with a flexed small finger.

Radial (C5-C8) Wrist drop (weak wrist extensors) and weak triceps are common presenting findings. Sensory loss involves the back of the hand. Injury may occur at the axilla (e.g., with crutch use) or the elbow ("bridegroom's palsy"), or it may be caused by diabetes or lead exposure.

Radicular Pain/ Dysesthesias

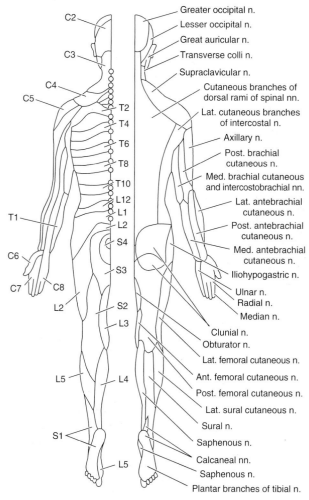

Figure 17. Posterior view of dermatomes and cutaneous projections of peripheral nerves. (Adapted from: Carpenter MB. Sutin J. Human Neuroanatomy. 8th ed. Baltimore: Williams & Wilkins, 1983.)

Axillary   Reduced arm abduction results from deltoid weakness, with decreased sensation over the deltoid. It is associated with shoulder dislocation, humeral neck fracture, and use of crutches.

Brachial plexus   Aching in the shoulder or scapula with pain shooting in an ulnar distribution, paresthesias in a T1 distribution, and Raynaud's phenomenon may be found. Up-

Radicular Pain/ Dysesthesias

per plexus injury (Erb-Duchenne) of C5-6 roots with forced depression of the shoulder leaves the arm limp at the side in a "waiter's tip" position. Lower plexus injury (Klumpke's) of C8 and T1 roots caused by violent upward pull of the arm or shoulder dislocation produces a claw hand and decreased ulnar sensation. A Pancoast tumor is suggested by suprascapular neuropathy with severe shoulder pain, weakness/atrophy of the supraspinatus and infraspinatus muscles, and a Horner's syndrome in two thirds **(Plate 120).**

Serratus anterior The main finding is a winged scapula.

Thoracic outlet syndrome It presents with symptoms of weakness of the intrinsics of the hands and decreased sensation of the palmar aspect of the fourth and fifth fingers. Arterial findings may also be produced by rib compression, leading to a pulse/blood pressure decrement or distal emboli.

Reflex sympathetic dystrophy Proximal pain (e.g., shoulder tendinitis) leads to distal burning, lancinating, and nondermatomal pain/dysesthesias. There is abnormal temperature (hot early, cold late), color (red early, cyanotic late), and sweating (dry early, moist late). Other findings include hyperesthesia, smooth atrophic skin, and limited joint motion.

Syringomyelia The patient has pain in the arm with dissociated sensory loss, atrophy of muscles, and loss of reflexes in the arms with pyramidal signs below the lesion. A Horner's syndrome may be present.

Sciatic (L4-S3) It supplies the hamstrings and all muscles below the knee. Symptoms are most often caused by compression of a single root by a herniated disc, but multidermatomal pain may be caused by entrapment in the sciatic notch by the pyriformis muscle. There will be local tenderness and Tinel's.

Lateral femoral cutaneous (L2,3) This is a pure sensory nerve producing numbness and burning over the anterolateral thigh (meralgia paresthetica). Injury occurs at the point the nerve passes over the anterior superior iliac spine. Symptoms increase when the patient lies flat.

Common peroneal Injury produces foot drop with a slapping gait and scuffing of the toe of the shoe. There is weakness of dorsiflexion of the great toe and sensory loss between the first and second toes. The usual cause is pressure over the lateral aspect of the knee.

Femoral Hip flexion and knee extension will be affected (dorsal L2, 3, 4), with quadriceps wasting, and weakness of hip flexion and knee jerk. Causes include diabetes, tumor, polyarteritis, and pelvic trauma.

Obturator Thigh adductors (ventral L2, 3, 4) may be damaged during labor or affected by diabetes or a pelvic mass.

Facial (CN VII) The onset of Bell's palsy is often heralded by facial pain and demonstrated by paralysis of both the upper and lower face. Central lesions spare the forehead musculature. Other affected areas include the lacrimal gland, stapedius (causing hyperacusis), and taste in the anterior two thirds of the tongue. Most cases are idiopathic but may be caused by Ebstein-Barr virus, a cerebellopontine angle tumor, or a brainstem plaque in multiple sclerosis. The latter two are usually associated with other brainstem signs. Bilateral seventh nerve palsy should suggest sarcoidosis or Lyme disease **(Plates 106, 119, 127, 128, 169, 171).**

Trigeminal (CN V, second or third division) Injury or inflammation causes symptoms of paroxysmal, excruciating, lancinating pain in the face. Pain may be elicited by touch or chewing. It may be caused by herpes simplex infection of the trigeminal ganglion, tumor, or demyelinating disease (especially in younger patients) **(Plate 132).**

DIFFERENTIAL OVERVIEW

- ❏ Generalized (grand mal)
- ❏ Partial (focal)
- ❏ Complex partial (temporal lobe)
- ❏ Absence (petit mal)
- ❏ Vasovagal syncope
- ❏ Myoclonic
- ❏ Akinetic (drop attacks)
- ❏ Psychomotor
- ❏ Pseudoseizures

DIAGNOSTIC APPROACH

When the patient is found unresponsive, the differential is seizure versus syncope. Interviewing witnesses is crucial to ascertain the diagnosis. Seizures can be distinguished by color (cyanosis in seizure, pallor in syncope), aura, injury from falling, protracted tonic-clonic activity, tongue biting, urinary incontinence, and slow recovery of consciousness (seizure). Confusion, headache, and drowsiness are sequelae of seizure whereas physical weakness and a clear sensorium occur with syncope. Seizures often have a promontory aura, such as an odor, and syncope has a prodrome of tunnel vision. Seizures are followed by eye closure, rotation of the head side-to-side, and prolonged, motionless unresponsiveness.

General precipitating factors include sleep deprivation, systemic disease, metabolic/electrolyte disorder, alcohol use, or drug use. Elicit a history of febrile seizures or prior head trauma. Common causes of recurrent seizures in previously controlled patients include alcohol use, intercurrent infection, and missed medication doses.

A neurological examination will indicate whether there is an underlying structural problem as evidenced by mild hemiparesis, reflex asymmetry, or extensor plantar response. Seizures are more common in slowly growing cerebral lesions, such as low-grade glioma or meningioma.

CLINICAL FINDINGS

Generalized (grand mal) In a tonic-clonic seizure, apnea, plethora, tongue biting, incontinence, and violent, rhythmic muscular contractions occur. These are followed by postictal lethargy and confusion. Systemic causes include high fever, alcohol or drug withdrawal, hyponatremia, metabolic acidosis, and renal or hepatic failure. Local causes include scar from trauma, neoplasm, or vasculitis of the central nervous system.

Partial (focal) Eye deviation occurs away from the side of a frontal focus. A Jacksonian seizure begins with clonic movement in the thumb or corner of the mouth and spreads to adjacent motor groups. If it is unilateral, the patient is awake.

Complex partial Temporal lobe seizures are most often characterized by auras and loss of awareness of the environment with repetitive behaviors or movements. Auras may be hallucinations (olfactory, gustatory, visual, or auditory), spatial distortions, deja vu or jamais vu, or affective changes (anxiety, rage). Repetitive motor acts typically include lip smacking, undressing, or speaking incoherently. Movements are purposeful but poorly coordinated. The seizures can be sensory, vertiginous, autonomic, dysphasic, deja vu, affective, illusions (macroscopia or microscopia), or structured hallucinations. In a patient with fever and confusion, herpes simplex encephalitis should be considered.

Absence (petit mal) These seizures are characterized by staring or ceasing ongoing behavior for 5–10 seconds, while fluttering the eyelids or twitching the face. There may be minor automatisms, such as licking the lips or shuffling the feet. These symptoms may be reproduced by the alkalosis of hyperventilation.

Vasovagal syncope Nonsustained (less than 15 seconds) clonic jerking with loss of consciousness may be seen.

Myoclonic Rhythmic motor jerks occur with cerebral anoxic injury or metabolic encephalopathy.

Akinetic (drop attacks)   Marked by loss of postural tone with petit mal activity, these seizures are difficult to distinguish from syncope.

Psychomotor   These may cause feelings of fear and rage or disturbing dreams.

Pseudoseizures   Atypical motor activity, lack of a postictal state, and secondary gain are common clues. Seizures occur in the presence of an audience. Movements are often exaggerated, there is no tongue biting, and plantar reflexes are normal.

DIFFERENTIAL OVERVIEW

TIA/Stroke
❏ Middle cerebral artery stroke
❏ Anterior cerebral artery stroke
❏ Posterior cerebral artery stroke
❏ Watershed stroke
❏ Thalamic lacune
❏ Vertebrobasilar ischemia
❏ Pontine lacune
❏ Pontine stroke
❏ Midbrain stroke
❏ Pure motor hemiplegia
❏ Ataxic hemiparesis
❏ Lateral medullary stroke
❏ Temporal lobe stroke

Hemorrhage
❏ Subarachnoid hemorrhage
❏ Cerebellar hemorrhage
❏ Thalamic hemorrhage
❏ Pontine hemorrhage
❏ Putaminal hemorrhage

DIAGNOSTIC APPROACH

A TIA proceeds to stroke in 10–40%. Risk is especially high in "crescendo TIA," which is usually caused by an ulcerated carotid plaque. Amaurosis fugax ("a shade coming down" or transient monocular loss of vision) is a classic presentation. Amaurosis fugax, an anterior circulation event, should be distinguished from transient hemianopsis, a posterior circulation event **(Plate 238).**

Carotid artery stenosis is characterized by an ipsilateral diminished pulse and bruit. Symptoms are often in the middle cerebral artery distribution. Symptoms may occur with relative hypotension in the presence of a fixed stenosis.

Consider cardiac emboli in the presence of atrial fibrillation, recent anterior myocardial infarction, endocarditis, prosthetic valve, or atrial myxoma. Strokes from these causes are usually not preceded by TIAs **(Plates 22, 23, 24).**

Lacunar infarcts are neurologically circumscribed and occur in the setting of poorly controlled hypertension.

Migraine is recognized by headache after the neurological symptoms, epiphenomena such as anorexia/nausea and photophobia, and occurrence in younger patients.

A posterior communicating artery aneurysm may produce symptoms that result from compression of the oculomotor nerve or a "herald bleed" with transient severe headache and neck stiffness, preceding a major hemorrhage.

CLINICAL FINDINGS

Middle cerebral artery stroke   Hemiparesis and cortical sensory loss that is greater in the arm and face than in the leg are found along with aphasia or nondominant hemisphere dysfunction. The eyes deviate conjugately toward the side of the lesion. Partial middle cerebral syndromes due to emboli include sensorimotor paresis with little aphasia, conduction aphasia, or Wernicke's aphasia without hemiparesis.

Anterior cerebral artery stroke   Presentations include paralysis, apraxia, and cortical sensory loss in the leg only. Frontal lobe findings such as incontinence, slow mentation with perseveration, and grasp and suck reflexes are found.

Posterior cerebral artery stroke   It produces homonymous hemianopsia without motor paresis, prominent sensory loss, alexia without agraphia, inability to name colors, and recent memory loss.

Stroke Syndromes Chapter 110

Watershed stroke   There is proximal arm weakness with distal sparing and transcortical aphasia.

Thalamic lacune   A pure sensory stroke occurs with sensory loss in the face, arm, and leg without hemiplegia.

Vertertobasilar ischemia   Transient vertigo, slurred speech, ataxia, diplopia, homonymous hemianopsia, and alternating or bilateral numbness around the face or lips may occur.

Pontine lacune   Slurred speech with clumsiness and mild weakness of one arm (clumsy hand/dysarthria) occur.

Pontine stroke   A medial pons lesion produces weakness and internuclear ophthalmoplegia. A lateral or tegmental pons lesion produces sensory loss and cerebellar signs.

Midbrain stroke   Weber's syndrome consists of mydriasis, ptosis, ophthalmoplegia, and contralateral hemiplegia.

Pure motor hemiplegia   Paralysis of the face, arm, and leg without sensory loss is found with a pontine or internal capsule lacune. If a right hemiplegia is present, there is no aphasia. If a left hemiplegia is present, there are no parietal lobe findings.

Ataxic hemiparesis   Ataxia and weakness of one leg occur in a pontine or internal capsule lacune.

Lateral medullary stroke   Wallenberg's syndrome presents with facial numbness, limb ataxia, Horner's, and supraorbital pain with contralateral pinprick and temperature loss. Vertigo, nausea, hiccups, hoarseness, dysphagia, and diplopia are also found.

Temporal lobe stroke   Visual distortions (e.g., micropsia), *deja vu* sensation, or recurrent fear may be experienced.

Subarachnoid hemorrhage   The classic presentation is sudden onset of a severe headache during activity, associated with an altered level of consciousness and nuchal rigidity. Focal neurological findings are not present unless intracerebral hemorrhage has also occurred. A posterior communicating artery aneurysm may have an associated third nerve palsy. An anterior communicating artery lesion may be associated with frontal lobe dysfunction. A middle cerebral artery aneurysm may have aphasia or nondominant findings.

Cerebellar hemorrhage   Headache, vomiting, and inability to walk are cardinal features. Strength and sensation are usually normal. There is gaze paresis toward the affected side, and there may be a sixth nerve palsy. Nystagmus and limb ataxia are only occasionally present.

Thalamic hemorrhage   Both eyes look down toward the nose and have small, nonreactive pupils. There is marked sensory loss with or without hemiplegia.

Pontine hemorrhage   A patient with this type of hemorrhage will be comatose with pinpoint pupils that react to strong light. The eyes are midposition with no movement to the doll's eyes maneuver. There is quadriparesis with upgoing toes.

Putaminal hemorrhage   It presents with hemiplegia, headache, field cut, and eye deviation to the side of the hemorrhage and away from the hemiplegia.

Syncope

PLATES 42, 43, 44, 45, 188

DIFFERENTIAL OVERVIEW

Orthostatic/Autonomic
❏ Neurally mediated hypotension
❏ Volume depletion
❏ Cough syncope
❏ Anemia
❏ Autonomic insufficiency

Cardiac/Obstructive
❏ Myocardial infarction
❏ Pulmonary embolism
❏ Aortic stenosis
❏ Hypertrophic obstructive cardiomyopathy
❏ Aortic dissection
❏ Cardiac tamponade
❏ Left atrial myxoma

Cardiac/Dysrhythmic
❏ Complete heart block
❏ Sick sinus syndrome
❏ Tachyarrhythmia
❏ Carotid sinus hypersensitivity

Neurologic
❏ Vertebrobasilar ischemia
❏ Hypoglycemia
❏ Unwitnessed seizure
❏ Subclavian steal syndrome

Psychologic
❏ Hyperventilation
❏ Hysterical faint

DIAGNOSTIC APPROACH

The cause of syncope is usually evident after a careful history and physical exam. Identification of cardiac causes is critical because they portend a poor prognosis (1-year mortality 18–33%). Syncope with chest pain mandates that aortic dissection, myocardial infarction, and pulmonary embolism be ruled out.

Focus on preceding events and witness description. Position prior to syncope is a useful insight (e.g., standing versus sitting versus lying). Syncope with exertion suggests aortic stenosis, hypertrophic obstructive cardiomyopathy, or bradycardia. Events after the syncope are also important, such as confusion, lethargy, headache or neurological symptoms, which suggest a seizure.

Consider syncope as the cause of unexplained trauma (e.g., hip fracture, MVA).

CLINICAL FINDINGS

Neurally mediated hypotension Also known as vasovagal syncope or common fainting, this phenomenon is autonomic, a paradoxical reflex initiated when ventricular preload is reduced by venous pooling. Syncope is often precipitated by perceived threat, fear, emotional stress, or pain. Premonitory symptoms such as lightheadedness and queasiness usually precede the syncope, and persistent weakness usually follows. If observed, the patient is pale with beads of perspiration on the forehead. There is often yawning, cold hands and feet, and a weak and slow radial pulse. There may be a few seizure-like movements at the time of the faint, but no loss of bowel or bladder function occurs. Syncope may occur with micturition, cough, Valsalva, ocular stimulation, or heat-induced vasodilatation.

Syncope

Volume depletion   Lightheadedness or syncope occurs on arising to standing, due to diuretics, diarrhea, vomiting, or blood loss. Significant orthostatic vital sign changes will be present.

Cough syncope   Syncope occurs following a severe or protracted cough.

Anemia   Pallor, absence of flushing of the palmar creases with extension of the hand, and orthostatic lightheadedness are clues **(Plate 188).**

Autonomic insufficiency   Syncope follows exertion. The heart rate fails to increase with a decrease in blood pressure. Other autonomic findings such as pupillary unreactiveness, urinary incontinence, diarrhea, and impotence may be present.

Myocardial infarction   The episode is often preceded by an unstable angina pattern of increasing frequency of chest pressure and decreasing level of activity required to precipitate it. The pain is deep, heavy, and substernal with radiation into the left shoulder, neck, or arm. Lightheadedness and syncope are associated with diaphoresis and low blood pressure.

Pulmonary embolism   Syncope may be a presenting sign of massive pulmonary embolism. Look for associated signs of pleuritic chest pain, acute dyspnea, hemoptysis, and leg swelling **(Plate 42).**

Aortic stenosis   Signs of hemodynamic significance include a low volume and delayed carotid upstroke (pulsus parvus et tardus), a long and loud murmur that travels through the second heart sound and is located at the upper right sternal border with radiation into the neck, and an absence of A2.

Hypertrophic obstructive cardiomyopathy   A systolic murmur increases dramatically in intensity with standing.

Aortic dissection   There is sudden onset of maximally severe tearing pain, which travels in location with the progression of the dissection and often radiates between the shoulder blades. The patient will often appear quite restless and be constantly in motion in an attempt to find a comfortable position. Asymmetry of pulses is a critical clue. Blood pressure may be normal in the presence of gray cyanosis. There is often a history of hypertension, blunt chest trauma, or Marfan's **(Plates 43, 44, 45).**

Cardiac tamponade   Tamponade is marked by muffled heart sounds or pericardial friction rub, pulsus paradoxus, and a narrow pulse pressure.

Left atrial myxoma   A variable diastolic murmur and the presence of systemic emboli are clues to this rare condition.

Complete heart block   This usually manifests as a slow yet strong pulse, with cannon a waves observed in the jugular veins. Survey for AV nodal blocking drugs.

Sick sinus syndrome   Syncope usually occurs with prolonged sinus pauses of 8–10 seconds.

Tachyarrhythmia   Syncope is precipitated by rates greater than 180 per minute, as seen in AV node reentry or bypass tract. Palpitations are often reported, and syncope may occur when the patient is supine.

Carotid sinus hypersensitivity   With a hypersensitive carotid sinus, carotid massage will produce a long period of asystole. Symptoms may occur with wearing a tight collar or turning the head and may be aggravated by digoxin.

Vertebrobasilar ischemia   Dizziness or vertigo, numbness of the ipsilateral face and contralateral limbs, diplopia, dysarthria, and dysphagia occur. Actual syncope is unusual.

Hypoglycemia   Syncope is gradual in onset, with early restlessness, confusion, and anxiety. Low glucose tends to cause an altered level of consciousness rather than complete syncope.

Unwitnessed seizure   Seizure can be recognized by an aura, postictal symptoms, tongue biting, and incontinence.

Subclavian steal syndrome   Syncope and basilar neurological symptoms begin following arm exercise. There will be a blood pressure differential between the arms and a subclavian bruit.

Hyperventilation   There is a smothering feeling along with perioral or acral paresthesias. Tetany occasionally occurs.

Hysterical faint   A dramatic and graceful faint to the floor or couch occurs with an audience present, and the patient describes the episode in an emotionally detached manner ("la belle indifférence"). Nausea, diaphoresis, and pallor will be absent.

Tremor/Involuntary Movements

PLATES 2, 6, 19, 20, 108, 119, 127, 128, 132

 DIFFERENTIAL OVERVIEW

Tremor
- ❏ Anxiety
- ❏ Physiologic tremor
- ❏ Essential tremor
- ❏ Parkinson's disease
- ❏ Cerebellar disease
- ❏ Hyperthyroidism
- ❏ Opiate withdrawal
- ❏ Myoclonus
- ❏ Multiple sclerosis
- ❏ Amyotrophic lateral sclerosis

Involuntary Movements
- ❏ Tics
- ❏ Drugs
- ❏ Systemic lupus erythematosus
- ❏ Rheumatic fever
- ❏ Chorea gravidarum
- ❏ Huntington's disease
- ❏ Tourette's syndrome
- ❏ Wilson's disease

DIAGNOSTIC APPROACH

A *postural tremor* is characterized by fine regular movement of the fingers or hands with the arms outstretched. It is not present at complete rest. Anxiety, benign essential tremor, hyperthyroidism, or medications (alcohol, caffeine, lithium, beta agonists, or phenytoin) may cause it. Proximal postural tremors involving the shoulder, pelvis, and neck are due to cerebellar lesions.

An *intention or action tremor*, characterized by irregular jerking brought out by movement, can be caused by cerebellar disorders such as multiple sclerosis and alcoholic or paraneoplastic cerebellar degeneration (lung or ovarian cancer). Hereditary ataxias also follow this pattern.

A *rest tremor* occurs with Parkinson's disease, phenothiazines, severe essential tremor, Wilson's disease, mercury poisoning, and general paresis.

Choreiform movements are brief, irregular, jerky, nonrhythmic muscle contractions. *Ballismus* is a large amplitude jerk that produces flinging of the limb. It is commonly unilateral (hemiballismus). *Athetosis* is a continuous, sinuous, writhing movement of the digits, limbs, trunk, face, or tongue. Dystonia is a slow, involuntary twisting spasm. *Tics* are patterned coordinated movements that appear suddenly and intermittently.

CLINICAL FINDINGS

Anxiety A psychological stimulus is evident. It is accompanied by sweating, tachycardia, and diarrhea.

Physiologic tremor This occurs as a fine tremor with a frequency of 8–12 Hz and is most noticeable while the patient is holding a fixed position. It may be increased by anxiety, caffeine, lithium, or tricyclic antidepressants.

Essential tremor Absent at rest and clearly present in the outstretched arms, it is accentuated by tasks requiring precision (e.g., writing) and alleviated by alcohol. Handwriting is therefore large and irregular, and the patient may have difficulty drinking from a cup. Essential tremor is of greater amplitude and slower frequency than physiologic tremor. A head tremor and quavering voice may develop. A family history and gradual progression are usually present.

Tremor/Involuntary Movements

Parkinson's disease   It is marked by a rest tremor in a relaxed supported limb, which diminishes with use. The "pill-rolling" tremor of thumb and index finger occurs at a frequency of 3–8 Hz. The tremor does not occur in isolation but is accompanied by cogwheel rigidity, bradykinesia, masked facies, stooped posture, micrographia, retropulsion with standing, and decreased voice volume.

Cerebellar disease   As the limb approaches the target, the tremor progressively increases in amplitude. It is multiplanar, large, slow (2–4 Hz), and worsened by alcohol. It may be found in multiple sclerosis, cerebellar infarction, degenerative disorders of the spinocerebellar pathways, and polyneuropathy.

Hyperthyroidism   A fine tremor of the outstretched fingers is associated with other signs of hyperthyroidism (lid lag, tachycardia, silky skin) **(Plates 19, 20).**

Opiate withdrawal   Tremor will be present in the hands, lips, and tongue. There will be a history of opiate use and often confusion or delirium.

Myoclonus   It appears as brief, lightning-like muscular jerks. Asterixis is a form of this tremor, characterized by a rhythmic flapping of the hands at full extension. This is characteristic of metabolic disorders such as hepatic or uremic encephalopathy.

Multiple sclerosis   Charcot's triad of intention tremor, nystagmus, and scanning speech is a classic presentation. Optic neuritis or atrophy and internuclear ophthalmoplegia are clues **(Plates 119, 127, 128).**

Amyotrophic lateral sclerosis   Early in the disease there is a subacute onset of asymmetric weakness, with visible atrophy and fasciculations. The tongue will appear twitching, scalloped, and atrophic. Corticospinal tract involvement will produce an upgoing plantar reflex (Babinski sign) **(Plate 132).**

Tics   These are usually benign although it is often difficult to distinguish pathologic causes. Eye blinking and facial grimaces are common manifestations.

Drugs   Phenothiazines and levodopa may produce dystonia or chorea, such as an acute dystonic reaction with neck torsion. Long-term use may also produce tardive dyskinesia, with lip smacking and tongue protrusion **(Plate 91).**

Systemic lupus erythematosus   Chorea occurs with cerebral arteritis. Malar rash, serositis, arthritis, and fever are clues to the underlying diagnosis.

Rheumatic fever   Sydenham's chorea occurs in children and young adults in the context of rheumatic fever, recognized by the syndrome of fever, arthritis, carditis, pharyngitis, and erythema marginatum. Movements of the face, tongue, and extremities are absent at rest and exaggerated by movement. Fluctuation of grip strength is characteristic. Hypotonia is present. Speech and swallowing may be distorted **(Plate 108).**

Chorea gravidarum   It occurs in pregnant women who have a history of rheumatic fever **(Plate 108).**

Huntington's disease   A slowly progressive chorea of dominant inheritance, it appears after age 40. An associated manifestation is mental deterioration with delusions.

Tourette's syndrome   Motor and vocal tics, including coprolalia (swearing), are essential and distinctive features.

Wilson's disease   The tremor will be flapping or wing-beating, with coarse to-and-fro movements, flexing and extending the wrist. It may appear like Parkinson's, but it occurs in young adults and is accompanied by cirrhosis and a golden iridic (Kayser-Fleischer) ring **(Plates 2, 6).**

Section VIII

Skin

Dyspigmentation

◼ DIFFERENTIAL OVERVIEW

Hyperpigmentation
❏ Chloasma
❏ Drugs
❏ Cafe-au-lait
❏ Heavy metals
❏ Addison's disease
❏ Ectopic ACTH syndrome
❏ Hemochromatosis
❏ Porphyria cutanea tarda
❏ Pellagra
❏ Whipple's disease
❏ Biliary cirrhosis
❏ Metastatic melanoma

Hypopigmentation
❏ Tinea versicolor
❏ Postinflammatory
❏ Chemical
❏ Vitiligo
❏ Piebaldism
❏ Tuberous sclerosis

CLINICAL FINDINGS

Chloasma   A mask-like brown pigmentation develops during pregnancy or with oral contraceptives.

Drugs   Busulfan, cyclophosphamide, and arsenic can induce melanin formation. Arsenic produces a "raindrop" appearance and hyperkeratosis of the palms. Long-term chlorpromazine, minocycline, or amiodarone can produce blue-gray discoloration in sun-exposed skin and conjunctivae. Chloroquine complexes with melanin to produce a gray to blue-black discoloration of the shins, face, and hard palate **(Plate 5)**.

Cafe-au-lait   Lesions are 0.5–12 cm in diameter, flat, uniformly brown, and have an irregular border like a coastal map. Patients with type I neurofibromatosis usually have 6 or more spots, with associated findings of axillary freckling, pigmented iris hamartomas (Lisch nodules), and flesh-colored neurofibromas **(Plate 121, 122)**.

Heavy metals   Gold (chrysiasis) produces a brown to blue-gray discoloration, accentuated in sun-exposed areas, which may also deposit in the sclera. Silver (argyria) produces a blue-gray color. Heavy metals do not cause mucosal hyperpigmentation.

Addison's disease   Diffuse hyperpigmentation is found, with accentuation in the palmar and plantar creases, oral mucosa, and around scars **(Plates 12, 13)**.

Ectopic ACTH syndrome   Hyperpigmentation develops in association with medullary carcinoma of the thyroid and small cell carcinoma of the lung.

Hemochromatosis   The skin becomes a bronze color, in patients with diabetes, congestive heart failure, or liver dysfunction **(Plate 65)**.

Porphyria cutanea tarda   Hyperpigmentation occurs in sun-exposed areas and is associated with vesicles and erosions **(Plate 193)**.

Pellagra   A dirty brownish discoloration, with a varnish-like scale, develops in sun-exposed areas **(Plate 67)**.

Whipple's disease   Generalized hyperpigmentation is associated with diarrhea, weight loss, arthritis, and lymphadenopathy.

Biliary cirrhosis   Photoaccentuated, dark brown skin is associated with pervasive pruritus, jaundice, and tendon xanthomas **(Plates 48, 66)**.

Metastatic melanoma   Slate-blue color and black urine occasionally develop with advanced disease.

Tinea versicolor   Patches are sprinkled over the trunk like snow, appearing hypopig-

231

mented compared with melanotic skin. Wood's lamp examination reveals a golden flu-orescence **(Plate 197).**

Postinflammatory   Hypopigmentation occurs following a dermatitis and in active discoid lupus lesions **(Plate 93).**

Chemical   Hypopigmentation usually begins on the hands and is a result of contact with phenols, rubber derivatives, or germicides.

Vitiligo   Symmetric areas of complete pigment loss appear around orifices and on flexor and extensor surfaces. Other autoimmune diseases are often present, such as pernicious anemia, thyroid disease, or Addison's disease.

Piebaldism   Congenital hypopigmentation of the trunk and midextremities, with a white forelock, is characteristic.

Tuberous sclerosis   An ash leaf spot measuring 1–3 cm in size is present at birth. Other findings include adenoma sebaceum adjacent to the nasal alae and ungual fibromas **(Plates 124, 125, 126).**

Exanthem

◼ DIFFERENTIAL OVERVIEW

Central
- ❏ Drug eruption
- ❏ Pityriasis rosea
- ❏ Epstein-Barr virus
- ❏ Varicella
- ❏ Rubeola
- ❏ Rubella
- ❏ Erythema infectiosum
- ❏ Ehrlichiosis
- ❏ Meningococcemia
- ❏ Typhoid fever

Peripheral
- ❏ Erythema multiforme
- ❏ Rocky Mountain Spotted Fever
- ❏ Acute HIV
- ❏ Secondary syphilis

Confluent Erythema/Desquamation
- ❏ Scarlet fever
- ❏ Toxic shock syndrome

DIAGNOSTIC APPROACH

Erythematous macules and papules are morbilliform, usually due to drugs or viral infection. Blanching erythema is scarlatiniform.

CLINICAL FINDINGS

Drug eruption   Morbilliform eruptions occur in at least 5% of patients receiving penicillins, sulfonamides, captopril, phenytoin, or gold. Associated signs include fever, pruritus, and transient lymphadenopathy **(Plate 182).**

Pityriasis rosea   Oval, salmon-colored macules with a collarette of scale are distributed in a fir-tree pattern on the trunk **(Plate 196).**

Epstein-Barr virus   A maculopapular rash develops with the use of ampicillin in a patient with typical signs of infectious mononucleosis, i.e., fever, severe fatigue, exudative pharyngitis, anterior and posterior cervical adenopathy, and splenomegaly **(Plates 229, 230).**

Varicella   Crops of maculopapules evolve into erythematous vesicles and then crust. The hallmark of varicella infection is lesions in various stages of evolution. The patient has a low-grade fever and malaise **(Plate 140).**

Rubeola   Measles has a prodrome of coryza, cough, and conjunctivitis. Koplik's spots (1–2 mm white specks surrounded by an erythematous halo on the buccal mucosa opposite the molars) occur at the time of a second fever spike. The rash begins at the hairline and spreads downward, occurring as small pink macules that become confluent, then brown, then desquamate **(Plate 136).**

Rubella   German measles begins with faint pink macules on the forehead and face, which spread downward. The rash is associated with postauricular and posterior cervical lymphadenopathy and prominent arthralgias **(Plate 137).**

Erythema infectiosum   Fifth disease, a Parvovirus infection, is characterized by erythema on the cheeks ("slapped cheeks"), followed by a reticular pattern on the extremities **(Plate 138).**

Ehrlichiosis   This is manifest as abrupt-onset of fever, chills, headache, and a maculopapular or petechial rash following a tick bite.

Meningococcemia   A macular rash may occur early in the course before the rapid development of angular purpura (purpura fulminans), meningeal signs, and vascular collapse **(Plate 32).**

233

Exanthem

Typhoid fever   An evanescent macular blanching rose spot may appear on the trunk of a patient and is associated with prominent and prolonged fever, hepatosplenomegaly, and relative bradycardia **(Plate 60).**

Erythema multiforme   Violaceous red discs with cyanotic or blistering centers, called iris/target lesions, develop on the extensor surfaces and mucous membranes. Fever and lymphadenopathy are also prominent. Precipitants include viruses (e.g., HSV), streptococcal infections, deep mycoses, drugs (sulfonamides, salicylates, tetracyclines, antirheumatics), and connective tissue diseases (e.g., lupus) **(Plate 181).**

Rocky Mountain Spotted Fever   There is a sudden onset of severe headache, rigors, prostration, deep myalgias, and high fever (as high as 104°) following a tick bite. Irregular pink macules begin on the palms and soles, spreading centrally and becoming deeper red and maculopapular over 2–3 days. Conjunctival petechiae and splenomegaly are frequently found **(Plate 139).**

Acute HIV   A maculopapular rash occurs along with fever, chills, arthralgias, myalgias, abdominal cramps, diarrhea, and/or aseptic meningitis. The rash may be present on the palms or soles and have desquamation or a hemorrhagic/necrotic center. It begins 3–6 weeks after exposure and lasts 2–3 weeks. An exposure history (blood transfusion, sexual contact, shared needle) within the right time frame is key.

Secondary syphilis   A maculopapular rash may occur in early secondary syphilis, followed by a papulosquamous ("copper penny") eruption that often involves the palms and soles. The primary chancre may still be present in 15%. An aseptic meningitis picture as well as findings of generalized lymphadenopathy (including a characteristic epitrochlear node) and painless silver-grey mucosal erosions on the glans, vulva, and mouth are useful clues **(Plate 80).**

Scarlet fever   In the setting of acute pharyngitis, a diffuse erythema develops, beginning on the neck and upper trunk with red perifollicular puncta. Associated findings include a white-coated tongue with red papilla (white strawberry tongue), palatine petechiae, facial flush with circumoral pallor, and linear petechiae in the anticubital fossa. Desquamation of the palms and soles occurs 5–20 days later **(Plates 142, 143).**

Toxic shock syndrome   Produced by a staph or strep exotoxin, or a staph endotoxin, clinical manifestations are fever; diffuse erythema; hypotension; hyperemia of the mucous membranes of the vagina, oropharynx, and conjunctivae; multiorgan dysfunction; and desquamation within 1–2 weeks **(Plate 144).**

DIFFERENTIAL OVERVIEW

❏ Menopause
❏ Alcohol/toxic
❏ Rosacea
❏ Palmar erythema
❏ Niacin
❏ Monosodium glutamate
❏ Carcinoid
❏ Pheochromocytoma
❏ Toxic shock syndrome
❏ Medullary thyroid carcinoma
❏ Scombroid
❏ Mastocytosis

DIAGNOSTIC APPROACH

Approximately 5% of cases of new-onset flushing will be caused by carcinoid and are therefore identifiable by associated findings. The carcinoid syndrome with flushing will occur in 30–60% of cases of small bowel carcinoid but only rarely (<5% of cases) in bronchial or appendix carcinoid.

CLINICAL FINDINGS

Menopause   "Hot flashes" may occur spontaneously or may be brought on by hot drinks, alcohol, or emotional upset. Representing a sudden triggering of the cutaneous heat loss mechanism, these flashes often cause profuse perspiration.

Alcohol/toxic   Flushing may occur with alcohol alone—probably caused by acetaldehyde accumulation—in Asians, Eskimos, and American Indians. A disulfiram reaction of flushing, nausea, tachycardia, and dyspnea may occur on alcohol ingestion and has also been reported with use of metronidazole, chlorpropamide, griseofulvin, quinacrine, and some cephalosporins. Occupational exposure to organic solvents such as chloroethylene, carbon disulfide, and dimethylformamide can also cause flushing with dizziness upon ingestion of alcohol.

Rosacea   Hereditary predisposition to flushing with alcohol, spicy foods, or heat leads over time to the development of facial telangiectasias and red papules.

Palmar erythema   Localized flushing in the palm is associated with pregnancy, liver disease, thyrotoxicosis, rheumatoid arthritis, high output states, and pancreatic cancer **(Plate 117)**.

Niacin   Flushing of the face and upper trunk occurs when plasma niacin levels rapidly rise. It may be prevented by aspirin; thus, flushing is presumed to be prostaglandin-mediated.

Monosodium glutamate   Food containing MSG produces transient flushing associated with tightness and pressure in the head, neck, and upper torso; headaches; and drowsiness.

Carcinoid   The carcinoid syndrome consists of flushing (often a violaceous hue), diarrhea, tachycardia, hypotension, and wheezing. A small bowel carcinoid can cause right-sided valvular thickening leading to tricuspid insufficiency or pulmonic stenosis. Left-sided valvular heart disease may develop with a bronchial carcinoid. The flush may be provoked by alcohol as well as foods rich in tyramine such as red wine and cheeses **(Plate 4)**.

Pheochromocytoma   Flushing is associated with paroxysmally high blood pressure and fainting.

Toxic shock syndrome   This is marked by diffuse erythema of the skin, mucous membranes, and conjunctivae, along with fever and hypotension, caused by a staph or strep exotoxin **(Plate 144)**.

235

Medullary thyroid carcinoma   Paroxysmal flushing is mediated by calcitonin.

Scombroid   After eating fresh tuna or bonito, the body and conjunctivae flush profusely, and headache, dizziness, nausea, and burning in the mouth develop.

Mastocytosis   It presents similarly to carcinoid but has dermatographism and splenomegaly **(Plate 186).**

Chapter 116

Hair Loss/Growth

◼ DIFFERENTIAL OVERVIEW

Alopecia
- ❏ Androgenetic
- ❏ Telogen effluvium
- ❏ Drugs/hair loss
- ❏ Anagen effluvium
- ❏ Alopecia areata
- ❏ Tinea capitis
- ❏ Traction
- ❏ Hypothyroidism
- ❏ Seborrheic dermatitis
- ❏ Discoid lupus
- ❏ Systemic lupus erythematosus
- ❏ Lichen planus
- ❏ Scleroderma
- ❏ Dietary deficiency
- ❏ Trichotillomania
- ❏ Syphilis

Hirsutism
- ❏ Idiopathic hirsutism
- ❏ Drugs/hair growth
- ❏ Hypertrichosis
- ❏ Hyperprolactinemia
- ❏ Polycystic ovary disease
- ❏ Cushing's syndrome
- ❏ Adrenal tumor
- ❏ Ovarian tumor
- ❏ Ovarian hyperthecosis

DIAGNOSTIC APPROACH

Nonscarring alopecia includes androgenetic, telogen effluvium, trichotillomania, traction, aerata, and syphilis. *Scarring* alopecia is characterized by fibrosis and inflammation and loss of follicles, occurring with inflammatory dermatoses, deep infections, neoplasms, burns, and genodermatoses. Broken hair shafts are seen in fungal infections, traction, and trichotillomania.

Most hirsutism is familial. If a woman with hirsutism has normal menses, a family history of hirsutism, no virilization, and gradual onset, no further evaluation is needed.

Androgen effects are more commonly defeminization with amenorrhea, decrease in breast size, or loss of female body contours than virilization. Other signs include acne, increased libido, clitoromegaly, temporal hair loss, deepened voice, and increased muscle mass. Acute onset of hirsutism/virilization suggests an androgen-producing adrenal or ovarian tumor or exogenous androgen ingestion.

CLINICAL FINDINGS

Androgenetic A typical pattern is a frontoparietal receding hairline or diffuse thinning over the crown with retention of frontal hair. In women, it may result from pathologic androgen excess, accompanied by hirsutism, virilization, or oligomenorrhea. Severe vertex balding (androgenetic) is a marker for cardiovascular risk, with a relative risk of 3.4 of cardiovascular mortality.

Telogen effluvium Diffuse thinning occurs with loss of mature hairs having a club-shaped base. It occurs 2–3 months after an acute illness (especially with fever), rapid weight loss, or pregnancy. A transverse white nail line (Beau's line) may also be seen as nail growth is affected. Hair can be readily pulled out (approximately half of those grasped).

Drugs/hair loss Antineoplastic drugs, heparin, warfarin, allopurinol, propylthiouracil, vitamin A, quinine, lithium, beta-blockers, colchicine, amphetamines, and thallium have all been associated with hair loss.

Hair Loss/Growth Chapter 116

Anagen effluvium   This is typical with chemotherapy (daunorubicin, fluorouracil, and cyclophosphamide) or heavy metal toxicity. The hair loss pattern may be diffuse and moth-eaten or complete. There is tapered narrowing of the hair fiber with breakage, producing diagnostic "arrow ends."

Alopecia areata   The hair is completely lost in a circumscribed circular patch without inflammation or scar, with "exclamation point" hairs at the edge. Remaining hairs within the patch are depigmented. Nail pitting occurs. A family or personal history of autoimmune disease is often found, with concurrent vitiligo or hypothyroidism being the most common.

Tinea capitis   The alopecia/rash typically has a raised erythematous border with a clear center. The area will fluoresce on examination with a Wood's lamp. The appearance may also vary from discrete patches with "black dots" (broken hairs) to a boggy plaque with pustules (kerion).

Traction   Patterned hair loss accompanies the use of tight braids or rollers. Hairs are short and broken.

Hypothyroidism   The hair becomes coarse, brittle, and diffusely thin, with thinning of the lateral eyebrows **(Plates 16, 18).**

Seborrheic dermatitis   Hair loss occurs with scaling and weeping, and there will be patches behind the ears, in the nasolabial fold, in the eyebrows, and on the midchest.

Discoid lupus   Scarring is seen in the bald patches. Follicles are absent **(Plate 93).**

Systemic lupus erythematosus   Nonscarring alopecia occurs with erythema, scaling, and broken hairs, often localized to the frontal scalp as short "lupus hairs" **(Plate 91).**

Lichen planus   Scarring alopecia is associated with white lace on the buccal mucosa and violet, flat-topped papules on the wrists.

Scleroderma   This appears as a linear forehead scar with a violaceous edge ("coup de sabre") **(Plate 99).**

Dietary deficiency   Zinc, biotin, iron, and protein deficiency can each cause diffuse hair loss **(Plate 189).**

Trichotillomania   Typically it appears as a "tonsure" pattern with a rim of hair around the edges of the scalp. Hair shafts are twisted and broken.

Syphilis   "Moth-eaten" alopecia appears as scattered, poorly circumscribed patches in 20% of cases of secondary syphilis. It is accompanied by fever, sore throat, and adenopathy **(Plate 81).**

Idiopathic hirsutism   A familial trait, in young adult women, 25% have noticeable facial hair, 33% have hair along the linea alba (male escutcheon), and 17% have periareolar hair. Weight gain can accelerate hirsutism. Menopause increases terminal hair growth on the face.

Drugs/hair growth   Oral contraceptives with androgenic progestins, phenytoin, minoxidil, diazoxide, penicillamine, glucocorticoids, and exogenous anabolic steroids in female athletes all cause hirsutism.

Hypertrichosis   Hair is vellus (fine, downy) and grows evenly over the body, not just in androgen-responsive areas. Causes include anorexia nervosa, hypothyroidism, dermatomyositis, porphyria cutanea tarda, malnutrition, and drugs.

Hyperprolactinemia   Galactorrhea and amenorrhea are the principal symptoms, but 25% also have hirsutism. Drugs that cause hyperprolactinemia can also cause hirsutism, including metoclopramide, methyldopa, phenothiazines, thioxanthenes, reserpine, estrogens, and opiates **(Plate 15).**

Polycystic ovary disease   This presents with peripubertal onset of hair growth, menstrual irregularities, obesity and infertility. Ovaries are usually enlarged (2–5 times normal size) and cystic, but may be normal sized.

Cushing's syndrome   Hirsutism occurs in 80% of cases, and is characteristically vellus, on the face and shoulders. Cardinal features of Cushing's are hypertension, central obesity, moon facies, striae, proximal muscle weakness, and abundant, easy bruising. Virilization along with the hirsutism suggests an adrenocortical carcinoma **(Plates 10, 11).**

Adrenal tumor   There may be a palpable abdominal mass.

Ovarian tumor   Most cases have a palpable adnexal mass.

Ovarian hyperthecosis   Hirsutism is found in association with acanthosis nigricans and insulin resistance.

Chapter 117

Leg Ulcer

◼ DIFFERENTIAL OVERVIEW

- ❏ Venous insufficiency
- ❏ Arterial insufficiency
- ❏ Diabetes/neuropathy
- ❏ Decubitus
- ❏ Hypertension
- ❏ Squamous cell cancer
- ❏ Carbuncle
- ❏ Vasculitis
- ❏ Pyoderma gangrenosum
- ❏ Syphilis
- ❏ Fistula
- ❏ Blood disorders
- ❏ Brown recluse spider bite

DIAGNOSTIC APPROACH

Painful necrosis in a cold foot is a result of ischemia. Painless necrosis at a pressure area (MTP heads, heels, toes) is caused by neuropathy.

In a young patient with ischemic leg ulcers, hemoglobinopathy and hereditary spherocytosis need to be considered.

Ulcerations of the fingertips can be caused by Raynaud's syndrome, especially in scleroderma, and by ergots or bleomycin **(Plate 36)**.

CLINICAL FINDINGS

Venous insufficiency   Varicosities, "flare sign" with a splay of venules, chronic edema, and brownish hyperpigmentation are present. Stasis ulcers occur most frequently above the medial malleolus where the vascular supply is poor. The ulcer base has granulation tissue with a yellow-green exudate **(Plate 151)**.

Arterial insufficiency   The leg is pale and cool, with diminished or absent pulses, hairless atrophic skin, and dystrophic nails. Ischemic ulcers most often occur on the sides of the feet, heels, toes, and nailbeds. Claudication, or rest pain diminished by dangling the feet, is present **(Plates 25, 152)**.

Diabetes/neuropathy   Ulcers develop from the combination of peripheral neuropathy predisposing to trauma and vascular insufficiency leading to poor healing. Punched-out ulcerations on the sole of the foot are common—especially under the metatarsal heads **(Plates 153, 166)**.

Decubitus   Ulcers occur in bedridden or semiambulatory patients over bony prominences, such as the malleolus or heel.

Hypertension   Painful, blue-red plaques with a purpuric halo progress to ulcers. They appear most often over the lateral malleolus **(Plate 37)**.

Squamous cell cancer   The edges of the ulcer are irregular, everted, and hard **(Plate 165)**.

Carbuncle   It begins as a red pustule; then the center ulcerates, with purulent drainage.

Vasculitis   Ulcers begin as palpable purpura or hemorrhagic vesicles, which progress to painful ulcers, surrounded by livedo reticularis. The ulcers heal slowly. Usual causes include lupus, with antiphospholipid syndrome, scleroderma, or cryoglobulinemia **(Plates 34, 97, 110)**.

Pyoderma gangrenosum   A central purplish area is surrounded by an intense erythema with exquisite tenderness. When the central zone sloughs, there is an ulcer with a characteristic violet undermined edge, a ragged and heaped-up border, and surrounding halo. Inflammatory bowel disease is the underlying diagnosis in more than 50%. Other causes include chronic active hepatitis B, rheumatoid arthritis, chronic myelogenous leukemia, polycythemia vera, and myeloma **(Plate 58)**.

Syphilis   A chancre is painless with oval, sloping edges and bloodstained discharge. The

239

ulcer is painless and hard to palpation. If on the leg, it will occur on the proximal thigh from contiguous spread **(Plate 79).**

Fistula   Exuberant granulation tissue around the orifice indicates a foreign body or bone infection.

Blood disorders   Ulcers occur in sickle cell anemia, polycythemia vera, dysproteinemia, leukemia, and thalassemia **(Plate 26).**

Brown recluse spider bite   A bite develops a necrotic center and then ulcerates **(Plate 149).**

◼ DIFFERENTIAL OVERVIEW

Pigmented
- ❏ Nevus
- ❏ Seborrheic keratosis
- ❏ Atypical nevi
- ❏ Melanoma

Colorful
- ❏ Cherry angioma
- ❏ Basal cell carcinoma
- ❏ Erythema nodosum
- ❏ Lichen planus
- ❏ Xanthoma
- ❏ Kaposi's sarcoma
- ❏ Sarcoidosis
- ❏ Blue nevus
- ❏ Amyloidosis
- ❏ Lymphoma cutis
- ❏ Polyarteritis nodosa
- ❏ Bacillary angiomatosis
- ❏ Sweet's syndrome
- ❏ Bowen's disease
- ❏ Cutaneous tuberculosis

Non-pigmented
- ❏ Epidermoid inclusion cyst
- ❏ Lipoma
- ❏ Acrochordon
- ❏ Dermatofibroma
- ❏ Ganglion cyst
- ❏ Verruca vulgaris
- ❏ Molluscum contagiosum
- ❏ Milia
- ❏ Rheumatoid nodule
- ❏ Tophus
- ❏ Squamous cell carcinoma
- ❏ Keratoacanthoma
- ❏ Neurofibroma
- ❏ Neuroma
- ❏ Cutaneous metastasis
- ❏ Calcinosis cutis
- ❏ Adenoma sebaceum

DIAGNOSTIC APPROACH

Violaceous papules and plaques occur in cutaneous sarcoidosis, lymphocytoma cutis, and cutaneous lupus. When in a linear array, sporotrichosis and Mycobacterium marinum should be suspected.

Findings useful in differentiating atypical from benign nevi are as follows:

Papules/Nodules

Finding	Atypical Nevi	Benign Nevi
Color	Variable mix of tan, brown, red, pink Look different nevus to nevus	Uniformly tan or brown
Shape	Irregular borders, pigment bleeds into surrounding skin	Round, sharp, crisp borders Flat or elevated
Size	>6 mm, may be >10 mm	<6 mm
Number	Often numerous (>100)	10–40 scattered over body
Location	Sun-exposed areas, especially back	Sun-exposed areas above waist, not scalp, breast, buttocks

CLINICAL FINDINGS

Nevus Uniformly round brown lesions, they are either flat or raised, with smooth borders.

Seborrheic keratosis Typically, they are brown plaques with a "stuck-on" appearance and a rough, greasy surface. A sudden increase in number with inflammation may be seen in association with internal malignancy (Leser-Trelat syndrome).

Atypical nevi Larger than common moles, these nevi have borders that are irregular and ill-defined. The color is variegated, tan to dark brown, often on a pink background. Atypical nevi are at increased risk for subsequently developing into melanoma (**Plate 163**).

Melanoma Hallmarks are an irregular border that sometimes has a notch and variegation in color and pigmentation pattern. The background color is usually jet black instead of brown. Admixed red, blue, gray, pink, and purple colors help to differentiate them from benign nevi. A previous blistering sunburn (episodic intense sun exposure), red hair with fair skin, and a family history of melanoma are important risk factors (**Plate 160**).

Cherry angioma They are small, red-purple, and round.

Basal cell carcinoma It appears as a translucent papule with fine superficial telangiectasias. As it enlarges, it may ulcerate in the center. It occurs in sun-exposed areas in individuals who spend time outdoors, such as farmers and sailors (**Plate 164**).

Erythema nodosum Lesions are initially red, but they may become blue as they resolve. They occur primarily over the shins and are tender to touch. There may be systemic symptoms, such as fever and arthralgias, even without underlying disease. Associated conditions include sarcoidosis, streptococcal and upper respiratory infections, inflammatory bowel disease, tuberculosis, drugs (oral contraceptives, sulfonamides, aspartame, and iodides), cat-scratch fever, and infectious diarrhea (**Plate 171**).

Lichen planus They are lilac pink, flat-topped, shiny polygonal papules on the flexor surfaces. Fine white lines traverse them (Wickham's striae).

Xanthoma Eruptive xanthomas are crops of yellow papules with an erythematous halo over the buttock or extensor surfaces, occurring in hypertriglyceridemia, as in uncontrolled diabetes. Tendon xanthomas occur on the Achilles and finger extensor tendon surfaces, in conjunction with hypercholesterolemia (**Plates 47, 48, 66**).

Kaposi's sarcoma These purple, nodular lesions occur in patients with HIV infection (**Plate 200**).

Sarcoidosis Lesions are red-brown, waxy papules or deeply indurated lesions (lupus pernio). Typical locations are periorbital, nose, mouth, and scalp. Additional findings include prominent lymphadenopathy, scarring alopecia, and parotid or lacrimal gland enlargement (**Plates 169, 170**).

Blue nevus These dome-shaped lesions commonly occur on the backs of the hands.

Amyloidosis Pink translucent lesions, especially in the periorbital and perioral regions, occur in primary amyloidosis. "Pinch purpura" and macroglossia may also be found (**Plates 131, 157**).

Lymphoma cutis Lesions are infiltrated pink to red-purple papules and plaques and are sometimes arcuate. They occur most often in non-Hodgkin's lymphoma and may precede the diagnosis (**Plate 159**).

Polyarteritis nodosa Painful subcutaneous nodules and ulcers arise within an area of red-purple reticular pattern.

Bacillary angiomatosis Multiple red, hemangioma-like lesions uncommonly occur in an HIV-positive patient **(Plate 199).**

Sweet's syndrome Painful red to red-brown plaques and nodules appear on the head, neck, and upper extremities. Of these, 10% are associated with cancer, most commonly acute myelogenous leukemia **(Plate 158).**

Bowen's disease Lesions develop as a chronic, nonhealing, slowly enlarging erythematous patch with a sharp but irregular outline, representing squamous cell carcinoma in situ.

Cutaneous tuberculosis It develops as a red-brown plaque on the face, with a yellow-brown color on diascopy. There is active tuberculosis elsewhere, usually pulmonary **(Plate 175).**

Epidermoid inclusion cyst Mobile, rubbery, and compressible, it has a central pore. Multiple cysts on the face occurring at an early age suggest Gardner's syndrome.

Lipoma It feels soft, mobile, and lobulated and has indistinct borders. The lobulation can be felt when the lesion is compressed between the thumb and forefinger of one hand while the surface is stroked with the other.

Acrochordon A skin tag is a soft, pedunculated lesion at the flexor surface, especially in the neck, axilla, and groin.

Dermatofibroma It is a firm, skin-colored to brownish (due to hemosiderin) nodule less than 1 cm in diameter. The lesion retracts below the surface with lateral pressure (dimple sign).

Ganglion cyst Adjacent to a synovial joint, especially on the volar wrist, the lump is fixed and firmly compressible and feels cystic.

Verruca vulgaris The top is rough and irregular. Skin lines are disrupted as they pass through the lesion. There may be small black dots, representing thrombosed capillaries.

Molluscum contagiosum Multiple, 2–5 mm, pearly flesh-colored nodules with an umbilicated center appear.

Milia Tiny, firm, whitish papules appear primarily on the face.

Rheumatoid nodule Nodules appear over pressure points in 20% of patients with rheumatoid arthritis, 6% with Still's disease, and transiently in rheumatic fever **(Plate 89).**

Tophus This firm nodule around the joints of the hand, on the helix of the ear, or in the olecranon and prepatellar bursa, has a characteristic waxy, yellow appearance when the overlying skin is stretched **(Plate 100).**

Squamous cell carcinoma Arising from an actinic keratosis, it appears as a flesh-colored nodule, which slowly enlarges, ulcerates, and crusts **(Plate 165).**

Keratoacanthoma This dome-shaped, rapidly enlarging nodule with a central keratin plug is often confused with squamous cell cancer.

Neurofibroma These soft papules or nodules exhibit the "button-hole" sign; that is, they invaginate into the skin with pressure, like a hernia. They may be found singly in otherwise healthy patients, but in persons with von Recklinghausen's disease, they appear in association with multiple cafe-au-lait spots and 1-mm yellow-brown Lisch nodules in the iris **(Plate 121).**

Neuroma Multiple papules occur on the eyelids, lips, distal tongue, or oral mucosa in patients with MEN (multiple endocrine neoplasia, type 2b) syndrome.

Cutaneous metastasis Hard nodules usually occur late in the course of malignancy.

Calcinosis cutis This lesion is calcium-hard and may drain chalky contents through ulceration **(Plate 96).**

Adenoma sebaceum Skin-colored papules around the nose are classic for tuberous sclerosis **(Plate 124).**

Patterned Erythema Chapter 119

▨ DIFFERENTIAL OVERVIEW

Figurate
- ❏ Tinea corporis
- ❏ Urticaria
- ❏ Erysipelas
- ❏ Erythema migrans
- ❏ Secondary syphilis
- ❏ Livedo reticularis
- ❏ Erythema multiforme
- ❏ Cutaneous larva migrans
- ❏ Granuloma annulare
- ❏ Erythema marginatum
- ❏ Erythema gyratum repens

Photodistribution
- ❏ Sunburn
- ❏ Drugs
- ❏ Polymorphous light eruption
- ❏ Systemic lupus erythematosus
- ❏ Porphyria cutanea tarda
- ❏ Pellagra

DIAGNOSTIC APPROACH

Sun-exposed areas of the face, the "V" of the neck (but not under the chin), and the dorsum of the hands and feet are common distributions for photodermatitis.

CLINICAL FINDINGS

Tinea corporis   It appears as a slowly expanding lesion with an active, scaling, erythematous border and central clearing.

Urticaria   Transient and migratory, there are well-marginated polycyclic wheals, with raised red serpiginous borders and clear centers. They may merge into extensive wheals **(Plate 183)**.

Erysipelas   A circumscribed crimson area appears on the face with a smooth, shiny appearance, and then it rapidly expands. It is tender and warm to touch, and the patient is febrile **(Plate 180)**.

Erythema migrans   A single annular lesion develops 3–30 days after a bite from a tiny tick. This lesion gradually expands to greater than 10 cm, heralding Lyme disease. Associated symptoms include fever, headache, photophobia, arthralgias, and malar rash **(Plate 106)**.

Secondary syphilis   The most common setting for annular lesions is on the face. They are distinguished by a central hyperpigmentation.

Livedo reticularis   It appears with a lacy pattern of blue-purple on the legs. It is seen with cold exposure and connective tissue diseases (polyarteritis nodosa, lupus, rheumatoid arthritis, and dermatomyositis). A similar pattern in red may be caused by heat (erythema ab igne) **(Plates 31, 35)**.

Erythema multiforme   The pathognomic manifestation is the iris or target lesion, which usually appears on extensor surfaces. Sulfonamides are the classic precipitant although connective tissue disease and infections may also be the cause **(Plate 181)**.

Cutaneous larva migrans   An intensely pruritic, serpiginous, red, raised track advances on the foot of a patient who has acquired an animal hookworm by walking barefoot outdoors **(Plate 177)**.

Granuloma annulare   The border is made of flesh-colored or red-brown papules. It usually occurs on the extremities, but a disseminated form may occur in patients with diabetes.

Erythema marginatum   The classic rash of rheumatic fever consists of pink-red, tran-

Chapter 119

Patterned Erythema

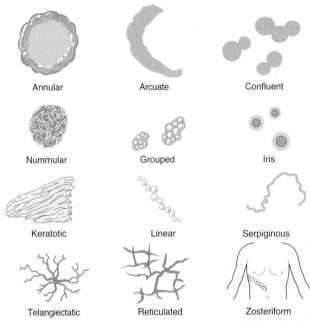

Annular	Arcuate	Confluent
Nummular	Grouped	Iris
Keratotic	Linear	Serpiginous
Telangiectatic	Reticulated	Zosteriform

Figure 18. Descriptors of skin lesions. (Adapted from: Swartz MH. Textbook of Physical Diagnosis. 2nd ed. Philadelphia: W.B. Saunders, 1994, p. 83.)

sient, flat truncal lesions. Associated symptoms such as fever, arthritis, chorea, and congestive heart failure are important clues **(Plate 108)**.

Erythema gyratum repens It consists of mobile concentric arcs and wavefronts resembling wood grain. This is rare but important to recognize because it signals occult internal malignancy **(Plate 72)**.

Sunburn It is readily suspected and its distribution is determined by the lie of the clothing.

Drugs Sulfonamides, tetracyclines, food or medicine coloring agents, phenothiazines, thiazides, sulfonureas, quinolones, and griseofulvin are common causes. The reaction is characterized by a prompt intense burning and erythema, which is more intense than the usual sunburn, followed by desquamation and hyperpigmentation **(Plate 7)**.

Polymorphous light eruption Exquisitely light sensitive, papules and vesicles erupt and coalesce in the spring, but tolerance builds in the summer.

Systemic lupus erythematosus Lupus may begin as an exaggerated sunburn or urticaria with sun exposure. Fever, fatigue, or arthralgias accompany it **(Plate 91)**.

Porphyria cutanea tarda It presents in the third or fourth decade with fragile bullae and erosions on the dorsum of the hands, dark urine (with an orange-red fluorescence under examination using a Wood's lamp when acidified), and mottled periorbital hyperpigmentation. Precipitating factors include alcohol and estrogens **(Plate 193)**.

Pellagra Niacin deficiency is rare, but may occur in alcoholics or patients with a staple diet of corn, presenting as an erythematous, vesicular dermatitis and progressing to an intense hyperpigmentation, desquamation, leathery skin, and a powdery scale in sun-exposed areas **(Plate 67)**.

Pruritus

Chapter 120

PLATES 21, 26, 30, 41, 48, 64, 66, 198

◼ DIFFERENTIAL OVERVIEW

- ❑ Eczema
- ❑ Atopic dermatitis
- ❑ Lichen simplex chronicus
- ❑ Diabetes
- ❑ Environmental
- ❑ Drugs
- ❑ HIV
- ❑ Neoplasm
- ❑ Uremia
- ❑ Psychogenic
- ❑ Cholestatic jaundice
- ❑ Polycythemia vera

DIAGNOSTIC APPROACH

The most pruritic dermatoses are atopic, lichen planus, urticaria, dermatitis herpetiformis, cutaneous T cell lymphoma, and scabies.

In patients with no skin lesions except excoriations, 15% have a systemic disorder such as uremia, cholestasis, lymphoma, or polycythemia vera.

CLINICAL FINDINGS

Eczema   Lesions usually begin with dry skin and pruritus, but soon develop into round crusting/scaling patches. Common locations include extensor surfaces, hands, and the trunk.

Atopic dermatitis   Dry, very itchy skin causes rubbing or scratching, which may cause excoriations and eczematous lesions. Common locations include flexor surfaces and the neck.

Lichen simplex chronicus   Recognized by deepening of normal skin lines and scratch marks. The nails will become polished smooth.

Diabetes   Pruritus occurs as an early symptom along with urinary frequency.

Environmental   Exposures such as sunburn, poison ivy, or fiberglass can cause pruritus.

Drugs   An allergic reaction is usually accompanied by a maculopapular rash or urticaria. Cholestasis occurs with tolbutamide, phenothiazines, erythromycin, estrogen, progesterone, and testosterone. Narcotics may cause a histamine release.

HIV   Pruritus occurs with normal skin, papules, or folliculitis.

Neoplasm   Presentations include pruritus without visible lesions, itching with hyperpigmentation, and erythroderma at the lateral malleolus. The most common neoplasm to present with pruritus is lymphoma; for example, Hodgkin's disease causes a severe burning pruritus in 30% of cases.

Uremia   Pruritus is usually present in chronic renal failure but not acute, probably because it is caused by secondary hyperparathyroidism with a resultant rise in histamines **(Plates 21, 41, 198).**

Psychogenic   Pruritus is usually more prominent at night when other stimuli are lacking. It also may occur with delusions of ectoparasites.

Cholestatic jaundice   Pruritus is related to the accumulation of bile salts in the skin. Most notably occurring in primary biliary cirrhosis, it may be increased by concurrent oral contraceptive use. Clinical jaundice is readily apparent **(Plates 48, 64, 66).**

Polycythemia vera   Pruritus is exacerbated after a hot shower or bath while the patient is cooling off. The patient will be plethoric with a "prickling" sensation, splenomegaly, and a headache **(Plates 26, 30).**

Chapter 121

Purpura/Petechiae/ Excessive Bleeding

DIFFERENTIAL OVERVIEW

Purpura
- ❏ Trauma
- ❏ Senile purpura
- ❏ Drugs
- ❏ Vasculitis
- ❏ Vitamin K deficiency
- ❏ Psychogenic purpura
- ❏ Cholesterol emboli
- ❏ Warfarin necrosis
- ❏ Scurvy
- ❏ Thrombotic thrombocytopenic purpura
- ❏ Henoch-Schonlein purpura
- ❏ Amyloidosis

Petechiae
- ❏ Autoimmune thrombocytopenia
- ❏ Bacteremia
- ❏ Hypersplenism

Excessive Bleeding
- ❏ Over-anticoagulation
- ❏ Thrombocytopenia
- ❏ von Willebrand's disease
- ❏ Circulating anticoagulant
- ❏ Disseminated intravascular coagulation
- ❏ Hemophilia

DIAGNOSTIC APPROACH

Petechiae result from platelet or vascular abnormalities. Petechiae on the lower extremities or mucous membranes are usually caused by thrombocytopenia. Tender, elevated petechiae plus abnormalities in other organs suggests vasculitis **(Plates 110, 187).**

Platelet defect disorders produce petechiae and ecchymoses occurring immediately after local trauma. Bleeding is superficial, occurring in the skin, the mucous membranes, the nose, and the gastrointestinal and genitourinary tracts. Bleeding does not occur with normal platelets until the count falls to less than 50,000, and the threshold for important bleeding is 20,000. Oozing blood around catheters suggests DIC, vitamin K deficiency, or platelet abnormalities.

Large-area bruising occurs with vitamin K-dependent factor deficiency, but not with hemophilia. Plasma protein disorders produce bleeding in deep tissues, such as joints, muscle, and retroperitoneum. The onset of such bleeding can be delayed for hours after trauma.

Viruses associated with thrombocytopenia include HSV, CMV, EBV, VZV, HIV, HBV, rubella, mumps, and enteroviruses.

Palpable purpura is seen with autoimmune or infectious (e.g., meningococcemia, endocarditis) vasculitis. Infectious emboli have an irregular outline whereas lesions of leukocytoclastic vasculitis are circular **(Plates 23, 110, 155).**

CLINICAL FINDINGS

Trauma Local ecchymoses will be well-circumscribed. Patients frequently present with ecchymosis for which they cannot recall trauma.

Senile purpura Sharply demarcated bruises occur on the extensor forearms in the elderly or patients on steroids. The skin is thinned and loose.

Drugs Heparin and warfarin have intended anticoagulant effects, but excess may produce widespread ecchymoses in response to trivial trauma. Penicillin, quinidine, quinine, phenytoin, trimethoprim, furosemide, gold salts, carbamazepine, and methyldopa may cause autoimmune thrombocytopenia. Chemotherapeutic agents, thiazides, and estrogens may produce myelosuppression. Aspirin and NSAIDs inhibit platelet aggregation but usually only produce mild clinical bleeding, such as easy bruising or oozing following tooth extractions. Drug hypersensitivity reactions (sulfonamides, penicillin, tetracycline, quinidine, guanethidine, phenothiazines, and propylthiouracil) may produce palpable purpura.

Vasculitis   Recognized as palpable purpura or petechiae that do not blanch, they arise in dependent areas. The skin often burns or itches. Vesicles and necrotic ulcerations may also develop. Precipitants include drug hypersensitivity reactions, connective tissue diseases (rheumatoid arthritis or systemic lupus erythematosus), or infections such as hepatitis C, which causes cryoglobulinemia. There will usually be concomitant signs of systemic vasculitis such as fever or arthralgias **(Plates 34, 110).**

Vitamin K deficiency   Deficiency is found with inadequate dietary intake, malabsorption, and chronic liver disease. The latter patients are especially predisposed to upper gastrointestinal hemorrhage from varices or alcohol-induced gastritis.

Psychogenic purpura   These patients have spontaneous painful ecchymoses surrounded by erythema and edema as well as other pronounced psychoneurotic complaints.

Cholesterol emboli   A purpuric livedo reticularis, cyanosis, and ultimately ischemic ulcerations occur in the legs and feet of patients with extensive atherosclerosis. The onset often coincides with aortic catheterization **(Plate 25).**

Warfarin necrosis   A reaction to warfarin may occur, which starts with painful erythema, progresses to purpura, and ultimately develops into necrosis in areas of subcutaneous fat **(Plate 195).**

Scurvy   Vitamin C deficiency is associated with painful perifollicular hemorrhages with corkscrew hairs, ecchymoses, bleeding into the muscles, and oozing from the gums **(Plate 68).**

Thrombotic thrombocytopenic purpura   A febrile patient who is in a toxic state presents with abdominal pain and prominent fluctuating neurologic signs.

Henoch-Schonlein purpura   Purpura appears over the lower extremities and buttocks, along with manifestations such as urticaria, edema, fever, headache, anorexia, arthralgias, colicky abdominal pain with melena, and hematuria. It is unusual in adults.

Amyloidosis   Pink, translucent periorbital lesions easily develop purpura when the skin is pinched ("pinch purpura") **(Plate 157).**

Autoimmune thrombocytopenia   The sudden appearance of crops of hydrostatic petechiae (on the lower extremities) follows a viral exanthem, upper respiratory illness, or mononucleosis-like syndrome. It may also be a presenting finding of HIV infection or lupus **(Plates 91, 187).**

Bacteremia   Endocarditis-associated petechiae appear in the mucous membranes and extremities, including splinter hemorrhages in the nail beds. Gonococcemia lesions on the extremities become pustular and then hemorrhagic and necrotic. Meningococcemia lesions develop rapidly, are broad and hemorrhagic, and predominate on the trunk. Rocky Mountain Spotted Fever lesions begin as pink macules on the wrists, soles, ankles, and palms and spread centripetally. By the fourth day, they become petechial and papular and then hemorrhagic and ulcerated **(Plates 22, 23, 24, 32, 75, 139).**

Hypersplenism   Thrombocytopenia with splenic enlargement occurs in states of passive congestion (e.g., portal hypertension or congestive heart failure) and with splenic sequestration due to antibody-coated platelets.

Over-anticoagulation   Suspect in a patient on warfarin.

von Willebrand's disease   It is an autosomal dominant trait; thus, determining if there is a family history of a bleeding disorder is helpful. Clinical bleeding may occur only after major surgery or trauma, or it may occur spontaneously from the mucosa of the nose, gastrointestinal tract, or genitourinary tract.

Circulating anticoagulant   Common causes of a circulating inhibitor of a procoagulant protein include lupus, the postpartum state, rheumatoid arthritis, AIDS, and penicillin. These produce abnormal coagulation tests and arterial or venous thromboses more often than clinical bleeding **(Plates 91, 92).**

Purpura/Petechiae/ Excessive Bleeding

Disseminated intravascular coagulation   The clinical presentation includes simultaneous bleeding from multiple sites and livedo reticularis and acrocyanosis due to microthrombi. Purpura fulminans occurring with gram-negative sepsis presents with extensive skin hemorrhage leading to necrosis. DIC occurs most commonly in the setting of obstetrical catastrophe, sepsis, massive trauma, or metastatic cancer. Heat stroke, transfusion reaction, and snakebite can also cause it **(Plate 33).**

Hemophilia   Family history, recurrent hemarthroses, and excessive bleeding following common hemostatic stresses such as dental extractions, childbirth, or minor surgery are prominent features. Bleeding into joints, muscles, mucous membranes, or the genitourinary tract may occur with trivial injury.

Scaling Rash

Chapter 122

PLATES 80, 103, 105, 151, 196, 197

◪ DIFFERENTIAL OVERVIEW

❏ Eczema
❏ Atopic dermatitis
❏ Seborrheic dermatitis
❏ Tinea versicolor
❏ Pityriasis rosea
❏ Psoriasis
❏ Contact dermatitis
❏ Tinea corporis
❏ Tinea manuum
❏ Stasis dermatitis
❏ Drugs
❏ Lichen planus
❏ Astatic eczema
❏ Secondary syphilis
❏ Reiter's
❏ Bowen's disease
❏ Cutaneous T-cell lymphoma

CLINICAL FINDINGS

Eczema   Red, poorly defined patches appear on the neck and flexor surfaces and thicken with excoriations caused by excessive scratching. Coin-like (nummular) lesions are common on the lower legs.

Atopic dermatitis   Pruritus/scratching lead to eczematous lesions. A personal or family history of atopy (asthma, allergic rhinitis) is elicited. An extra fold of skin below the lower eyelid is a common finding.

Seborrheic dermatitis   Red, scaly patches with an indistinct outline develop in the scalp, eyebrows, nasolabial crease, behind the ears, in the ear canal, over the sternum, and in intertriginous areas.

Tinea versicolor   A finely scaled macular eruption appears over the trunk. Hypopigmented macules may occur on dark skin; hyperpigmented macules occur on light skin **(Plate 197)**.

Pityriasis rosea   Salmon-pink, oval lesions have their long axis following the cleavage lines of the skin. Lesions have a collarette of fine scale around the perimeter. They are distributed on the trunk and proximal extremities, sparing the palms (involved in secondary syphilis). There is usually a herald patch, which is the initial and largest lesion **(Plate 196)**.

Psoriasis   Pink-red, sharply demarcated plaques have a silvery micaceous scale. They occur on the elbows, knees, scalp, and gluteal crease. There is often nail dystrophy with pitting, onycholysis, and yellow discoloration. Guttate psoriasis—a widespread eruption of small, scaling lesions—may be brought on by streptococcal infection, lithium, beta-blockers, rapid steroid taper, or acute HIV infection. It spares the face, palms, and soles **(Plates 103, 105)**.

Contact dermatitis   Well-demarcated lesions develop in areas of thin, exposed skin. Lesions are in a localized distribution, reflecting the contact exposure.

Tinea corporis   Red annular lesions have an active scaling border with central clearing. The inner thigh is a typical location.

Tinea manuum   One hand is gray-red with scaling within the palmar creases, with associated scaling and nail dystrophy on both feet.

Stasis dermatitis   The lower extremities are edematous, red, and scaling. A brownish discoloration develops due to hemosiderin; it occurs especially over the medial ankle **(Plate 151)**.

Drugs   Pityriasis rosea–like lesions may be seen with beta-blockers, captopril, clonidine, gold, griseofulvin, isotretinoin, metronidazole, and penicillin. Lichenoid eruptions can be produced by gold, antimalarials, thiazides, quinidine, phenothiazines, sulfonylureas, furosemide, methyldopa, griseofulvin, beta-blockers, and captopril.

Lichen planus   Lesions appear as violet-colored, polygonal, and flat-topped papules, traversed by a network of thin gray-white lines (Wickham's striae). They occur in the flexor aspects of the wrists, ankles, and glans penis. The oral mucosa also has lacy white plaques or erosions. The plaques are only scaly on the legs.

Astatic eczema   Fine cracks like those in porcelain develop in the dry skin on the lower legs of elderly patients.

Secondary syphilis   Scattered red-brown papules with thin scale often involve the palms or soles. Associated findings that assist diagnosis are systemic symptoms such as fever, malaise, and lymphadenopathy; recent (4–8 weeks previously) chancre; annular plaques on the face; alopecia; or broad-based and moist condyloma lata **(Plate 80).**

Reiter's   Psoriasiform lesions occur in a patient with arthritis, urethritis, and/or uveitis.

Bowen's disease   A single, well-demarcated plaque with variable scale develops in a patient with a known history of arsenic exposure, or exposure manifest as palmar hyperkeratosis.

Cutaneous T-cell lymphoma   Retiform (net-like) psoriatic lesions occur without the typical distribution, increase in palpability, and do not respond to topical steroids. The earliest lesions are macular, scaly, and red, admixed with yellow (poikiloderma).

◼ DIFFERENTIAL OVERVIEW

- ❏ Acne rosacea
- ❏ Actinic damage
- ❏ Essential/venous hypertension
- ❏ Cherry angioma
- ❏ Senile angioma
- ❏ Pregnancy
- ❏ Cirrhosis
- ❏ Systemic lupus erythematosus
- ❏ Dermatomyositis
- ❏ Scleroderma
- ❏ Kaposi's sarcoma
- ❏ Poikiloderma
- ❏ Port wine stain
- ❏ Cavernous hemangioma
- ❏ Venous lake
- ❏ Carcinoid
- ❏ Ataxia-telangiectasia
- ❏ Hereditary hemorrhagic telangiectasia
- ❏ Glomus tumor

DIAGNOSTIC APPROACH

Linear telangiectasias are simple red or blue lines that disappear with diascopy. They are common with actinic damage, rosacea, carcinoid, ataxia-telangiectasia, or cutaneous inflammation (such as discoid lupus).

Spider angiomata have a central pulsating punctum seen with diascopy, radial legs, and a halo of pallor caused by a vascular steal phenomenon.

Periungual nailfold telangiectasias, resembling glomeruli on tenfold magnification, are found in lupus, scleroderma, and dermatomyositis.

CLINICAL FINDINGS

Acne rosacea   Linear facial telangiectasias are associated with flushing, erythema, papulopustules, and rhinophyma.

Actinic damage   Damage occurs in sun-exposed areas and is associated with hyperpigmentation and keratoses.

Essential/venous hypertension   Occurring as linear telangiectasias in netlike sheets on the legs, they are more common in women.

Cherry angioma   They appear in the third decade as 1-3-mm, red, soft, globular lesions that blanch when the surrounding skin is stretched.

Senile angioma   Raspberry red and raised, they do not empty or blanch. They increase in number and size with age.

Pregnancy   Spider angiomas occur in the upper half of the body, and venous stars occur on the legs.

Cirrhosis   Spider angioma occur on the chest and upper back. Other stigmata of cirrhosis are usually present, such as ascites, a prominent venous pattern on the abdomen, and palmar erythema **(Plates 61, 62)**.

Systemic lupus erythematosus   Tortuous nailbed telangiectasias look like glomeruli when magnified. They occur in association with classic lupus findings such as malar rash and Raynaud's phenomenon **(Plates 36, 91, 113)**.

Dermatomyositis   Periungual telangiectasias, nailfold erythema, ragged cuticles, and fingertip tenderness develop. A violet/heliotrope eyelid rash and Gottron's papules on the extensor surfaces of the fingers are characteristic findings.

Scleroderma   Mat (interconnected) telangiectasias appear on the face along with dilated nailbed telangiectasias. The skin on the face and hands develops a shiny, bound-down appearance **(Plate 97)**.

Telangiectasias/Angiomas

Kaposi's sarcoma A purple papule/plaque appears in a patient with HIV infection **(Plate 200).**

Poikiloderma It appears as a patch of skin with reticulated hypo or hyperpigmentation, wrinkling due to epidermal atrophy and telangiectasias. Causes include ionizing radiation, dermatomyositis, and xeroderma pigmentosum.

Port wine stain The patches are broad, pale pink to deep purple, and rarely cross the midline. A trigeminal distribution may signal intracranial angioma, especially with ipsilateral ocular abnormalities (Sturge-Weber syndrome).

Cavernous hemangioma Large strawberry hemangiomas are more prominent at birth and tend to fade with age.

Venous lake It is a bluish lesion on the lower lip. On the scrotum it is called angiokeratoma when accompanied by hyperkeratosis.

Carcinoid Episodes of recurrent flushing of the head and neck lead to facial telangiectasias that may mimic acne rosacea **(Plate 4).**

Ataxia-telangiectasia Linear telangiectasias appear on the bulbar conjunctiva during childhood and eventually on the ears, cheeks, and flexural areas.

Hereditary hemorrhagic telangiectasia Telangiectasias appear in adulthood on the mucous membranes and nail beds. They are dark red, slightly palpable, arteriovenous malformations. When the overlying skin is stretched, an eccentric punctum with radiating legs may be seen. They are associated with epistaxis, gastrointestinal hemorrhage, and pulmonary AV fistulas with hypoxemia **(Plate 55).**

Glomus tumor It appears as a bluish-red, rounded, tender papule under the nail.

◼ DIFFERENTIAL OVERVIEW

- ❏ Ingestants
- ❏ Drugs
- ❏ Inhalants
- ❏ Hymenoptera venom
- ❏ Dermatographism
- ❏ Pressure urticaria
- ❏ Cholinergic urticaria
- ❏ Cold urticaria
- ❏ Solar urticaria
- ❏ Infection
- ❏ Urticarial vasculitis
- ❏ Hereditary angioedema

DIAGNOSTIC APPROACH

Urticaria appears as transient, mutable wheals with red raised serpiginous borders and clear centers. These often coalesce. Urticaria is experienced by 10–20% of the population at some time. Angioedema is well-demarcated localized edema **(Plates 183, 185)**.

The appearance may be helpful. Gyrate hives (erythema gyratum) are associated with internal malignancy. Hives without pseudopods suggest allergy. Small lesions with erythematous flares suggest cholinergic urticaria. Urticarial lesions unchanged for 24 hours suggest vasculitis—especially if associated with scaling or purpura.

CLINICAL FINDINGS

Ingestants   Particularly culpable causes are nuts, strawberries, shellfish, chocolate, and eggs. Drugs and chemicals may also be ingested with food, such as penicillin in meat or milk, tartrazine dye in pills, metabisulfites in salad bar food or wine, or yeast in beer.

Drugs   Drugs such as penicillin, aspirin, or NSAIDs may cause urticaria on an allergic basis. Opiates, thiamine, and pilocarpine may cause urticaria via stimulation of histamine release from mast cells **(Plate 183)**.

Inhalants   Mold, dust, and pollens are common inhalant causes.

Hymenoptera venom   Stings may cause reactions ranging from intensely local to generalized anaphylaxis, depending upon the individual's sensitivity.

Dermatographism   Demonstrated as a linear wheal induced by briskly stroking the skin, it occurs normally in up to 4% of the population **(Plate 186)**.

Pressure urticaria   Urticaria occurs at points of chronic pressure, such as the waist (belt), feet (running), or hands (manual work).

Cholinergic urticaria   These 1-2 mm, papular wheals with surrounding erythema appear in response to exercise or a hot bath. They may be associated with parasympathetic symptoms of cramps, diarrhea, headache, or diaphoresis.

Cold urticaria   Induction of urticaria with cold exposure could be benign or a sign of cryoglobulinemia. Occasionally, cold urticaria may progress to vascular collapse in cold water **(Plate 34)**.

Solar urticaria   Urticaria forming in a photodistribution may be a response to a portion of the UV light spectrum or a sign of erythropoietic porphyria **(Plate 7)**.

Infection   Urticaria may be initiated by viral infection, especially with Ebstein-Barr virus or hepatitis B virus. In hepatitis B, it occurs as part of the prodromal phase along with fever and arthralgias. Bacterial infection (dental abscess, sinusitis, or prostatitis), parasitic infection (strongyloides, ascariasis, trichuriasis, giardiasis, or trichomoniasis), or cutaneous infection (Candida and dermatophytes) can also cause urticaria.

Urticaria/Angioedema

Urticarial vasculitis   Vasculitis lesions last more than 24 hours and have a central petechiae. They burn rather than itch. If associated with arthralgias and cramping abdominal pain, they could reflect occult lupus or a complement deficiency. Similar
symptoms may occur with serum sickness or as a hepatitis B prodrome.

Hereditary angioedema   It occurs as recurrent episodes of well-demarcated local
edema, especially in the face and upper airway **(Plate 185).**

PLATES 59, 73, 75, 109, 140, 141, 181, 190, 191, 192, 193, 194, 210, 212, 213

◼ DIFFERENTIAL OVERVIEW

Vesicles
- ❑ Herpes simplex
- ❑ Contact dermatitis
- ❑ Varicella/zoster
- ❑ Dyshidrotic eczema
- ❑ Scabies
- ❑ Erythema multiforme
- ❑ Coxsackievirus
- ❑ Dermatitis herpetiformis

Bullae
- ❑ Friction blister
- ❑ Bullous impetigo
- ❑ Diabetic bullae
- ❑ Fixed drug eruption
- ❑ Frostbite
- ❑ Porphyria cutanea tarda
- ❑ Staphylococcal scalded skin syndrome
- ❑ Toxic epidermal necrolysis
- ❑ Coma bullae
- ❑ Pseudoporphyria
- ❑ Pemphigus vulgaris
- ❑ Bullous pemphigoid
- ❑ Variegate porphyria

Pustules
- ❑ Acne vulgaris
- ❑ Rosacea
- ❑ Folliculitis
- ❑ Furuncle
- ❑ Candida
- ❑ Gonococcemia
- ❑ Pustular psoriasis
- ❑ Ecthyma gangrenosum

DIAGNOSTIC APPROACH

Vesicles are less than 5 mm in diameter, and bullae are larger. If bullae, petechiae, purpura, or necrosis are present, look for an "allergen" such as HSV, strep, deep fungal infection, collagen disease (especially lupus), or occult neoplasm.

Erythema multiforme (EM) can be differentiated from a drug reaction by a dusky violet color and petechiae at the center of the lesion. A target or iris lesion is also characteristic of EM.

Staphylococcal scalded skin syndrome can be differentiated from toxic epidermal necrolysis by superficial blisters and absence of oral lesions.

Multidermatomal or disseminated zoster in a young adult should suggest HIV infection.

CLINICAL FINDINGS

Herpes simplex   Lesions appear as grouped vesicles on an erythematous base. Systemic illness, characterized by fever, malaise, headache, and myalgias, is common in primary infection. Common sites of occurrence include the oral mucosa, vermilion border of the lip, the external genitalia, and the finger by inoculation (herpetic whitlow). Tender regional adenopathy is also found. Persistent ulcerative HSV lesions are common with HIV **(Plates 73, 210).**

Contact dermatitis   The hallmark is a circumscribed pattern that reflects the mode of

Vesicles/Bullae/Pustules

contact. A linear appearance is seen with contact with a plant such as poison ivy.

Varicella/zoster   The initial lesions are vesicles on an erythematous base; these coalesce. Varicella can be recognized by lesions present simultaneously in several stages (vesicles, bullae, crusting). An outbreak of zoster is preceded by a dysesthesia, and it occurs in a unilateral dermatomal distribution **(Plates 140, 141).**

Dyshidrotic eczema   Deep, very pruritic microvesicles appear on the sides of the fingers.

Scabies   Burrows appear as small linear vesicles in the axilla, flexor wrists, interdigital fingers, waist, and genitalia. The skin is excoriated.

Erythema multiforme   Primary lesions are pink-red macules and edematous papules, which develop a dusky violet color or occur as petechiae, which develop central vesicles. Target /iris lesions are also characteristic although not universally present. Lesions occur preferentially on the hands, palms, soles, extensor forearms, and mucous membranes. Hemorrhagic crusts of the lips are often seen. Common causes include drugs, HSV (7–12 days after the primary lesion), M. pneumoniae, EBV, coxsackievirus, and influenza virus **(Plate 181).**

Coxsackievirus   In hand, foot, and mouth disease, oval gray vesicles with a red halo appear on the sides of the fingers, ankles, and tongue **(Plates 212, 213).**

Dermatitis herpetiformis   There is intense pruritus with a distinctive burning or stinging component. The primary lesion is a papule, papulovesicle, or urticarial plaque, symmetrically distributed over the extensor surfaces. Gluten sensitivity, although usually present, is otherwise subclinical **(Plate 59).**

Friction blister   They are easily identifiable as painful bullae at the site of friction/trauma, such as on the heel during a long hike.

Bullous impetigo   It appears as honey-colored crusts and purulent blisters on a weeping red base.

Diabetic bullae   Tense bullae filled with clear fluid may arise on normal skin. The lesions appear on the distal extremities, and these may be several centimeters in diameter.

Fixed drug eruption   Blisters with an erythematous base recur stereotypically in the same location with repeated drug exposure, commonly on the orogenital mucosa.

Frostbite   Hemorrhagic bullae are characteristic, as is the history **(Plate 192).**

Porphyria cutanea tarda   In sun-exposed areas, such as the hands and face, minor trauma may lead to erosions and tense vesicles. These heal with scarring and often form milia (2-3 mm white or yellow papules). Malar hypertrichosis and hyperpigmented, sclerotic plaques also occur. Precipitating agents include alcohol, estrogen, iron, and chlorinated hydrocarbons **(Plate 193).**

Staphylococcal scalded skin syndrome   It begins as redness and tenderness in the face, neck, trunk, and intertrigonal zones, and is followed by short-lived flaccid bullae. Crusting then develops, especially around the mouth.

Toxic epidermal necrolysis   Bullae arise on widespread areas of erythema and then slough. Friction applied to normal skin causes separation and bunching of the epidermis (Nikolsky's sign). Drugs are the most common cause, including phenytoin, penicillin, sulfonamides, barbiturates, allopurinol, NSAIDs, and phenolphthalein **(Plate 194).**

Coma bullae   These occur classically with barbiturate coma, from the patient lying motionless **(Plate 190).**

Pseudoporphyria   Clinically similar to porphyria cutanea tarda, it is caused by photosensitivity induced by furosemide, tetracycline, nalidixic acid, dapsone, naproxen, or pyridoxine.

Pemphigus vulgaris   Lesions consist of flaccid blisters that rupture easily, leaving denuded areas that crust and enlarge readily. Nikolsky's sign is also present. In more than half, lesions begin in the mouth, but also commonly occur on the scalp, face, neck, axilla, and trunk **(Plate 194).**

Bullous pemphigoid   Tense, thick-walled blisters develop on normal-appearing or erythematous skin. They are distributed over the abdomen, groin, flexor surfaces, and oral mucosa. As bullae rupture, they leave flaccid erosions without crust. Hundreds may appear within days **(Plate 191).**

Variegate porphyria   It has the skin signs of porphyria cutanea tarda and the systemic findings of acute intermittent porphyria.

Chapter 126

Visible Paraneoplastic Phenomena

DIFFERENTIAL OVERVIEW

- ❏ Cutaneous metastases
- ❏ Hyperpigmentation
- ❏ Cryoglobulinemia
- ❏ Acanthosis nigricans
- ❏ Acquired lanugo hair
- ❏ Generalized pruritus
- ❏ Carcinoid flush
- ❏ Dermatomyositis
- ❏ Seborrheic keratosis
- ❏ Neuromas
- ❏ Mucocutaneous nevi
- ❏ Palmar and plantar hyperkeratosis
- ❏ Thrombophlebitis migrans
- ❏ Amyloidosis
- ❏ Sweet's syndrome
- ❏ Erythema gyratum repens
- ❏ Necrolytic migratory erythema
- ❏ Acquired pachydermoperiostosis

CLINICAL FINDINGS

Cutaneous metastases   Hard nodules in the scalp will have spread from lung, breast, or genitourinary cancers. Umbilical (Sister Mary Joseph) nodules appear with intraabdominal malignancy.

Hyperpigmentation   Small cell carcinoma can produce circulating MSH-like polypeptides, causing diffuse hyperpigmentation.

Cryoglobulinemia   Hemorrhagic bullae or ulcers appearing in acral regions after cold exposure are seen in plasma cell dyscrasias (or more commonly in hepatitis C) **(Plate 34)**.

Acanthosis nigricans   Hyperpigmented, velvety, hyperkeratotic patches in the body folds, especially axilla, nipples, and umbilicus, are associated with adenocarcinoma of the stomach and less frequently with cancer of the pancreas, colon, lung, breast, uterus, ovary, rectum, and bile ducts. It may precede the clinical appearance of malignancy in 20%. Other causes, such as diabetes with insulin resistance, are more common **(Plate 168)**.

Acquired lanugo hair   Downy hair appearing on the face and trunk may signal cancer of the bronchus, gallbladder, bladder, or rectum. More common causes are anorexia nervosa and Cushing's syndrome.

Generalized pruritus   Pruritus associated with lymphoma (both Hodgkin's and non-Hodgkin's) and leukemia begins with local burning, which develops into intense pruritus.

Carcinoid flush   A deep red to purple flush appears over the face and neck, is associated with abdominal pain, diarrhea, edema, palpitations, wheezing, and dizziness, and is precipitated by food rich in tyramine or alcohol. It is seen in GI carcinoid tumors once metastatic to the liver **(Plate 4)**.

Dermatomyositis   Heliotrope, ranging from a violet suffusion to a rash on the eyelids, and purplish Gottron's papules over the knuckles have an association with gastrointestinal, breast, lung, and genitourinary cancers and lymphoma, especially in patients older than 60 years of age **(Plates 94, 95)**.

Seborrheic keratosis   The sudden development of a large number of inflamed/pruritic seborrheic keratoses (Leser-Trélat) is associated with carcinoma of the stomach, breast and lung, as well as lymphoma **(Plate 126)**.

Neuromas   Pink nodules on the lips, eyelids, nares, and anterior two-thirds of the tongue are found in MEN III syndrome and in those with thyroid cancer and pheochromocytoma.

Mucocutaneous nevi Peutz-Jeghers is associated with gastrointestinal malignancies occurring before the ligament of Treitz **(Plate 56)**.

Palmar and plantar hyperkeratosis Tylosis is associated with esophageal cancer and chronic arsenic poisoning **(Plates 71, 133)**.

Thrombophlebitis migrans Recurrent episodes of thrombophlebitis, which are especially suspicious because they occur in the absence of precipitating factors, in unusual locations, or while on anticoagulation medications, signal an underlying adenocarcinoma of the pancreas, lung, colon, or stomach.

Amyloidosis An enlarged tongue and waxy, purpuric periorbital plaques are visible manifestations of amyloidosis. Secondary amyloidosis may be caused by multiple myeloma **(Plates 131, 157)**.

Sweet's syndrome Painful bright red to red-brown plaques appear on the head, neck, and upper extremities. A minority are associated with cancer, most commonly acute myelogenous leukemia **(Plate 158)**.

Erythema gyratum repens Serpiginous bands with marginal desquamation resemble burled wood and are associated with breast and lung cancer **(Plate 72)**.

Necrolytic migratory erythema Bright erythematous areas with serpiginous outlines on the buttocks, intertriginous folds, and flexural aspects of the legs are characteristic of glucagonoma. Central blister formation occurs and is followed by hyperpigmentation with healing **(Plate 8)**.

Acquired pachydermoperiostosis Increased sebaceous activity with thickening of the skin on the forehead and scalp gives a leonine facial appearance. The palms thicken, and the fingers become clubbed. These findings are associated with cancer of the bronchus, stomach, esophagus, thymus and with mesothelioma **(Plate 52)**.

Section IX
Head/Neck

Anisocoria

◼ DIFFERENTIAL OVERVIEW

- ❏ Angle closure glaucoma
- ❏ Trauma
- ❏ Essential anisocoria
- ❏ Drugs
- ❏ Horner's syndrome
- ❏ Uveitis
- ❏ Adie's pupil
- ❏ Cavernous sinus thrombosis
- ❏ Uncal herniation
- ❏ Argyll-Robertson pupils

DIAGNOSTIC APPROACH

Iritis or pilocarpine can cause abnormal *miosis* (constriction). If light and convergence responses are normal, encephalitis, brain abscess, or neoplasm must be considered.

Abnormal *mydriasis* (dilation) may be caused by atropine, glaucoma or cranial third nerve palsy. If light and convergence reactions are normal, stimulation of the cervical sympathetic nerves must be considered. Causes include aortic aneurysm, mediastinal Hodgkin's disease, and lung cancer.

CLINICAL FINDINGS

Angle closure glaucoma   The pupil is large, and the anterior chamber is shallow, transmitting tangential light poorly (**Plate 217**).

Trauma   A direct blow produces a dilated pupil that does not react to either light or accomodation (**Plates 221, 222**).

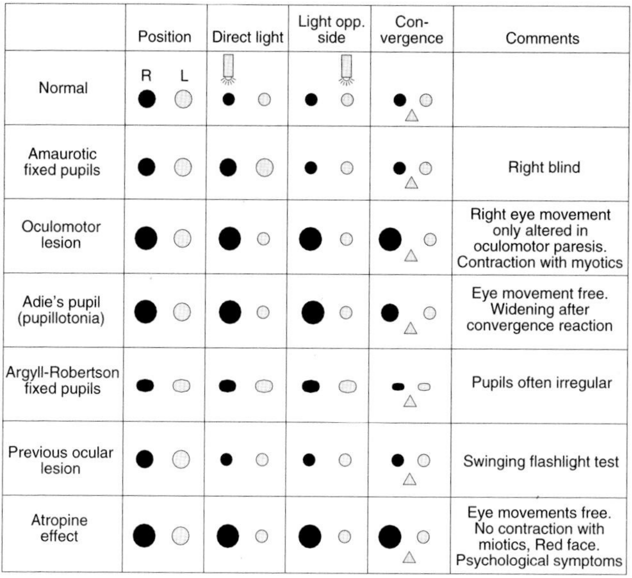

	Position	Direct light	Light opp. side	Convergence	Comments
Normal	R L				
Amaurotic fixed pupils					Right blind
Oculomotor lesion					Right eye movement only altered in oculomotor paresis. Contraction with myotics
Adie's pupil (pupillotonia)					Eye movement free. Widening after convergence reaction
Argyll-Robertson fixed pupils					Pupils often irregular
Previous ocular lesion					Swinging flashlight test
Atropine effect					Eye movements free. No contraction with miotics, Red face. Psychological symptoms

Figure 19. Pupillary reaction disorders. (Adapted from: Mumemthaler M. Neurology. 8th ed. Stuttgart: Thieme, 1986.)

Anisocoria

Essential anisocoria   The relative difference in pupil size remains the same regardless of ambient illumination. Use old photos of the pupil for comparison.

Drugs   Dilation occurs with unilateral application of atropine or homatropine. Constriction occurs with pilocarpine.

Horner's syndrome   The classic presentation is miosis (small pupil) with ipsilateral ptosis, anhidrosis, and enophthalmos. It may be seen with an apical (Pancoast) lung tumor, multiple sclerosis, posterior inferior cerebellar artery syndrome, or internal carotid artery aneurysm **(Plate 120).**

Uveitis   The eye will be red with a limbic (ciliary) flush adjacent to the iris. Anisocoria is a result of ciliary spasm **(Plate 86).**

Adie's pupil   Acutely, there is a large immobile pupil. Later, with refixation near to far, the affected pupil dilates more slowly than the normal one. There may be vermiform contraction of the pupil and hypersensitivity to dilute pilocarpine.

Cavernous sinus thrombosis   Unilateral exophthalmos, chemosis, severe retro-orbital headache, and multiple extraocular palsies are important clues.

Uncal herniation   A dilated, fixed pupil, may occur with a rapidly expanding intracranial mass, such as a subdural or epidural hematoma occurring after head trauma. Consciousness is usually altered, and decorticate posturing with apnea often occurs.

Argyll-Robertson pupils   Pupils are small, irregular, and unequal in diameter. They constrict on accomodation but not when exposed to direct bright light. Usually associated with neurosyphilis, Argyll-Robertson pupils are also seen in patients with midbrain tumors or diabetes **(Plate 118).**

Diplopia/Nystagmus

◨ DIFFERENTIAL OVERVIEW

Diplopia
- ❏ Alcohol
- ❏ Diabetes
- ❏ Brainstem ischemia/lesion
- ❏ Grave's disease
- ❏ Multiple sclerosis
- ❏ Ophthalmoplegic migraine
- ❏ Myasthenia gravis
- ❏ Wernicke's encephalopathy
- ❏ Zygoma fracture
- ❏ Basilar meningitis
- ❏ Posterior communicating artery aneurysm
- ❏ Cavernous sinus thrombosis
- ❏ Syphilis
- ❏ Guillain-Barré variant
- ❏ Botulism

Nystagmus
- ❏ Labyrinthitis
- ❏ Multiple sclerosis
- ❏ Oculogyric crisis
- ❏ Cerebellar lesion
- ❏ Brainstem lesion
- ❏ Frontal lesion
- ❏ Occipital lesion
- ❏ Dorsal midbrain lesion
- ❏ Heavy metal intoxication
- ❏ Congenital

DIAGNOSTIC APPROACH

CN III paresis: The lateral rectus and superior oblique are unopposed, turning the eye outward and downward. Acute lesions may be peripheral (diabetic or ischemic) or central (posterior communicating artery aneurysm or cavernous sinus lesions). Both have ptosis, absent eye elevation, and adduction, but peripheral lesions have normal pupil size and movement ("pupillary sparing"). Central lesions produce a pupil that is dilated and unresponsive to light or accomodation. Unilateral third nerve palsy with contralateral superior rectus palsy and bilateral partial ptosis, and bilateral third nerve palsy always represent central lesions. Unilateral external ophthalmoplegia with normal contralateral superior rectus function, unilateral internal ophthalmoplegia, and unilateral ptosis represent peripheral lesions.

CN IV paresis: Superior oblique weakness produces vertical diplopia. The patient tilts his or her head to the opposite side to lessen the displacement.

CN VI paresis: Lateral rectus palsy produces weakness in abduction and horizontal diplopia.

Acute monocular diplopia is usually imaginary, but it can occur with corneal aberrations, cataract, or foveal traction.

True nystagmus is characterized by rapid regular oscillations around a fixed point not just with lateral gaze but also when the eyes are looking forward. A few beats of nystagmus at extremes of gaze are not pathologic. Nystagmus of ocular causes has a pendular motion whereas disease in the central nervous system produces fast and slow components.

Internuclear ophthalmoplegia occurs when the oculomotor and abducens nerves (CN III and VI) are disconnected at the medial longitudinal fasciculus. When conjugate gaze is attempted, one eye will not adduct medially and the abducting eye (lateral gaze) will show nystagmus. This finding is seen in persons with multiple sclerosis and pontine vascular lesions.

Diplopia/Nystagmus

CLINICAL FINDINGS

Alcohol   Diplopia occurs with acute intoxication.

Diabetes   The third nerve is typically affected with sparing of pupillary fibers.

Brainstem ischemia/lesion   Vertebrobasilar transient ischemia is associated with vertigo, numbness of the ipsilateral face and contralateral limbs, dysarthria, and dysphagia in addition to the diplopia. A third nerve lesion with contralateral tremor results from a lesion of the red nucleus. A third nerve lesion with contralateral spastic hemiparesis is caused by a ventral lesion involving the corticospinal tract (Weber's syndrome). A brainstem lesion characteristically produces vertical nystagmus, which is more marked when the patient gazes toward the side of the lesion. An abducens nucleus lesion produces an ipsilateral gaze palsy with ipsilateral absent "doll's eyes" and calorics.

Grave's disease   Exophthalmos and lid lag are present as are general symptoms of hypermetabolism. Primary position strabismus and incomplete eye movements may be present **(Plate 19)**.

Multiple sclerosis   Important clues are optic neuritis, internuclear ophthalmoplegia, and a prior history of sensory neurological lesions. Charcot's triad of nystagmus, intention tremor, and scanning speech is a classic presentation **(Plates 119, 127, 128)**.

Ophthalmoplegic migraine   Unilateral headache, nausea, and visual phenomena such as scintillating scotoma are clues to a migraine.

Myasthenia gravis   Diplopia fluctuates. An isolated fourth or sixth nerve palsy is associated with unilateral or bilateral ptosis. The pupillary reaction is normal **(Plate 219)**.

Wernicke's encephalopathy   Paresis of the abducens nerve, horizontal diplopia, and nystagmus occur in a malnourished alcoholic patient.

Zygoma fracture   Following facial trauma, the inferior oblique muscle may become trapped leading to paresis of upward gaze. Ataxia, confusion, and polyneuropathy are additional findings **(Plate 222)**.

Basilar meningitis   Unilateral or bilateral sixth nerve palsies are an early sign. Cancer, tuberculosis, sarcoidosis, or cryptococcosis may cause this syndrome.

Posterior communicating artery aneurysm   Most patients have intense headache, stupor or coma, and complete (central) third nerve paralysis.

Cavernous sinus thrombosis   Retro-orbital headache is followed by polyneuropathic ophthalmoplegia (III, IV, V, VI), proptosis, and chemosis **(Plate 227)**.

Syphilis   An Argyll-Robertson pupil accommodates but does not react. A self-limited genital chancre is usually recalled **(Plate 118)**.

Guillain-Barré variant   Bilateral polyneuropathic ophthalmoplegia is associated with areflexia and ataxia.

Botulism   Diplopia is a common presenting symptom. Concomitant features include bilateral ptosis, mydriasis, dysphagia, dysphonia, vomiting, limb cramping, and generalized muscle weakness. Consumption of possibly contaminated canned food within 6–36 hours is a key clue.

Labyrinthitis   Nystagmus responds to positional changes of the head (Barany maneuver) with a latency of response of 3–10 seconds and is fatigable. Rotatory nystagmus is typical.

Oculogyric crisis   Tonic upgaze is seen in Parkinson's disease, and tonic downgaze, in phenothiazine reaction.

Cerebellar lesion   Irritative lesions produce coarse movement toward the side of the lesion, and fine movement away from it. There is no latency with head movement and little vertigo.

Frontal lesion   There is tonic deviation ipsilateral to the lesion and saccadic palsy contralateral to the lesion. Calorics are normal.

Occipital lesion   There is ipsilateral pursuit palsy with normal calorics.

Dorsal midbrain lesion   It presents with paralysis of upgaze, large Argyll-Robertson pupils, no vertical pursuit, and lid retraction. Causes include thalamic hemorrhage, metabolic encephalopathy, pineal tumor, and syphilis.

Heavy metal intoxication   Nystagmus occurs in intoxication, particularly with manganese or lead **(Plate 134)**.

Congenital   Nystagmus is present from childhood, and the macula is hypopigmented.

Chapter 129

Ear Pain/Discharge

▚ DIFFERENTIAL OVERVIEW

Ear Pain
- ❏ Acute otitis media
- ❏ Acute otitis externa
- ❏ Eustachian dysfunction
- ❏ Temporomandibular joint arthritis
- ❏ Traumatic tympanic membrane rupture
- ❏ Foreign body, external auditory canal
- ❏ Erysipelas
- ❏ Herpes zoster oticus
- ❏ Dental abscess
- ❏ Frostbite
- ❏ Relapsing polychondritis
- ❏ Malignant otitis externa
- ❏ Acute mastoiditis
- ❏ Nasopharyngeal cancer

Ear Discharge
- ❏ Otitis externa
- ❏ Eczematoid dermatitis
- ❏ Low-viscosity cerumen
- ❏ Otitis media with perforation
- ❏ Foreign body
- ❏ Psoriasis
- ❏ Herpes zoster oticus

DIAGNOSTIC APPROACH

If ear pain is present without ear findings, consider referred pain from the tonsils, teeth, trachea, or temporomandibular joint. Ear pain may be an early sign of nasopharyngeal carcinoma. Lesions of the anterior portion of the tongue refer pain in front of the ear whereas the posterior one-third of the tongue refers pain to within the ear.

CLINICAL FINDINGS

Acute otitis media   The sine qua non is erythema of the tympanic membrane. It is usually also opaque and bulging, with the light reflex and bony landmarks obscured. It does not move with pneumoscopy **(Plate 233)**.

Acute otitis externa   There is pain with traction on the pinna. The external auditory canal is edematous and crusty, and has a serous to purulent discharge, with itching as a prominent symptom **(Plate 234)**.

Eustachian dysfunction   This is commonly known as serous otitis. It results in blockage that usually causes a mild pain, which is characterized as a pressure sensation, occurring in the setting of an upper respiratory infection or seasonal allergies. The tympanic membrane is not red but may have dullness due to fluid behind it. Sometimes, an air-fluid level or bubbles can be seen, or decreased mobility with insufflation occurs.

Temporomandibular joint arthritis   Pain radiates into the masseter, which may be tender. There is often a click or crepitance over the TMJ, and symptoms are worsened by opening the mouth. A history of bruxism may be elicited.

Traumatic tympanic membrane rupture   It commonly occurs with introduction of a foreign body or a blow to the ear. Blood issues from the ear. Careful attention to the tympanic membrane will reveal the disruption although distortion of the landmarks may make it difficult to get your bearings.

Foreign body, external auditory canal   It is readily visible on ophthalmoscopy.

Erysipelas   The pinna is bright red and tender, and the redness may extend onto the adjacent face. Periauricular lymphadenitis is present **(Plate 237)**.

Herpes zoster oticus   Vesicles and crusting are present in the external auditory canal.

Tinnitus, decreased hearing, vertigo, and ipsilateral facial palsy occur **(Plate 235).**

Dental abscess   The lower molars refer pain to the ear. There will be concussion tenderness over the affected tooth and usually a swollen jaw.

Frostbite   Following cold exposure, the ear is red, edematous, and painful.

Relapsing polychondritis   The key finding is that the inflammation and redness spare the earlobe. Associated findings include inflammation of the cartilage of the nose or thyroid cartilage and/or symmetrical polyarthritis **(Plate 236).**

Malignant otitis externa   It occurs in diabetics, with severe ear pain, green and purulent discharge, and fleshy or friable granulation tissue at the junction of the cartilage and bony canal.

Acute mastoiditis   There is exquisite tenderness and swelling behind the ear.

Nasopharyngeal cancer   Deep pain referred to the ear occurs especially in nasopharyngeal cancer growing near the origin of the eustachian tube; however, referred pain may originate in the tongue, tonsils, palate, or larynx.

Eczematoid dermatitis   Because this dermatitis is very pruritic, the patient will have a history of frequent scratching or swabbing in the ear.

Low-viscosity cerumen   The ear is not itchy or tender, and there is often a history of liquid introduced externally.

Otitis media with perforation   A bright red perforated tympanic membrane can be seen if the fluid is gently swabbed or lavaged out. Copious otorrhea with slight maceration or a red canal suggests chronic otitis media with perforation. A pulsating mucopurulent discharge, the "lighthouse sign," may be seen.

Psoriasis   Silver scales on an erythematous base are evident elsewhere on the body, usually in the scalp or behind the ear **(Plate 105).**

Chapter 130

Epistaxis

◪ DIFFERENTIAL OVERVIEW

❑ Trauma
❑ Sinusitis
❑ Uncontrolled hypertension
❑ Excessive anticoagulation
❑ Septal ulceration
❑ Bleeding diathesis

DIAGNOSTIC APPROACH

Anterior epistaxis originates in the septal vascular plexus. Bleeding comes from one naris and is easily reduced with external pressure. The bleeding site can be seen on visual inspection.

Posterior epistaxis originates in the sphenopalatine or ethmoid artery. Bleeding is brisk and continually swallowed, and it may occasionally present as melena. Blunt nasal trauma is the most common cause.

CLINICAL FINDINGS

Trauma   Low-humidity air or old age can predispose persons to epistaxis with forceful blowing. Out of shame, the patient may disguise the history of digital trauma or being punched in the nose.

Sinusitis   Unilateral facial fullness, pressure, or tenderness and purulent, bloody nasal discharge and fever are key signs.

Uncontrolled hypertension   This is a less common cause of epistaxis than is usually assumed, but it is easily confirmed by blood pressure measurement.

Excessive anticoagulation   In a patient taking therapeutic warfarin, this may be a signal event, helping avert a more serious bleed.

Septal ulceration   Intranasal cocaine may cause ulceration or perforation. Wegener's granulomatosis is a rare cause of ulceration **(Plate 111).**

Bleeding diathesis   Petechiae or purpura and a history of easy bleeding with surgery or minor injury are often found **(Plate 187).**

▇ DIFFERENTIAL OVERVIEW

❏ Grave's disease
❏ Familial
❏ Orbital asymmetry
❏ Orbital cellulitis
❏ Lithium
❏ Cavernous sinus thrombosis
❏ Orbital hemorrhage/emphysema
❏ Intracavernous carotid artery aneurysm
❏ Arteriovenous fistula
❏ Carotid-cavernous sinus fistula
❏ Orbital tumor
❏ Pituitary apoplexy
❏ Meningioma

DIAGNOSTIC APPROACH

The patient may present with exposure keratitis, resulting from an inability to close the eyelid fully, or with diplopia resulting from unilaterally impaired extraocular movement. By standing behind the patient, tilting the head back, and viewing down the brow ridge, as little as 2 mm of eye protrusion can be detected.

Unilateral pulsating proptosis can be caused by an AV fistula between the internal carotid and the cavernous sinus in a basilar skull fracture, to an aneurysm of the ophthalmic artery, or to a rapidly enlarging and highly vascular orbital neoplasm. These vascular lesions produce a pulsating tinnitus and a dimming of vision.

CLINICAL FINDINGS

Grave's disease   Eye phenomena may range from a mild stare (a look of alarm or surprise); to lid lag and proptosis; to marked protrusion, edema, limitation of extraocular movements, and optic nerve compression. Other signs of hyperthyroidism such as an enlarged thyroid with a bruit, tachycardia, and symptoms of hypermetabolism are usually evident, but the degree of proptosis does not parallel the degree of hyperthyroidism **(Plate 19).**

Familial   The patient will have had bulging eyes all his or her life and often has relatives with a similar appearance.

Orbital asymmetry   The illusion of exophthalmus may be produced by severe unilateral myopia, facial nerve paresis, or enophthalmos of the opposite eye.

Orbital cellulitis   Usually a result of direct extension of a sinusitis, this cellulitis causes prominent and rapidly evolving erythema, lid edema, proptosis, chemosis, retro-orbital pain, and fever **(Plate 227).**

Lithium   This is easily recognized by the patient's therapeutic use of lithium to treat bipolar illness.

Cavernous sinus thrombosis   The eyes are protruded with the lids red and engorged. There is ophthalmoplegia, hypesthesia of the upper face, and a dilated fixed pupil. Mental status changes occur in 50% and meningismus in 40%. The precipitating cause is sinusitis, periorbital cellulitis, or a furuncle **(Plate 227).**

Orbital hemorrhage/emphysema   Sudden protrusion follows strenuous physical effort. Ecchymoses do not appear initially.

Intracavernous carotid artery aneurysm   Retro-orbital pain occurs in combination with diplopia and third, fourth, or sixth cranial nerve paresis. A giant aneurysm may compress the chiasm, producing visual field defects.

Arteriovenous fistula   Findings include a pulsating globe and a bruit that decreases with ipsilateral carotid compression.

Carotid-cavernous sinus fistula   It presents with a diffusely congested orbit with exophthalmos, prominent episcleral vessels, and elevated intraocular pressure. Ophthal-moplegia with supertemporal gaze and a palpable orbital pulsation with a bruit are additional findings.

Orbital tumor   There is painless, progressive proptosis and visual loss.

Pituitary apoplexy   Apoplexy presents acutely with severe retro-orbital pain, cranial nerve defects, and a central scotoma.

Meningioma   An orbital ridge meningioma can deform the bony structure, causing proptosis and unilateral visual loss.

Eye Pain

Chapter 132

PLATES 86, 128, 208, 217, 222, 223, 224, 225, 227

▨ DIFFERENTIAL OVERVIEW

❑ Conjunctivitis
❑ Corneal abrasion
❑ Foreign body
❑ Sinusitis
❑ Migraine
❑ Acute glaucoma
❑ Orbital cellulitis
❑ Zoster prodrome
❑ Orbital fracture
❑ Keratitis
❑ Scleritis
❑ Iritis
❑ Optic neuritis
❑ Temporal arteritis

DIAGNOSTIC APPROACH

A foreign body sensation occurs with a foreign body, corneal abrasion, or keratoconjunctivitis sicca. Itching is associated with allergic and vernal conjunctivitis. Photophobia occurs with iritis and herpes simplex keratitis. Deep pain suggests acute glaucoma or posterior scleritis. Pain on eye movement is found with optic neuritis, sinusitis, and influenza.

CLINICAL FINDINGS

Conjunctivitis There is a mild burning, grittiness, and foreign body sensation, accompanied by conjunctival erythema and discharge **(Plates 223, 224, 225)**.

Corneal abrasion There is a prominent foreign body sensation, reflex blinking, and lacrimation, and a denuded area visible with fluorescein or slit lamp.

Foreign body There is usually a well-localized sensation of something in the eye, with abundant tearing.

Sinusitis Pain centers over the maxillary or frontal sinuses or the bridge of the nose.

Migraine This condition is recognized by its stereotypic repetitive nature, visual aura/scotoma, and nausea.

Acute glaucoma Ocular aching radiates to the frontal and temporal regions. Visual acuity is decreased and halos appear to surround lights. The anterior chamber is shallow to tangential light, the globe is firm and tender, the pupil is midposition and fixed, and the cornea is hazy **(Plate 217)**.

Orbital cellulitis Cellulitis presents in a toxic patient as a rapidly advancing periorbital inflammation with proptosis and diplopia **(Plate 227)**.

Zoster prodrome Pain is perceived over the entire distribution of the ophthalmic division of the trigeminal nerve, with a neuritic quality (burning, numb, lancinating).

Orbital fracture The color will be purplish from the outset, not beefy red like a black eye. There may be a limitation in extraocular movements if an ocular muscle is entrapped. Bilateral black eyes suggest basilar skull fracture **(Plate 222)**.

Keratitis There is a loss of corneal luster, and central defects are visible with fluorescein. Herpes simplex keratitis has a characteristic branching (dendritic) pattern on the corneal surface **(Plate 208)**.

Scleritis Presenting with deep, dull pain and localized scleral redness, it is often associated with connective tissue disease.

Iritis There is a dull ache and photophobia. The pupil is irregular, the anterior chamber is cloudy, and the limbus surrounding the iris is injected **(Plate 86)**.

Optic neuritis Neuritis begins with eye pain aggravated by movement and abnormal color vision with a central scotoma. The involved eye has an afferent pupillary defect (normal consensual but decreased direct light response). The optic disc may appear normal or similar to early papilledema except that retinal venous pulsations are present. Optic neuritis may be the presenting manifestation of multiple sclerosis in 10–15% of cases **(Plate 128).**

Temporal arteritis   A tender, ropy temporal artery and jaw claudication in an elderly patient are important corroborative clues.

Facial/Dental/ Temporomandibular Pain

PLATES 88, 222

DIFFERENTIAL OVERVIEW

❏ Maxillary sinusitis
❏ Dental infection
❏ Temporomandibular joint dysfunction
❏ Myofascial masseter pain
❏ Migraine
❏ Trigeminal neuralgia
❏ Frontal sinusitis
❏ Ethmoid sinusitis
❏ Sphenoid sinusitis
❏ Parotitis
❏ Parotid calculus
❏ Orbital fracture
❏ Mandibular fracture
❏ Maxillary fracture
❏ Myocardial infarction
❏ Connective tissue disease
❏ Temporal arteritis
❏ Cavernous sinus thrombosis

DIAGNOSTIC APPROACH

The V1 ophthalmic branch of the trigeminal innervates the forehead, cornea (corneal reflex), dorsum of the nose, and anterior cranial dura. The V2 maxillary branch innervates the upper lip, lateral nose, upper cheek, anterior temple, upper jaw and teeth, roof of the mouth, and middle cranial dura. The V3 mandibular branch innervates the lower lip, chin, posterior cheek, external ear, mucosa of the lower mouth, anterior two-thirds of the tongue, and parts of the anterior and middle cranial dura.

Pain provoked by hot, cold, or sweet foods is usually dental in origin. Neuralgia may produce a similar pain, but the pain will have a refractory period after an initial response. Pain increased by chewing suggests trigeminal neuralgia, temporomandibular joint pain, or jaw claudication. Pain increased by swallowing and taste is consistent with glossopharyngeal neuralgia. Objective sensory loss persisting after the pain is an important clue to organic disease.

Epidemiologic studies reveal that despite lack of symptoms, temporomandibular joint tenderness is common, occurring in 35% of asymptomatic people, clicking in 25%, crepitus in 8%, and jaw deviation in 15%.

CLINICAL FINDINGS

Maxillary sinusitis   The classic presentation is facial pressure/pain, purulent nasal discharge, and fever. The pain increases when the patient leans forward, and there is tenderness and warmth over the maxilla. A combination of maxillary pain with unilateral predominance and purulent nasal discharge has an Se 0.81, Sp 0.88, and LR 6.8 for sinusitis.

Dental infection   Infection is usually easily recognized by jaw pain, dental concussion tenderness, and gum swelling adjacent to the affected tooth.

Temporomandibular joint dysfunction   With temporomandibular joint inflammation, there will be tenderness directly over the joint and pain with opening and closing but no locking of the jaw. There may be crepitance but no click unless there is associated disc displacement. With disc displacement, there will be limitation of opening and closing of the jaw and deviation away from the affected side.

Myofascial masseter pain   There is a dull, aching jaw pain that increases with jaw movement. Jaw opening is limited. The muscles of mastication are tender. Clicks and crepitance are absent. There is usually a history of bruxism or repeated clenching of the jaw.

Facial/Dental/
Temporomandibular Pain

Migraine   Episodic unilateral pain is associated with aura, nausea, and hypersensitivity to light and/or noise.

Trigeminal neuralgia   It presents as a paroxysmal intense shooting or stabbing pain in a trigeminal distribution, and it is prompted by thermal or tactile stimuli. There is no objective sensory loss. The tongue may be furred on the affected side. Trigeminal zoster begins acutely with facial dysesthesia and pain, followed by crusting vesicles in a unilateral dermatomal distribution.

Frontal sinusitis   Frontal pain and tenderness are present and often hard to distinguish from a noninfectious frontal tension headache. Pitting edema and severe tenderness over the forehead suggest a contiguous osteomyelitis.

Ethmoid sinusitis   Central facial pain and nasal blockage are clues to diagnosis. Complications include orbital cellulitis and, rarely, cavernous sinus thrombosis.

Sphenoid sinusitis   Frontal, temporal, or occipital headache is common, and tenderness may occur over the vertex or mastoids.

Parotitis   A tender, warm, swollen gland may be palpated at the angle of the jaw. The ampulla of Stensen's duct, opposite the upper second molar, may be inflamed or pus may be expressed. Bilateral parotid enlargement may be seen with mumps, cirrhosis, or bulimia.

Parotid calculus   Parotid colic and recurrent swelling occur with eating. A stone may be palpated inferior to the zygoma.

Orbital fracture   A blow to the eye is followed by eyelid ecchymosis. Diplopia on vertical gaze indicates muscle entrapment **(Plate 222).**

Mandibular fracture   Following jaw trauma, there is a palpable step-off and the teeth do not seat together normally.

Maxillary fracture   With facial trauma, look for unilateral epistaxis, periorbital and subconjunctival ecchymoses, a flat cheek contour, a notch in the bony orbital rim, an anesthetic upper lip, diplopia, decreased transillumination of the maxillary sinus, and subcutaneous emphysema. With a LeFort I fracture, there will be a floating upper jaw with a midpalatal ecchymotic line. A LeFort II fracture produces a "dish face" with massive facial swelling, diplopia, and malocclusion. A LeFort III fracture causes mobility of the upper face on the cranial vault, with CSF rhinorrhea.

Myocardial infarction   Severe lower jaw or neck pain usually, but not always, occurs in association with chest pain.

Connective tissue disease   Inflammatory arthritis of the temporomandibular joint is associated with rheumatoid arthritis, systemic lupus erythematosus, ankylosing spondylitis, and Reiter's syndrome **(Plate 88).**

Temporal arteritis   Suspect this in a patient older than 50 years of age with jaw claudication, a tender ropy or nodular temporal artery, or transient visual loss.

Cavernous sinus thrombosis   An acute onset of photophobia, headache, ophthalmoplegia, chemosis, and proptosis occurs in a patient in an extremely toxic condition.

Flashing Lights/Scotoma   Chapter 134

PLATES 14, 15, 128, 215, 218, 238

DIFFERENTIAL OVERVIEW

- ❑ Vitreous opacities
- ❑ Migraine prodrome
- ❑ Glaucoma
- ❑ Cataract
- ❑ Amaurosis fugax
- ❑ Retinal detachment
- ❑ Optic neuritis
- ❑ Eclipse blindness
- ❑ Pituitary tumor
- ❑ Occipital cortex lesion

DIAGNOSTIC APPROACH

A scotoma is usually recognized by the patient as missing words when reading or as being unable to view part of the examiner's face. A dark cloud or spot blocking part of the visual field is a result of a preretinal opacity.

CLINICAL FINDINGS

Vitreous opacities   "Floaters" appear as dark spots that move with a slight delay across the field of vision after the eye is moved.

Migraine prodrome   Visual phenomena include scintillating scotoma, appearing similar to wavy lines made by heat rising off pavement, or brightly colored zigzag patterns, which suggest a prairie fire with a flaming periphery and dark center.

Glaucoma   Colored halos may surround lights, due to corneal edema **(Plate 218).**

Cataract   Spokes radiate from bright lights, and the vision is vaguely hazy.

Amaurosis fugax   There is a transient monocular blurring of vision. An embolism may be seen in a retinal arteriole bifurcation. A source is suggested by an ipsilateral carotid bruit or atrial fibrillation **(Plate 238).**

Retinal detachment   The occurrence of a sudden shower of flashing lights, especially in the periphery of vision, is a herald sign. A gray cloud will then occur over one part of the visual field. Visual outlines are blurred and may appear double or distorted. On fundoscopy, a portion of the retina looks gray or white and is difficult to bring into focus **(Plate 215).**

Optic neuritis   Neuritis produces a central scotoma with hyperemia of the optic disc. When resulting from multiple sclerosis, it is associated with other eye findings such as internuclear ophthalmoplegia (with horizontal conjugate pursuit, there is paresis of abduction of one eye and nystagmus of the other) **(Plate 215).**

Eclipse blindness   A fixed dark spot appears, due to a macular burn from staring at a bright light (e.g., the sun) without protection.

Pituitary tumor   A gradually enlarging central scotoma develops, often with endocrine findings such as acromegaly or galactorrhea **(Plates 14, 15).**

Occipital cortex lesion   A scotoma may occur, but the patient is often unaware of it. Its presence is indicated by the patient persistently bumping into objects and by visual field testing. Sometimes, positive phenomena are produced (i.e., colored lights).

◪ DIFFERENTIAL OVERVIEW

Sensorineural
❑ Presbyacusis
❑ Noise-induced loss
❑ Drugs
❑ Ménière's disease
❑ Eighth nerve injury
❑ Acoustic neuroma

Conductive
❑ Impacted cerumen
❑ Otitis media
❑ Middle ear effusion
❑ Perforation of tympanic membrane
❑ Otosclerosis
❑ Exostoses
❑ Developmental defect
❑ Glomus tumor

DIAGNOSTIC APPROACH

Conductive hearing loss presents with loss of low tones and vowels. Sensorineural hearing loss produces impaired high tone perception, with diminished speech discrimination—especially for female voices—and hearing ringing sounds (tinnitus). Hyperacusis (the sensation that sounds are overly loud to the point of discomfort) is associated with sensorineural cochlear hearing loss. Paracusis (words perceived more clearly in a noisy environment) is associated with conductive middle ear hearing loss.

The Weber test detects 5 dB of hearing loss. A tuning fork is placed in the midline. With conductive loss, it lateralizes to the affected ear, and with sensorineural loss, to the unaffected ear. The Rinne test (bone conduction > air conduction) detects a 20 dB hearing loss. Qualitative tests for high frequency loss include hearing a watch tick and hearing whispered speech from a distance of 2 feet.

Acute hearing loss occurs with infection, traumatic tympanic membrane rupture, or acute vascular event.

CLINICAL FINDINGS

Presbyacusis Bilateral symmetric hearing loss of gradual onset begins with high frequency loss with difficulty discriminating voices when there is distracting sound, such as conversation in a noisy room.

Noise-induced loss Chronic noise levels higher than 90 dB can produce a hearing loss beginning at high frequencies (4000 Hz). Acoustic trauma—for example, caused by a blast—produces immediate loss resulting from a ruptured tympanic membrane or disarticulation of the ossicles.

Drugs Aminoglycoside antibiotics, furosemide, ethacrynic acid, quinidine, and salicylates can all cause hearing loss.

Ménière's disease Perceived as an asymmetric, fluctuating low-frequency impairment, it is usually associated with tinnitus, fullness in the ear, and episodic vertigo.

Eighth nerve injury Hearing loss may be a sequela of meningitis, mumps, scarlet fever, or skull fracture (**Plate 142**).

Acoustic neuroma This presents as unilateral progressive hearing loss, vertigo, and notably poor speech discrimination. Look for neurofibromas or cafe-au-lait spots elsewhere.

Impacted cerumen Cerumen is apparent on examination of the external auditory canal, and hearing improves immediately after irrigation.

Otitis media The sine qua non is a red and painful tympanic membrane (**Plate 233**).

Middle ear effusion The tympanic membrane is dull but not red, and bubbles or an air-fluid level can be seen through it. The tympanic membrane will not move with exhalation against a closed mouth and nose nor with air insufflation into the ear. Symptoms of viral upper respiratory infection or allergy are usually present.

Perforation of tympanic membrane   A hole will be visible in the tympanic membrane. This is sometimes difficult to discern because the usual landmarks are so distorted. A history of barotrauma is most common.

Otosclerosis   Autosomally dominant, this appears in the second or third decade, marked by tinnitus and a reddish color of promontories visible through the tympanic membrane.

Exostoses   Bilaterally symmetric bony excrescences appear in the external auditory canal; these are often associated with repetitive cold water exposure (e.g., ocean swimming).

Developmental defect   Ossicular malformations are usually associated with atresia of the external auditory canal or deformation of the pinnae.

Glomus tumor   The patient presents with conductive hearing loss, spontaneous bleeding from the external auditory canal, and/or paralysis of cranial nerves IX, X, and XI (jugular foramen syndrome). The tumor can be seen as a reddish mass visible through the tympanic membrane.

Chapter 136

Hoarseness

◼ DIFFERENTIAL OVERVIEW

Acute
- ❑ Viral laryngitis
- ❑ Vocal overuse
- ❑ Vocal cord trauma
- ❑ Angioedema
- ❑ Epiglottitis

Chronic
- ❑ Smoking
- ❑ Recurrent vocal abuse
- ❑ Gastroesophageal reflux
- ❑ Vocal cord polyp
- ❑ Vocal cord nodule
- ❑ Laryngeal nerve injury
- ❑ Hypothyroidism
- ❑ Laryngeal carcinoma

DIAGNOSTIC APPROACH

Persistent or progressive hoarseness is the most suspicious finding.

A breathy voice occurs when the vocal cords do not approximate completely, due to a tumor, polyp, or nodule. A high, shaky voice resulting from decreased respiratory force may occur in elderly patients.

CLINICAL FINDINGS

Viral laryngitis   Other symptoms of upper respiratory infection, such as sore throat or cough, will usually be present.

Vocal overuse   Common causes include inhaling smoke or dust, irritant fumes, or shouting.

Vocal cord trauma   Onset follows intubation or a blow to the neck. Intubation injury may progress to ulceration with painful phonation. Trauma may progress to stridor with subcutaneous emphysema present if the larynx is fractured.

Angioedema   Transient edema without erythema occurs in the tongue, lips, periorbital region or gut, as well as the larynx. There is a sensation of swelling in the throat (**Plate 185**).

Epiglottitis   A sore throat out of proportion to the degree of pharyngeal erythema and progressing rapidly to stridor is a signal presentation.

Smoking   A raspy voice is caused by vocal cord thickening due to edema or inflammation in a chronic heavy smoker.

Gastroesophageal reflux   Heartburn and an acidic taste in the throat are clear indicators, but more subtle symptoms may include a nocturnal cough, frequent throat clearing, or sore throat.

Vocal cord polyp   Polyps arise in patients with hypothyroidism or chronic sinusitis and cause a low and gravelly voice.

Vocal cord nodule   Nodules occur when edematous cords have been used excessively.

Laryngeal nerve injury   Causes include viral neuritis, Pancoast lung tumor, esophageal cancer, neck surgery, and aortic aneurysm.

Hypothyroidism   The voice is deep and husky. Other signs such as goiter, periorbital edema, fatigue, and delayed relaxation of the ankle jerk reflex are found (**Plates 16, 17, 18**).

Laryngeal carcinoma   Dysphagia and pain occur before hoarseness unless the tumor involves the vocal cords. Other presentations include pain with swallowing, fetid breath, or an unexplained lymph node in the neck. Tobacco use and alcohol use are predisposing factors.

Loss of Vision Chapter 137

◼ DIFFERENTIAL OVERVIEW

Acute Loss
- ❏ Ophthalmic migraine
- ❏ Amaurosis fugax
- ❏ Retinal detachment
- ❏ Acute angle closure glaucoma
- ❏ Optic neuritis
- ❏ Papilledema
- ❏ Retinal artery occlusion
- ❏ Giant cell arteritis
- ❏ Trauma
- ❏ Toxic
- ❏ Occipital stroke
- ❏ Ischemic optic neuropathy
- ❏ Retinal hemorrhage
- ❏ Vitreous hemorrhage
- ❏ Central retinal vein occlusion

Gradual Loss
- ❏ Refractive error
- ❏ Intraocular hypertension
- ❏ Cataract
- ❏ Diabetic retinopathy
- ❏ Macular degeneration
- ❏ Cytomegalovirus retinitis
- ❏ Drugs
- ❏ Keratoconjunctivitis sicca
- ❏ Optic nerve compression
- ❏ Pituitary adenoma
- ❏ Choroidal melanoma
- ❏ Retinitis pigmentosa

DIAGNOSTIC APPROACH

Homonymous hemianopsia may be perceived as blurring or as trouble finding the start of a line of print. On closer inspection, visual loss in corresponding fields in both eyes will be detected. This usually results from a lesion in the suprageniculate pathway. The macula is usually spared in cortical lesions. Bitemporal hemianopsia is due to a chiasmal lesion such as a pituitary adenoma, anterior communicating artery aneurysm, cerebellar tumor with third ventricle hydrocephalus, or meningitis. Thiamine deficiency, methanol toxicity, or optic neuritis at the chiasm can cause true acute bilateral visual loss

An afferent pupillary defect (Marcus Gunn pupil) is diagnostic for a prechiasmal optic nerve lesion. Have the patient fixate on a far object, and then shine a bright light into his or her eyes. The initial (abnormal) response is dilation instead of brisk contraction.

Tunnel vision causes a patient to turn his or her head to avoid bumping into objects, and it can be outlined by visual field confrontation. Causes include glaucoma, retinitis pigmentosa, and quinine toxicity.

CLINICAL FINDINGS

Ophthalmic migraine The transient visual loss may or may not be accompanied by headache, but the patient usually has a history of migraine. Homonymous hemianopsia with flashing or scintillating zigzag lights at the periphery is perceived in both eyes.

Amaurosis fugax This is a classic sentinel sign for an impending stroke. Vision becomes grayer until no vision remains, and then returns after 1 minute, progressing from gray to clear. It is caused by a transient retinal artery embolism, usually by a platelet thrombus.

If seen, this may appear dull white within a vessel. An ipsilateral carotid bruit often is present **(Plate 238)**.

Retinal detachment   There is often a prodrome of flashing lights and a shower of vitreous floaters. Visual loss occurs as if a veil is being placed over the person or a shade is being pulled down. A gray billowing retina can be seen unless obscured by blood **(Plate 215)**.

Acute angle closure glaucoma   The eye is severely painful and red. The pupil is fixed and midposition. The anterior chamber is shallow and does not transmit tangential light well. The cornea becomes cloudy **(Plate 217)**.

Optic neuritis   Visual loss is progressive over hours or days. The optic nerve is hyperemic in the acute stages, having the appearance of papilledema, but spontaneous venous pulsations are present. There is often an afferent pupillary defect and internuclear ophthalmoplegia (weak ipsilateral adduction and contralateral nystagmus on abduction), as well as prominent impairment of macular and red vision. There is pain with eye movement, and the globe is tender. This is a common prologue to multiple sclerosis **(Plate 128)**.

Papilledema   Central vision is normal, but the periphery is constricted. The optic disc margins are blurred, the disc is hyperemic, and venous pulsations are absent **(Plate 129)**.

Retinal artery occlusion   All or part of a monocular visual field is affected. Visual acuity is reduced to light perception only or worse. In central retinal artery occlusion, the retina appears pale and edematous with a prominent "cherry red" macula, and there will be anisocoria. In branch occlusions, a brightly refractile yellow cholesterol embolus may be seen in a retinal artery **(Plate 239)**.

Giant cell arteritis   Visual loss occurs in the context of headache, ropy and tender temporal artery, jaw claudication, or proximal muscle weakness.

Trauma   Vision may be lost through an occipital concussion that produces edema or by a skull fracture into the sphenoid that affects the optic nerve.

Toxic   There is bilateral optic disc swelling with a central scotoma. Agents include ethambutol, methyl alcohol, ethylene glycol, and carbon monoxide.

Occipital stroke   Homonymous hemianopsia is the main manifestation.

Ischemic optic neuropathy   Visual loss involves the superior visual field and macula. The optic disc appears edematous with flame hemorrhages in one portion. This usually occurs in younger patients with diabetes or hypertension or in older patients with vascular disease.

Retinal hemorrhage   Easily seen as a red retinal plaque, it occurs in diabetes, glaucoma, and thrombocytopenia. **(Plate 214)**.

Vitreous hemorrhage   Hemorrhage occurs with retinal detachment, diabetes, and sickle cell anemia. The media is cloudy.

Central retinal vein occlusion   Visual loss is sudden but less pronounced. The fundus has a "squashed tomato" appearance with engorged tortuous veins and flame (nerve layer) hemorrhages **(Plate 240)**.

Refractive error   Myopia usually stabilizes by the time a patient reaches his or her twenties. By determining the number of diopters needed to focus on the retina one can assess the degree of the problem. With presbyopia, the decreased ability to accommodate reduces acuity with close reading.

Intraocular hypertension   Findings of chronic glaucomatous pressure effects include increased cup-to-disc ratio, nasalization of the vessels, and cribriform striations in a deep disc. Field loss begins with arcuate or sector-shaped scotoma, which enlarge. Central vision remains intact **(Plate 218)**.

Cataract   The patient has difficulty focusing and is visually irritated by oncoming headlights. The retina cannot be brought into clear focus on fundoscopy, and opacity may be seen when focusing the fundoscope more anteriorly.

Diabetic retinopathy   Neovascularization around the optic disc is the key finding. Diabetes can also cause blurred vision through an edematous lens **(Plate 166)**.

Macular degeneration   Central vision is impaired, but peripheral vision remains intact. Fundoscopy reveals macular drusen (small, yellow lesions clustered at the macula) and atrophy of the retinal pigment epithelium with prominent choroidal vessels, subretinal hemorrhage, and central fibrous scar **(Plate 216)**.

Loss of Vision

Cytomegalovirus retinitis   Occurring in a patient with HIV infection, retinitis causes a broad crystalline "crumbled cheese" retinal exudate, with hemorrhage at the advancing border **(Plates 202, 203).**

Drugs   Chloroquine and phenothiazines may affect the vision.

Keratoconjunctivitis sicca   There is a dry, gritty sensation in the eyes with decreased tearing. It often occurs in a patient with a connective tissue disease (Sjogren's syndrome).

Optic nerve compression   Compression may be suggested by functional pupillary abnormalities, visual field defects, or pallor/atrophy of the optic disc **(Plate 127).**

Pituitary adenoma   Loss of central vision occurs along with altered endocrine function, such as lactation in prolactinoma **(Plate 15).**

Choroidal melanoma   Symptoms include photopsia, an enlarging scotoma, and visual loss. On fundoscopy, a darkly pigmented retinal lesion can be seen **(Plate 161).**

Retinitis pigmentosa   Night blindness and tunnel vision are typical symptoms. Fundoscopy reveals pigment clumped at the periphery of the retina and constriction of retinal arterioles.

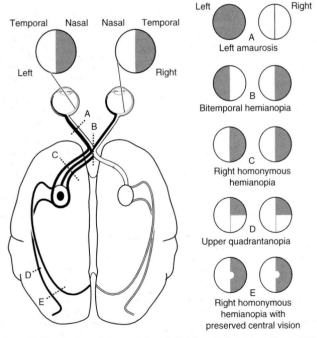

Figure 20. Visual pathway lesions and visual field defects. (Adapted from: Droste C, Von Planta M. Memorik Clinical Medicine. London: Chapman & Hall, 1997, p. 268.)

Chapter 138

Nasal Congestion/Discharge

PLATES 111, 169

▨ DIFFERENTIAL OVERVIEW

❑ Common cold
❑ Allergic rhinitis
❑ Vasomotor rhinitis
❑ Nasal polyp
❑ Sinusitis
❑ Drugs
❑ Deviated septum
❑ Intranasal foreign body
❑ Sarcoidosis
❑ Cerebrospinal fluid leak
❑ Wegener's granulomatosis

CLINICAL FINDINGS

Common cold   The onset is acute, causing a scratchy sore throat and cough. The nasal mucosa will appear red, boggy, and glassy. The nasal drainage will initially be clear but will later become colored (yellow-green).

Allergic rhinitis   Seasonal rhinitis is usually caused by inhaled pollens. Perennial rhinitis is caused by allergy to animals, dust, mites, or mold. The nasal mucosa will be bluish and pale. Acute allergic rhinitis is often associated with eye irritation and sneezing.

Vasomotor rhinitis   Congestion is prominent, but rhinorrhea, sneezing, and itching are not. Rhinitis medicamentosa occurs after 3–4 days of continuous use of a topical vaso-constrictor. There will be initial relief with its use that is then followed by rebound with worsened congestion. Vasomotor rhinitis may also be precipitated by cold, emotion, or sexual arousal.

Nasal polyp   Unilateral airflow will be obstructed and a polyp will be visible deep inside, beyond the turbinate, as a gray structure with the appearance of a skinned grape. There is an association between aspirin use, nasal polyps, and asthma, but the most common cause is chronic allergic rhinitis.

Sinusitis   Drainage will be purulent although colored drainage can be found in other conditions. There will be a sensation of facial fullness that worsens with bending forward, often accompanied by fever and a headache. On physical examination, there will be tenderness to concussion and pressure, overlying warmth, and fever. The sinuses will not transilluminate.

Drugs   Cocaine, beta-blockers, reserpine, and hydralazine can each cause nasal obstruction.

Deviated septum   Deviation causes chronic unilateral obstruction, which is readily observed with a nasal speculum.

Intranasal foreign body   There will be nasal obstruction associated with a chronic unilateral mucopurulent discharge with a foul odor.

Sarcoidosis   Sarcoidosis presents with bilateral nasal congestion in as many as 20% of cases. Systemic symptoms such as fever, fatigue, or weight loss; pulmonary symptoms such as cough or dyspnea; or skin manifestations such as erythema nodosum or purple, waxy plaques are clues to the underlying diagnosis **(Plate 169).**

Cerebrospinal fluid leak   Head trauma with a basilar skull fracture may go unrecognized. Clear nasal drainage tests positive for glucose using a urine dipstick.

Wegener's granulomatosis   Its earliest manifestation may be nasal obstruction, rhinorrhea, crusting, and chronic sinusitis with a fetid drainage. Development of a septal ulceration is classic **(Plate 111).**

DIFFERENTIAL OVERVIEW

Neck Mass
❏ Inflammatory lymphadenopathy
❏ Parotid swelling/tumor
❏ Intramuscular hematoma
❏ Lymphoma
❏ Metastatic nasopharyngeal cancer
❏ Branchial cleft cyst
❏ Thyroglossal duct cyst
❏ Supraclavicular adenopathy
❏ Aortic aneurysm
❏ Carotid aneurysm
❏ Ludwig's angina
❏ Pharyngeal pouch
❏ Carotid body tumor

Thyroid Enlargement
❏ Simple goiter
❏ Hashimoto's thyroiditis
❏ Grave's disease
❏ Drugs
❏ Subacute thyroiditis
❏ Thyroid cancer
❏ Infiltrative disease

DIAGNOSTIC APPROACH

Patients will often present for evaluation of a "neck mass" that is a normal structure such as the hyoid, and they will insist that it is new or asymmetric.

With thyroid enlargement, the mass will be low in the neck and extend across the midline. Occasionally, a prominent thyroid nodule will mimic a lymph node but is in an atypical location. The thyroid gland rises and falls with swallowing. The only other structure to do this is a thyroglossal duct cyst.

In a multinodular goiter, a malignancy should be suspected when there is a dominant nodule or cervical adenopathy.

CLINICAL FINDINGS

Inflammatory lymphadenopathy   Bilateral, enlarged, tender anterior cervical nodes are seen in streptococcal pharyngitis and infectious mononucleosis. Concomitant posterior cervical nodes are found with the latter. Unilateral tender adenopathy is seen in dental, sinus, ear, and facial skin infections **(Plate 230).**

Parotid swelling/tumor   The swelling will be present at the angle of the jaw. Bilateral swelling with fever, lacrimal gland inflammation, and uveitis occurs in patients with Hodgkin's, tuberculosis, lupus, and sarcoidosis. Isolated swelling can occur with mumps, HIV, or bulimia. A tumor appears as a discrete rubbery mass. Unilateral swelling occurs with ductal obstruction caused by a stone.

Intramuscular hematoma   Hematoma occurs with neck strain or trauma, as a rapidly appearing mass within a muscle body.

Lymphoma   It presents with firm, large (>2 cm), rubbery, nontender nodes, often contiguous in a chain. Fever, night sweats, and weight loss are helpful signs.

Metastatic nasopharyngeal cancer   Suspect cancer when there is a hard mass in the anterior cervical nodes in a person who smokes.

Branchial cleft cyst   It is a lateral cystic structure that may enlarge suddenly as a result of trauma or infection.

Neck Mass/ Thyroid Enlargement

Thyroglossal duct cyst   It appears as a fluid-filled mass in the midline, which transilluminates and elevates when the tongue is protruded.

Supraclavicular adenopathy   Right supraclavicular nodes are found in intrathoracic cancers. Left supraclavicular nodes are found in intraabdominal cancers **(Plate 63)**.

Aortic aneurysm   A pulsatile mass will appear in the supraclavicular space.

Carotid aneurysm   A pulsatile mass is palpated over the carotid.

Ludwig's angina   Because of infection from a dental source, the floor of the mouth and sublingual/submandibular space beneath the deep cervical fascia are swollen.

Pharyngeal pouch   The swollen area feels uncomfortable when the patient swallows. Stagnating food causes halitosis.

Carotid body tumor   It is present at the carotid bifurcation, with a transmitted pulse.

Simple goiter   Goiter presents as diffuse or multinodular thyroid enlargement in a clinically euthyroid person, most commonly a woman (5–10:1). Diffuse goiter occurs in adolescence or pregnancy, and multinodular goiter occurs in middle age. Iodine deficiency, soybeans, and iodides (seaweed) are dietary causes **(Plate 16)**.

Hashimoto's thyroiditis   Diffuse thyroid enlargement has a gradual onset. The gland is lobulated and rubbery and often has a prominent pyramidal lobe. The patient may be either euthyroid or hypothyroid on clinical evaluation. A family history of autoimmune endocrine disorders frequently exists **(Plate 16)**.

Grave's disease   An autoimmune goiter has a finely nodular "cobblestone" feel and is vascular with a bruit and thrill. The patient is usually overtly hyperthyroid, with signs of hyperthyroidism and infiltrative ophthalmopathy **(Plates 16, 19)**.

Drugs   Antithyroid drugs, iodides, lithium, sulfonamides, sulfonylureas, methylxanthines, and ethionamide can all cause thyroid enlargement.

Subacute thyroiditis   The enlarged, tender gland has a bruit.

Thyroid cancer   It begins as a hard focal nodule, often with firm regional lymphadenopathy. Local extension produces loss of movement of the thyroid with swallowing. The recurrent laryngeal nerve and carotid bundle may be involved early, but Horner's is a late finding.

Infiltrative disease   Riedel's thyroiditis produces a firm goiter, often mistaken for cancer, and pressure symptoms disproportionate to the size of the gland. It may be associated with retroperitoneal fibrosis or sclerosing cholangitis. The recurrent laryngeal nerve is involved early. Sarcoidosis, amyloidosis, and lymphoma can also produce this.

Oral Ulcers

Chapter 140

PLATES 69, 87, 178, 184, 209, 211, 213

◤ DIFFERENTIAL OVERVIEW

❑ Aphthous ulcers
❑ Angular cheilitis
❑ Herpes simplex
❑ Traumatic ulcers
❑ Impetigo
❑ Erythema multiforme
❑ Mucositis
❑ Lichen planus
❑ Squamous cell cancer
❑ Coxsackievirus A
❑ Herpes zoster
❑ Primary HIV
❑ Crohn's disease
❑ Behçet's syndrome
❑ Syphilis
❑ Acute leukemia
❑ Pemphigoid

CLINICAL FINDINGS

Aphthous ulcers   They occur on nonkeratinized mucosa as single lesions or clusters of shallow, painful ulcers with an erythematous halo and a white base. There are usually no systemic symptoms or lymphadenopathy. These ulcers stereotypically recur.

Angular cheilitis   Tender fissuring at the corner of the mouth can be caused by *Candida*, iron, or vitamin B12 deficiency **(Plate 69).**

Herpes simplex   An acute outbreak consists of labial vesicles that rupture and crust and intraoral vesicles that quickly ulcerate. The lesions are usually quite painful and associated with fever, malaise, pharyngitis, and tender cervical lymphadenopathy. Recurrent lesions usually occur at the vermilion border and are preceded by localized burning dysesthesias **(Plate 209).**

Traumatic ulcers   These ulcers occur at the bite margin or adjacent to dentures.

Impetigo   Perioral painful shallow erosions spread rapidly. They are red and weeping, with honey-colored crusts **(Plate 178).**

Erythema multiforme   The onset is rapid and progresses to systemic toxicity. Intraoral ruptured bullae surrounded by erythema become painful mucosal erosions with gray exudate. Hemorrhagic crusts appear on the lips. An extensive maculopapular rash develops on the extensor surfaces and is characterized by target and polycyclic lesions and persisting urticarial plaques. Target lesions on the hands and feet are pathognomonic **(Plate 184).**

Mucositis   Commonly occurring with chemotherapy, mucositis causes a burning with diffuse mucosal redness and shininess that progresses to painful ulcers. There may also be a yellow pseudomembrane or hemorrhagic crust.

Lichen planus   Lacy mucosal striae break down into painful erosions. This is often associated with drugs such as chloroquine, furosemide, gold, lithium, methyldopa, phenothiazines, propranolol, quinidine, spironolactone, tetracycline, or thiazides.

Squamous cell cancer   The ulcer is painless and indolent, failing to heal. It arises in an area of leukoplakia and has an elevated, indurated border.

Coxsackievirus A   Herpangina presents with fever, sore throat, and grayish-white vesicles with a red halo, which quickly ulcerate. Hand, foot, and mouth disease (A16) has similar pharyngeal lesions accompanied by other lesions in the forenamed distribution **(Plates 211, 213).**

Herpes zoster   A vesicular eruption with ulceration stops at the midline. Vesicles will also be present on the lower midface. Burning pain is characteristic.

Primary HIV   The most common presentation is a febrile mononucleosis-like illness. Acute gingivitis and ulceration may be part of the spectrum.

Crohn's disease   Oral ulcers may occur when intestinal disease is active, with symptoms of diarrhea, mucus, and blood.

Behçet's syndrome   Multiple aphthous ulcers of the mouth occur with uveitis and genital ulcers **(Plate 87).**

Syphilis   A primary chancre is a painless ulcer with an indurated copper border and unilateral lymphadenopathy. Secondary lesions are linear "snail track" ulcers and gray mucous patches on the lips, tonsils, and palate. There is concurrent generalized rash and fever. A tertiary gumma is a firm, broad, ulcerated plaque that may produce palatal perforation.

Acute leukemia   Gingival swelling and superficial ulceration occur; hyperplasia, hemorrhage, and necrosis ensue. Deep ulcers may occur elsewhere on the mucosa, and they often become secondarily infected.

Pemphigoid   Painful grayish-white collapsed vesicles or bullae ulcerate when on the gingiva. Bullae may also involve the eyes, urethra, vagina, or rectum.

Ptosis

Chapter 141

◼ DIFFERENTIAL OVERVIEW

❑ Horner's syndrome
❑ Diabetic mononeuritis
❑ Eyelid edema
❑ Myasthenia gravis
❑ Posterior communicating artery aneurysm

DIAGNOSTIC APPROACH

Observation of pupillary involvement is the key to differentiating oculomotor (CNIII) lesions (mydriasis) from Horner's syndrome (miosis).

CLINICAL FINDINGS

Horner's syndrome   Findings include a small pupil, enophthalmos (illusory, caused by retraction of the globe), and anhidrosis with mild vasodilation on the affected side. The ptotic eyelid can still be voluntarily raised **(Plate 120).**

Diabetic mononeuritis   There may be severe pain and ophthalmoplegia but there is usually pupillary sparing **(Plate 166).**

Eyelid edema   Usually conjunctival erythema exists although angioedema may occur without apparent inflammation **(Plate 185).**

Myasthenia gravis   Ptosis is bilateral and fluctuates, being worse later in the day. Sustained upward gaze produces gradual ptosis of the eyelids. Associated findings include dysconjugate eye movements with sustained horizontal gaze; hoarse, nasal, or slurred voice on prolonged phonation; and inability to sustain motor activity of the limbs **(Plate 219).**

Posterior communicating artery aneurysm   Ptosis is associated with pupillary dilation and abduction of the eye, with inability to turn the eye medially.

◼ DIFFERENTIAL OVERVIEW

- ❑ Viral conjunctivitis
- ❑ Allergic conjunctivitis
- ❑ Bacterial conjunctivitis
- ❑ Corneal abrasion
- ❑ Foreign body
- ❑ Subconjunctival hemorrhage
- ❑ Hordeolum
- ❑ Blepharitis
- ❑ Photophthalmia
- ❑ Acute angle closure glaucoma
- ❑ Chlamydial conjunctivitis
- ❑ Hypopyon
- ❑ Dacryocystitis
- ❑ Herpes simplex keratitis
- ❑ Iritis
- ❑ Scleritis
- ❑ Gonococcal conjunctivitis
- ❑ Keratoconjunctivitis sicca
- ❑ Measles
- ❑ Endophthalmitis

DIAGNOSTIC APPROACH

Decreased vision, pain, photophobia, and a history of trauma are important indicators of serious pathology.

In conjunctivitis, the anterior chamber is clear and the pupil active. There is great overlap in the clinical spectrum of bacterial and viral conjunctivitis. Ciliary flush—dilation of the fine capillaries around the iris border producing a violet-red halo—is a differentiating sign indicating anterior uveal inflammation caused by iritis/uveitis, a connective tissue disease, rather than by infection. It may also occur with acute glaucoma. The eye is tender in patients with scleritis, iritis, and glaucoma, but not in conjunctivitis.

CLINICAL FINDINGS

Viral conjunctivitis Watery or mucoid discharge, common cold symptoms, follicular swelling of the lid, and tender preauricular lymph nodes are helpful clues **(Plate 224).**

Allergic conjunctivitis Bilateral itching and tears are associated with seasonal allergic rhinitis and atopic dermatitis. Vernal conjunctivitis (papillary hypertrophy of the underside of the lid) may develop in soft contact lens wearers. Edema without erythema suggests allergy **(Plate 225).**

Bacterial conjunctivitis A unilateral mucopurulent discharge, with lids stuck together in the morning by a thick crust, is prominent. The conjunctival erythema is more intense than in viral or allergic conjunctivitis **(Plate 223).**

Corneal abrasion Superficial eye irritation, a foreign body sensation without any foreign particle apparent, and excessive tearing are present. A history of trauma or of discomfort persisting after removal of a foreign body is usually elicited. Slit lamp examination or a patch of fluorescence with fluorescein confirms the diagnosis.

Foreign body There is copious tearing with the sensation of a particle in the eye. The patient will be able to localize the source of the discomfort. If no foreign body is seen, evert the upper lid.

Subconjunctival hemorrhage A painless, fixed, blood-red quadrantic lesion often occurs with minor trauma. If the patient is taking anticoagulants, the lesion may signal overdose.

Hordeolum A painful, red, tender nodule appears at the lid margin (external) or under the lid (internal).

289

Blepharitis Redness and crusting along the lid margins may be associated with a conjunctivitis and loss of eyelashes. A clue is associated seborrheic dermatitis of the face or scalp.

Photophthalmia Redness occurs in the setting of excessive sun exposure or tanning booth use.

Acute angle closure glaucoma Symptoms are unilateral headache or eye pain with nausea, colored halos surrounding lights, and cloudy vision. The pupil is poorly reactive to light. The cornea is cloudy as a result of edema. The globe feels hard on palpation. The anterior chamber does not transmit light with tangential illumination (light reaches less than one-third of the way to the nasal iris) **(Plate 217)**.

Chlamydia conjunctivitis Early infection appears as conjunctivitis with small lymphoid follicles on the upper tarsal conjunctiva and a watery-to-mucoid discharge.

Hypopyon A yellow, ragged corneal ulcer develops and is followed by a pus in the anterior chamber, which layers out inferiorly **(Plate 226)**.

Dacryocystitis Swelling, redness, and tenderness develop at the inner canthus of the eye **(Plate 228)**.

Herpes simplex keratitis Ciliary flush and photophobia are present. A fine branching dendritic pattern or a broader geographic defect (also seen with zoster) is apparent with fluorescein staining **(Plate 208)**.

Iritis Deep pain, photophobia, blurred vision, and ciliary flush indicate iritis. When the ciliary body is involved (iridocyclitis), there are punctate precipitates on the inner surface of the cornea. A blue iris may become greenish as a result of vascular congestion. There may be contraction and irregularity of the pupil. Associated conditions include autoimmune disease (ankylosing spondylitis, Reiter's, Behçet's, Crohn's, sarcoidosis, or sprue) and infections (tuberculosis, syphilis, HSV, or Lyme disease) **(Plate 86)**.

Scleritis The eyes become tender and irritated with small purple corneal nodules on a red background. Inflammation often occurs in a quadrantic distribution. This may be seen in association with connective tissue disease (rheumatoid arthritis, lupus, PAN, Wegener's, or gout), allergic conditions, or psoriasis.

Gonococcal conjunctivitis Urethritis is usually present, and the affected eye is ipsilateral to the dominant hand. Swelling, chemosis, pain, and purulent discharge are more prominent than with bacterial conjunctivitis.

Keratoconjunctivitis sicca It occurs in geriatric patients, in patients who have connective tissue disease, or in those who have had corneal exposure owing to Bell's palsy. The eyes feel gritty and have a mucoid discharge.

Measles Conjunctivitis occurs 3–4 days before the rash, during the phase characterized by fever, malaise, cough, and Koplik spots **(Plate 136)**.

Endophthalmitis Infection occurs from hematogenous seeding in immunosuppressed or diabetic patients, producing ocular pain and visual loss **(Plate 154)**.

Retinal Phenomena

■ DIFFERENTIAL OVERVIEW

❑ Hypertension
❑ Diabetic retinopathy
❑ Glaucoma
❑ Cholesterol emboli
❑ Papilledema
❑ Pigmented crescent
❑ Macular degeneration
❑ Retinal detachment
❑ Acute optic neuritis
❑ Optic atrophy
❑ Retinal hemorrhage
❑ Chorioretinal exudates
❑ Lipemia retinalis
❑ Central retinal artery occlusion
❑ Central retinal vein occlusion
❑ Angioid streaks
❑ Hyperviscosity

CLINICAL FINDINGS

Hypertension   A significant AV crossing change is one that is two disc diameters out and that obliterates the venous column of blood. This is because of longstanding arterial muscular hypertrophy, and it will remain even after the hypertension is treated. Accelerated hypertension is most readily recognized by retinal hemorrhage, which is a marker for a similar pathophysiology in the brain **(Plates 37, 38).**

Diabetic retinopathy   Diabetic retinopathy most often involves microaneurysms, dot hemorrhages, and exudates. Neovascularization around the optic disc heralds retinal and vitreous hemorrhage, which leads to blindness **(Plate 166).**

Glaucoma   The optic cup-to-disc ratio is increased, and striations can be seen on the surface of the cup. The cup is several diopters deep, with vessels visibly rising over the lip of the disc **(Plate 218).**

Cholesterol emboli   A brightly refractile yellow embolus impacts at an arteriolar branch point. This is important to recognize as a marker of an ulcerated carotid plaque **(Plate 238).**

Papilledema   The optic disc becomes edematous, which is manifest as an indistinct disc margin, hyperemia, and absence of venous pulsations. The usual implication is raised intracranial pressure **(Plate 129).**

Pigmented crescent   This is a normal finding adjacent to the disc, and its appearance corresponds to the degree of skin pigmentation.

Macular degeneration   Macular drusen, atrophy of the retinal pigment with prominent choroidal vessels, subretinal edema or hemorrhage, and a central fibrous scar are typical findings **(Plate 216).**

Retinal detachment   The retina appears to billow in undulating folds. It is difficult to keep vessels in focus because they cross focal planes **(Plate 215).**

Acute optic neuritis   On examination it appears very similar to papilledema, but there is decreased visual acuity as opposed to an enlarged physiologic blind spot **(Plate 128).**

Optic atrophy   It appears as a porcelain-white disc with sharply demarcated edges **(Plate 127).**

Retinal hemorrhage   Retinal hemorrhage is found in accelerated hypertension, diabetes, pernicious anemia, DIC, leukemia, and subarachnoid hemorrhage. In endocarditis, a Roth spot (focal hemorrhage with a clear center) may be found **(Plate 214).**

Chorioretinal exudates   Cytomegalovirus retinitis in a patient with AIDS has an appearance of a yellow granular exudate with hemorrhage at the advancing border. These should be distinguished from the cotton-wool spots caused by HIV infection alone. White cotton-like lesions in a febrile immunocompromised patient suggest systemic candidiasis **(Plates 202, 203, 204, 205).**

291

Lipemia retinalis   The retina and retinal vessels have a pale/yellow appearance in hyper-triglyceridemia **(Plate 39).**

Central retinal artery occlusion   The optic disc is pale, the retina is edematous, the macula appears cherry-red, and there are "boxcar veins" **(Plate 239).**

Central retinal vein occlusion   Veins are tortuous and dilated, the retina is edematous and has flame hemorrhages, and the optic disc margin is blurred **(Plate 240).**

Angioid streaks   Dark linear streaking of the retina in pseudoxanthoma elasticum appears like ghosts of traversing vessels. This condition is associated with accelerated peripheral vascular and coronary artery disease **(Plate 50).**

Hyperviscosity   Tortuous sausage-link retinal veins are found in macroglobulinemia.

Chapter 144

Sore Throat

◼ DIFFERENTIAL OVERVIEW

- ❑ Rhinovirus
- ❑ Group A streptococci
- ❑ Ebstein-Barr virus
- ❑ Adenovirus
- ❑ Candida/thrush
- ❑ Herpes simplex virus
- ❑ Peritonsillar abscess
- ❑ Mycoplasma pneumoniae
- ❑ Coxsackievirus
- ❑ Primary HIV
- ❑ Epiglottitis
- ❑ Corynebacterium diphtheriae
- ❑ Leukemia

DIAGNOSTIC APPROACH

The most important consideration is whether the patient has a group A strep infection because prompt treatment prevents rheumatic fever. The findings of fever, tender anterior cervical adenopathy, and tonsillar exudate can be combined to make the diagnosis more or less likely: 0 findings (LR 0.3); 1–2 findings (LR 1.4); and all 3 findings (LR 8.0).

A prominent sore throat out of proportion to the degree of pharyngeal inflammation should raise the possibility of acute epiglottitis and acutely impending airway compromise.

Persistent unilateral tonsillar enlargement in a young adult without sore throat should raise the suspicion of lymphoma.

CLINICAL FINDINGS

Rhinovirus   The sore throat is mildly scratchy with nasal congestion, rhinorrhea, and nonproductive cough.

Group A streptococci   There is acute onset of a bright red throat with a tonsillar exudate, fever and tender anterior cervical adenopathy **(Plate 230)**.

Ebstein-Barr virus   There is a systemic illness with fever and prominent fatigue. The tonsils are usually quite large and covered with an exudate. Palatal petechiae, posterior cervical adenopathy, and splenomegaly are helpful clues although not always present **(Plates 229, 230)**.

Adenovirus   Infection causes a febrile pharyngitis and conjunctivitis that occurs in the summer.

Candida/thrush   A cottage cheese-like exudate appears on the throat, tongue, and buccal mucosa with the underlying mucosa becoming bright red. Precipitating factors include immune compromise, such as HIV, diabetes, or use of inhaled steroids for asthma **(Plate 206)**.

Herpes simplex virus   Infection presents as a vesicular and ulcerative pharyngitis/stomatitis. Often a typical vesicular "cold sore" will be present on the lip **(Plate 209)**.

Peritonsillar abscess   Abscess is recognized by the severity of the sore throat, high fever, toxic appearance of the patient, and trismus with drooling (unable to open the mouth or swallow). A unilateral bulging of the anterior tonsillar pillar may be fluctuant and displace the uvula. The patient has a muffled "hot potato" voice. Common carotid infection can lead to rupture, heralded by bleeding in the nose, mouth, or ear **(Plate 231)**.

Mycoplasma pneumoniae   Associated symptoms include a prominent dry cough or a syndrome of atypical pneumonia. Bullous otitis media, when present, is diagnostically helpful **(Plate 232)**.

Coxsackievirus   Vesicles and ulcers on the tonsillar pillars and soft palate appear similar to herpes **(Plate 211)**.

Primary HIV   Sore throat occurs in 70%. Characteristic features include an acute mono-like illness with fever, lymphadenopathy, diffuse maculopapular rash including involvement of the palms or soles, and mucocutaneous ulceration.

Epiglottitis The patient has a severe sore throat without erythema, appears acutely anxious, sits forward, and has stridor. The edematous uvula may project over the base of the tongue.

Corynebacterium diphtheriae An adherent bluish-white to green-gray membrane covers the tonsils and causes bleeding if removed. The patient is severely lethargic often with stridor. There is a "bull's neck" appearance due to submental and cervical adenopathy. The breath is said to smell like a "wet mouse."

Leukemia A nonspecific sore throat, asthenia, lymphadenopathy, and gum infiltrates are indicators.

■ DIFFERENTIAL OVERVIEW

❑ Hashimoto's thyroiditis
❑ Multinodular goiter
❑ Follicular adenoma
❑ Thyroid cyst
❑ Thyroid carcinoma
❑ Subacute thyroiditis

DIAGNOSTIC APPROACH

The major task of physical examination is the detection of nodules. A palpable nodule can be detected in 4–7% of adults, but these are present in approximately 50% on ultrasound or autopsy series. The history or physical examination should rarely dissuade one from proceeding to thyroid scan and/or fine needle aspiration.

Approximately 5% of nodules are cancer. High-risk (71%) features include the following: rapid growth, a very firm nodule, fixation, vocal cord paralysis, enlarged regional lymph nodes, distant metastases, and family history of medullary cancer. Moderate risk (14%) features are as follows: Age less than 20 years or greater than 60 years, history of neck irradiation (>100 cGy >15 years before), solitary nodule, diameter greater than 4 cm, and questionable fixation.

A thyroid nodule in a hyperthyroid patient is virtually never malignant, but a prominent or hard nodule in a multinodular goiter must be evaluated for cancer.

CLINICAL FINDINGS

Hashimoto's thyroiditis The gland is rubbery as a result of lymphocytic infiltration, diffusely enlarged, and bosselated. Symptoms of hypothyroidism coincide. The pyramidal lobe may be prominently enlarged.

Multinodular goiter The gland is irregular and not as firm as in Hashimoto's. Nodules may develop when colloid accumulates in hyperplastic cells (colloid cyst). Lithium, beets, and turnips are goitrogens **(Plate 16).**

Follicular adenoma Adenoma often presents as a solitary nodule that has grown slowly over years. Small adenomas are usually inactive although those larger than 3 cm may function autonomously and present with thyrotoxicosis. Reduction in size with suppressive therapy is the rule although this can also occur on occasion with thyroid cancer. Hemorrhage into a preexisting nodule may cause acute painful enlargement.

Thyroid cyst It transilluminates and may suddenly enlarge with pain because of hemorrhage.

Thyroid carcinoma A firm (hardness of an unripe apple), irregular, large (>2 cm) nodule that is fixed and fails to move with swallowing suggests cancer. The consistency of the tissue may not be a reliable sign of malignancy because papillary carcinomas that have undergone cystic degeneration may present as soft nodules. Additional clues are hard cervical adenopathy, hoarseness (caused by recurrent laryngeal compression), Horner's syndrome, or tenderness in a rapidly growing nodule. Anaplastic carcinoma occurs in elderly patients and has rapid local invasion. Medullary carcinoma occurs in the context of a familial MEN syndrome with pheochromocytoma.

Subacute thyroiditis Often occurring postpartum or following an upper respiratory infection, subacute thyroiditis causes symptoms of malaise and pain over the thyroid. The thyroid is finely nodular. Acutely, there is fever, and severe, often unilateral pain, which responds readily to salicylates. The patient is usually mildly thyrotoxic.

Tinnitus

◼ DIFFERENTIAL OVERVIEW

- ❑ Impacted cerumen
- ❑ Otitis media
- ❑ Eustachian dysfunction
- ❑ Presbyacusis
- ❑ Hypertension
- ❑ Drugs
- ❑ Ménière's
- ❑ Acoustic neuroma
- ❑ Vascular aneurysm
- ❑ Arteriovenous malformation
- ❑ Functional
- ❑ Glomus tumor

DIAGNOSTIC APPROACH

Pulsatile tinnitus occurs with hypertension, berry aneurysm, arteriovenous malformation, internal carotid stenosis, a tortuous carotid within the temporal bone, or glomus tumor. Myoclonus of the palate or stapedial or tensor tympani muscles can produce a rhythmic tinnitus that does not follow the pulse. Tinnitus that can be heard with a stethoscope is usually a result of a tumor, aneurysm, or arteriovenous malformation.

CLINICAL FINDINGS

Impacted cerumen   It is evident on otoscopic examination and confirmed by relief with irrigation.

Otitis media   The tympanic membrane is bright red **(Plate 233).**

Eustachian dysfunction   Associated with allergies or an upper respiratory infection, this dysfunction causes the patient's hearing to be muffled as if he or she is "hearing underwater," and the tympanic membrane is dull gray with bubbles or a fluid level behind it.

Presbyacusis   High-pitched tinnitus appears near the frequency of the greatest hearing loss. Sometimes sensory deprivation may induce faint auditory illusions of voices or music.

Hypertension   Pulsatile tinnitus can occur with elevated blood pressure.

Drugs   Salicylate toxicity (usually >4 gm/day), aminoglycosides, ethacrynic acid, furosemide, quinidine, cocaine, heavy metals, or methotrexate all can cause tinnitus.

Ménière's   A low-pitched roaring tinnitus is associated with fluctuating vertigo, hearing loss, and a sense of fullness in the ear.

Acoustic neuroma   This often presents with unilateral continuous or pulsatile tinnitus, with subsequent development of vertigo and unilateral hearing loss. Speech discrimination is especially impaired. Facial numbness often occurs.

Vascular aneurysm   Tinnitus can precede neurological phenomena. There may be an audible bruit, especially when the intrapetrous portion of the internal carotid is involved.

Arteriovenous malformation   A to-and-fro bruit may be heard when listening to the skull with the stethoscope.

Functional   Accentuation of normal head sounds is a likely cause, especially of tinnitus that is heard mostly at night. Depression and fatigue lower the threshold of tolerance.

Glomus tumor   Pulsatile tinnitus; conductive hearing loss; paralysis of cranial nerves IX, X, and XI; and spontaneous bleeding from the ear canal are signs. This tumor can sometimes be seen as a red mass through the tympanic membrane.

Chapter 147

Tongue Disorders

◼ DIFFERENTIAL OVERVIEW

Glossitis
- ❏ Vitamin B12 deficiency
- ❏ Folate deficiency
- ❏ Niacin deficiency
- ❏ Riboflavin deficiency
- ❏ Leukoplakia
- ❏ Scarlet fever
- ❏ Kwashiorkor
- ❏ Polyarteritis nodosa

Macroglossia
- ❏ Myxedema
- ❏ Angioedema
- ❏ Acromegaly
- ❏ Amyloidosis

Ulceration
- ❏ Aphthous ulcer
- ❏ Dental ulcer
- ❏ Candida
- ❏ Geographic tongue
- ❏ Herpes simplex
- ❏ Mucositis
- ❏ Syphilis
- ❏ Tongue cancer

DIAGNOSTIC APPROACH

Macroglossia is usually accompanied by serrated dental impressions on the tongue. It will elevate the tongue and cause the sublingual glands to bulge.

A "hairy tongue" usually follows systemic antibiotic use, especially in smokers.

CLINICAL FINDINGS

Vitamin B12 deficiency   The tongue is beefy red, smooth, edematous, and painful. Pinpoint dots occur as a result of hyperemic capillaries and atrophied papillae. Peripheral neuropathy is commonly concurrent (**Plate 69**).

Folate deficiency   It is similar in presentation to B12 deficiency but occurs more rapidly with nutritional depletion (e.g., alcoholics).

Niacin deficiency   Pellagra produces a burning sensation with hot or spicy food, without a visible abnormality early in the course. Later there is an increase in papilla and redness of the tongue's tip and sides, and then fiery redness and swelling with desquamation occur. It is associated with severe watery diarrhea, red skin eruptions, and confusion (**Plate 67**).

Riboflavin deficiency   When advanced, the tongue looks magenta. Associated findings include a "shark skin" nose and conjunctival injection.

Leukoplakia   Early lesions are thin, pearly, and crinkled especially on the lateral border of the tongue. A white-gray thickened epithelium without papillae appears later. Oral hairy leukoplakia is a sentinel finding of HIV infection and is caused by concurrent EBV infection (**Plate 207**).

Scarlet fever   A "strawberry tongue" occurs in a patient with a confluent rash that has the texture of fine sandpaper (**Plates 142, 143**).

Kwashiorkor   Glossitis occurs early and is later accompanied by generalized edema and ascites.

Polyarteritis nodosa   The patient presents with a diffusely inflamed, orange-red tongue that has a burning sensation.

Myxedema   In addition to tongue enlargement, facial and pretibial skin is coarse, the voice is low and husky, and the relaxation phase of the deep tendon reflexes is delayed **(Plate 18).**

Angioedema   Acute edema of tissues frequently includes the tongue. Similar findings may occur with food allergies (e.g., shellfish), drug reactions (penicillin), and serum sickness **(Plate 185).**

Acromegaly   Tissues are generally thickened, and tongue enlargement is associated with jaw protrusion, malocclusion, and teeth that are widely spaced and tilt outward **(Plate 14).**

Amyloidosis   Tongue enlargement occurs with enlargement of other viscera and with peripheral neuropathy **(Plate 131).**

Aphthous ulcer   There are recurrent, small, clean, painful ulcers.

Dental ulcer   It is found adjacent to a sharp tooth edge.

Candida   The tongue is bright red with cottage cheese–like material on the surface **(Plate 206).**

Geographic tongue   The surface has a changing demarcated pattern. This finding is present in serious illness with antibiotic use.

Herpes simplex   Confluent, shallow, painful ulcers on an erythematous base are typical.

Mucositis   The tongue and buccal mucosa are denuded and ulcerated. This condition is found with Stevens-Johnson syndrome, agranulocytosis, and cancer chemotherapy **(Plate 184).**

Syphilis   There will be a clean ulcer with indurated serpentine borders and a history of oral-genital exposure.

Tongue cancer   Cancer appears as a deep, malodorous ulcer, which bleeds easily and has indurated, rolled, everted edges. Pain is referred to the ear.

Color Plate Credit List

The author gratefully acknowledges the use of the following illustrations:

Plates 3, 6, 8, 10, 12, 16, 17, 19, 22, 24, 31, 32, 33, 35, 40, 44, 47, 49, 59, 70, 79, 80, 88, 92, 93, 94, 95, 97, 100, 105, 106, 109, 114, 121, 125, 126, 131, 135, 136, 137, 139, 140, 141, 144, 150, 156, 164, 169, 170, 171, 175, 176, 177, 179, 181, 182, 183, 185, 186, 189, 190, 191, 196, 197, 198, 200, 201, 206, 207, 209, 210, 212, 213, 237. Courtesy of Yale Dermatology Residents' Slide Collection, provided by Lisa Kugelman, MD and Douglas Grossman, MD.

Plates 1, 7, 9, 11, 20, 25, 26, 34, 46, 48, 52, 53, 54, 55, 56, 58, 64, 67, 75, 81, 85, 87, 89, 91, 96, 98, 99, 103, 104, 107, 110, 111, 112, 113, 116, 117, 124, 133, 138, 142, 143, 146, 148, 151, 155, 157, 158, 159, 160, 163, 167, 168, 172, 173, 180, 183, 184, 192, 193, 194, 195, 234, 235, 236. Courtesy of the Dartmouth Dermatology Slide Collection, provided by Steven Spencer, MD.

Plates 21, 23, 37, 38, 39, 45, 50, 86, 118, 122, 127, 128, 129, 154, 161, 166, 202, 204, 205, 208, 214, 215, 216, 217, 218, 221, 222, 223, 224, 225, 226, 227, 228, 239, 240. Courtesy of the Yale University Department of Ophthalmology and Visual Sciences and University of Iowa Department of Opthamology, provided by Peter Gloor, MD.

Plates 71, 149, 152, 153, 165. Courtesy of Douglas Grossman, MD.

Plate 238. David Smith, MD.

Specific acknowledgment is made for use of the following illustrations:

Plates 69, 120, 211, 230, 231, 232, 233. Benjamin B, Bingham B, Hawke M, Stammberger H. Color Atlas of Otorhinolaryngology. London, Martin Dunitz, 1995; distributed in United States by J.B. Lippincott Company.

Plates 4, 66. Braverman IM. Skin Signs of Systemic Disease, 3rd ed. Philadelphia, W.B. Saunders, 1998.

Plates 72, 187. Callen JP, Greer KE, Hood AF, Paller AS, Swinyer LJ. Color Atlas of Dermatology. Philadelphia, W.B. Saunders, 1998.

Plate 5, 147. Fitzpatrick TB, Johnson RA, Polano MK, Suurmond D, Wolff K. Color Atlas and Synopsis of Clinical Dermatology: Common and Serious Diseases, 2nd ed. New York, McGraw-Hill, 1992.

Plates 10, 15, 27, 42, 63, 65, 119, 132, Forbes CD, Jackson WF. Color Atlas and Text of Clinical Medicine, 2nd ed, 1997, Times Mirror International Publishers. By permission of Mosby International Ltd.

Plates 60, 90, 134. From Forbes CD, Jackson WF. Color Atlas and Text of Clinical Medicine, 2nd ed 1997, Times Mirror International Publishers.

Plates 162, 178. Habif TP. Clinical Dermatology: A Color Guide to Diagnosis and Therapy, 3rd ed. St. Louis, Mosby, 1996

Plates 14, 18, 28, 30. Hart FD. French's Index of Differential Diagnosis, 12th ed. Bristol, Wright, 1985.

Plates 74, 76, 77, 82, 83, 84. Holmes KK, Mardh P-A, Sparling PF, Wieser PJ. Sexually Transmitted Diseases, 2nd ed. New York, McGraw-Hill, 1990.

Plates 27, 29, 41, 51, 61, 102, 108, 145, 219, 229. Jamieson MJ, McHardy KC, Towler HMA, Chessel G, et al. Essential Clinical Signs. Edinburgh, Churchill-Livingstone, 1990.

Plate 2. Kelley WN, ed. Textbook of Internal Medicine, 3rd ed. Philadelphia, Lippincott-Raven Publishers, 1997.

Plate 13. Frothingham R. Images in clinical medicine: a medical mystery. New Engl J Med 1997; 337:1666.

Plate 43. Falk RH. Images in clinical medicine: the "thumb sign" in Marfan's syndrome. New Engl J Med 1995; 333:430.

Plate 62. Kovacs RG, Aguayo SM. Images in clinical medicine: superior vena cava syndrome. New Engl J Med 1993; 329:1007.

Plate 68. Kronauer CM, Bühler H. Images in clinical medicine: skin findings in a patient with scurvy. New Engl J Med 1995;332:1611.

Plate 101. Wuthrich DA, Lebowitz AL. Images in clinical medicine: tophaceous gout. New Engl J Med 1995;332:646.

Plate 115. Miles DW, Rubens RD. Images in clinical medicine: transverse leukonychia. New Engl J Med 1995;333:100.

Plate 199. Phillips TJ, Dover JS. Recent advances in dermatology. New Engl J Med 1992;326:174.

Plate 203. Mannis MJ, Macsai MS, Huntley AC. Eye and Skin Disease. Lippincott-Raven Publishers, 1996.

Plate 57. Schneiderman H, Eisenberg E. Bulimia: a dangerous variant of anorexia with oral physical signs. Consultant 1995;35:1695–1700.

Plate 123. Schneiderman H. Charot joint. Consultant 1995;35:1288.

Plate 130. Schneiderman H. Trident tongue of myasthenia gravis. Consultant 1993;34:367–368.

Plate 220. Schneiderman H. Battle sign and external assessment of head trauma. Consultant 1995;35:1529–1530.

Plate 188. Sheth TN, Choudhry NK, Bowes M, Detsky AS. The relation of conjunctival pallor to the presence of anemia. J Gen Intern Med 1997;12:103.

Plate 36. Used with permission from Arthritis Foundation ARA Clinical Slide Collection, 1981.

Plate 73. Courtesy of Upjohn Pharmaceuticals.

Plate 78. Used with permission from American Academy of Dermatology, Courses in Clinical Dermatology: Sexually Transmitted Diseases, 1980.

Plate 174. Courtesy of the Armed Forces Institute of Pathology.

Plates 224, 226. Used with permission from American Academy of Opthamology, External Disease and Cornea: A Slide-Script Program, 2nd ed. 1988.

Index

Page numbers followed by an "f" indicate figures; numbers preceded by "plate" indicate color plate numbers.

Index

Index

Index

B

Bacillary angiomatosis, plate 199
    papules/nodules in, 243
Back pain, low, 164–166
Bacteremia, petechiae in, 248
Bacterial conjunctivitis, plate 223
Bacterial endocarditis, palpable spleen in, 117
Bacterial prostatitis, 138
Bacterial vaginosis, 147
Baker's cyst
    knee pain in, 153
    ruptured, unilateral leg swelling in, 60
Ballismus, 227
Band keratopathy, plate 21
Bartholinitis, intercourse pain with, 136
Basal cell cancer, plate 164
    papules/nodules in, 242
Basilar meningitis, diplopia/nystagmus in, 266
Battle's sign, plate 220
Behçet's syndrome, plate 85, plate 87
    arthritis-dermatitis in, 158
    genital ulcer in, 129
    oral ulcers in, 287
Bell's palsy, facial appearances in, 6
Benign exertional headache, 208
Benign prostatic hypertrophy, 138
    urinary incontinence in, 144
Bennet's fracture, 184
Biceps tendon, ruptured distal, 161
Bicipital tendonitis, 180
Bigeminal pulse, 28
Biliary cirrhosis, plate 48
    dyspigmentation in, 231
    hepatomegaly in, 109
    primary, plate 66
        jaundice in, 112
Biliary colic, abdominal pain in, 93
Biliary disease, chest pain in, 24
Biot's breathing, 78
Bipolar disorder, 203
Bisferiens pulse, 28
Black color, 3
Black longitudinal streak, nail, 170
Black widow spider bite, 168
Bladder cancer, hematuria in, 131
Bladder distension
    abdominal distension in, 88
    abdominal/pelvic mass in, 89
Bladder outlet obstruction
    anuria/oliguria in, 123
    polyuria in, 137
Bleeding. *See also* Hemorrhage(s)
    excessive, 247–249
Bleeding diathesis, epistaxis in, 269
Blepharitis, 290
Blindness, eclipse, 277
Blister, friction, 257

Blood disorders, leg ulcer from, 240
Blood loss, anemia from, 26
Blood pressure, high, 45–46
Blue lunulae, 170, plate 6
Blue nevus, 242
Blue sclera, plate 3
Blue/gray color, 3
Blue-green nails, 170
Body mass index (BMI), 18
Bone marrow transplant, plate 135
Bony prominence, 160
Botulism
    deep tendon reflex in, 197
    diplopia/nystagmus in, 266
    dysphagia in, 105
Bouchard's nodes, plate 90
Bounding pulse, 28
Bowel obstruction
    large, abdominal pain in, 93
    small
        abdominal distension in, 88
        abdominal pain in, 93
        nausea and vomiting in, 115
Bowen's disease
    genital ulcer in, 129
    papules/nodules in, 243
    scaling rash in, 251
Brachial plexus, pain/dysesthesia in, 219—220
Bradycardia, 30
Brain abscess, headache in, 209
Brain tumor
    dementia in, 202
    headache in, 209
Brainstem ischemia/lesion, diplopia/nystagmus from, 266
Branchial cleft cyst, 284
Breast cancer, plate 51
    breast discharge in, 69
    breast mass in, 70
    prevention of, 19
    screening for, 19
Breast discharge, 69
Breast mass, 70
Breathing, patterned, 78
Broca's aphasia, 189
Bronchial adenoma, hemoptysis in, 76
Bronchial hyperreactivity, induced, 65
Bronchiectasis
    cough in, 72
    hemoptysis in, 75
    nail phenomena in, 171
Bronchitis
    cough in, 71
    hemoptysis in, 75
Bronchogenic cancer
    hemoptysis in, 75
    nail phenomena in, 170
Brown recluse spider bite, 240, plate 149

Index

Index

Index

Index

Index

Index

Index

Index

Index

Index

Index

Index

Index

Index

Index

Index

Index

Index

Index

Index

Index

Index

List of Plates

333

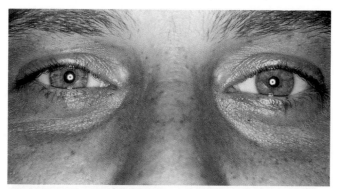

PLATE 1. Heterochromia iridium. *(Ch. 1)*

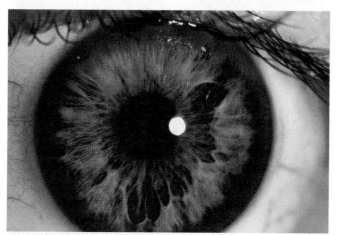

PLATE 2. Golden Kayser-Fleischer ring/Wilson's. *(Ch. 1, 101, 112)*

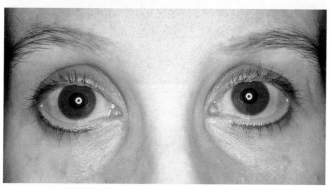

PLATE 3. Blue sclera/osteogenesis imperfecta. *(Ch. 1)*

Plates 4–6

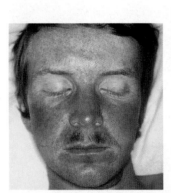
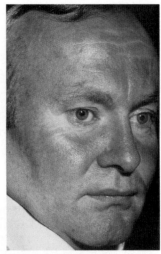

PLATE 4. (Left) Carcinoid flush. *(Ch. 2, 43, 49, 115, 123, 126)*
PLATE 5. (Right) Ceruloderma/amiodarone. *(Ch. 1, 19, 113*

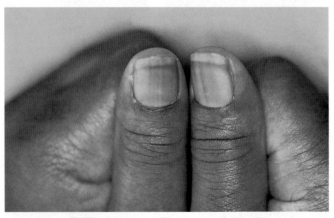

PLATE 6. Blue lunulae/AZT. *(Ch. 1, 19, 87, 101, 112)*

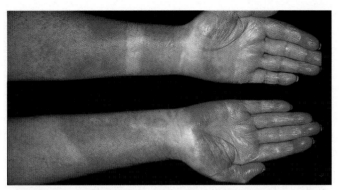

PLATE 7. Photodermatitis/quinidine. *(Ch. 119, 124)*

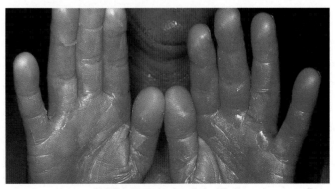

PLATE 8. Necrolytic migratory erythema/glucagonoma. *(Ch. 126)*

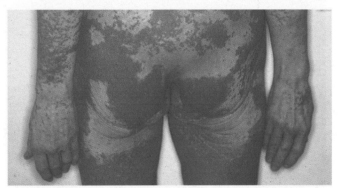

PLATE 9. Pityriasis rubra pilaris. *(Ch. 1)*

Plates 10–11

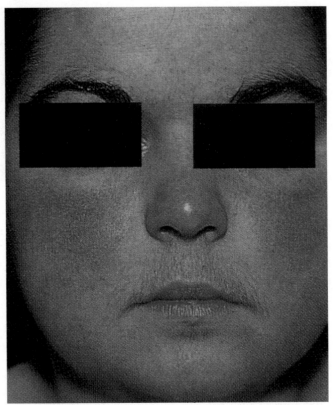

PLATE 10. Moon face/Cushing's. *(Ch. 3, 4, 5, 9, 23, 116)*

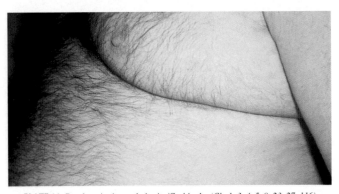

PLATE 11. Purple striae/truncal obesity/Cushing's. *(Ch. 1, 3, 4, 5, 9, 23, 27, 116)*

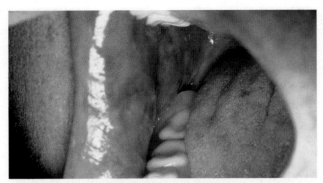

PLATE 12. Buccal hyperpigmentation/Addison's. *(Ch. 3, 4, 6, 25, 27, 48, 50, 57, 113)*

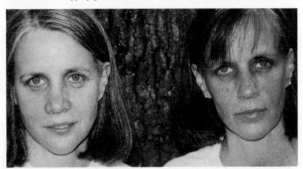

PLATE 13. Hyperpigmentation/wasting/Addison's (right) compared with healthy identical twin (left). *(Ch. 3, 4, 6, 25, 48, 50, 57, 113)*

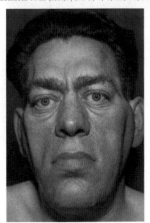
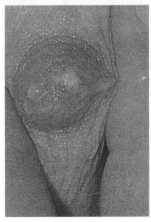

PLATE 14. (Left) Acromegaly. *(Ch. 2, 3, 82, 134, 147)*
PLATE 15. (Right) Galactorrhea/prolactinoma. *(Ch. 5, 33, 34, 73, 116, 134, 137)*

Plates 16–18

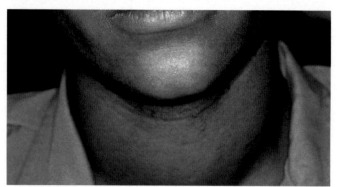

PLATE 16. Goiter. *(Ch. 3, 4, 8, 9, 14, 15, 16, 22, 51, 99, 102, 105, 116, 136, 139, 145)*

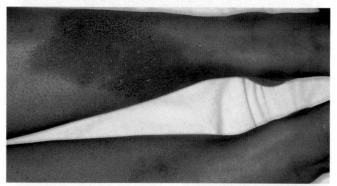

PLATE 17. Pretibial myxedema. *(Ch. 3, 4, 8, 9, 14, 15, 22, 51, 99, 102, 136)*

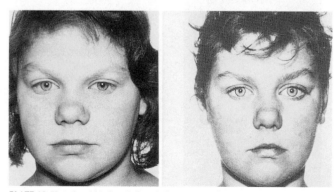

PLATE 18. Hypothyroid before (left) and after (right) treatment. *(Ch. 3, 4, 8, 9, 14, 15, 22, 51, 93, 99, 102, 105, 116, 136, 147)*

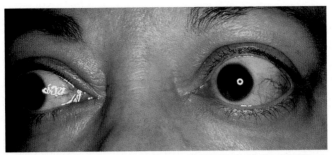

PLATE 19. Exophthalmos/Grave's. *(Ch. 2, 3, 6, 13, 15, 16, 26, 87, 95, 100, 105, 106, 112, 128, 131, 139)*

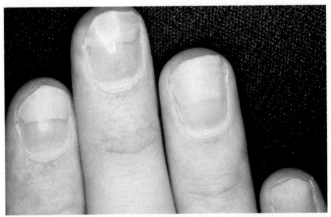

PLATE 20. Thyroid onycholysis/Grave's. *(Ch. 2, 3, 6, 87, 95, 112)*

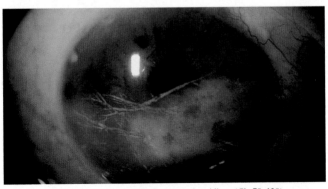

PLATE 21. Band keratopathy/hyperparathyroidism. *(Ch. 78, 120)*

Plates 22–24

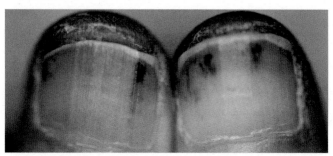

PLATE 22. Splinter hemorrhages/endocarditis. *(Ch. 2, 4, 5, 6, 15, 28, 41, 58, 65, 87, 110, 121)*

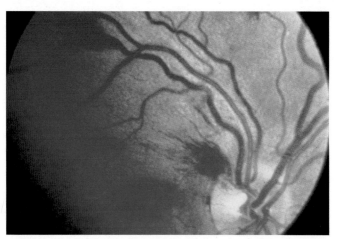

PLATE 23. Roth spots/endocarditis. *(Ch. 2, 4, 5, 6, 15, 28, 41, 58, 65, 87, 110, 121)*

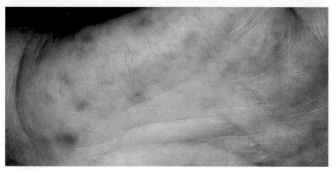

PLATE 24. Osler's nodes/endocarditis. *(Ch. 2, 4, 5, 6, 15, 28, 41, 58, 65, 87, 110, 121)*

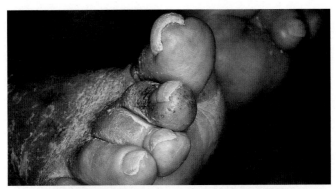

PLATE 25. Arterial embolism. *(Ch. 1, 11, 17, 46, 85, 106, 117, 121)*

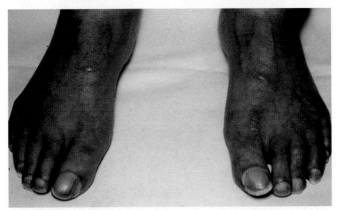

PLATE 26. Erythromelalgia/polycythemia vera. *(Ch. 1, 3, 17, 19, 58, 117, 120)*

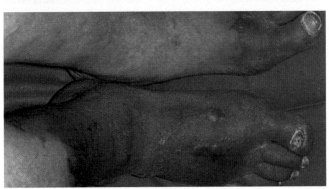

PLATE 27. Phlegmasia cerulea dolens. *(Ch. 1, 17)*

Plates 28–30

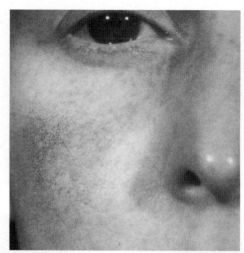

PLATE 28. Malar cyanotic flush/mitral stenosis. *(Ch. 3, 15, 20, 26, 36, 38)*

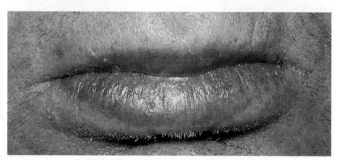

PLATE 29. Central cyanosis. *(Ch. 19, 20, 87)*

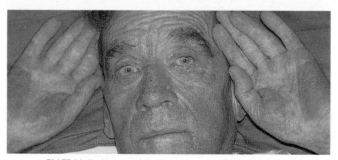

PLATE 30. Ruddy cyanosis/polycythemia vera. *(Ch. 3, 19, 58, 120)*

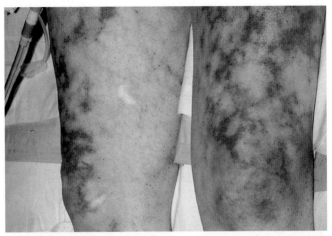

PLATE 31. Purpuric livedo/pneumococcal sepsis. *(Ch. 13, 27, 100, 119)*

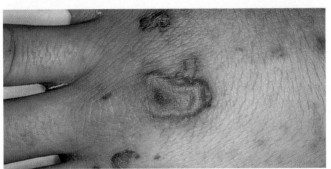

PLATE 32. Gun-metal gray purpura/meningococcemia. *(Ch. 1, 5, 27, 104, 114, 121)*

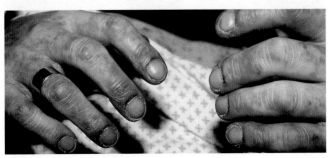

PLATE 33. Acral diffuse intravascular coagulation (DIC)/pneumococcal sepsis. *(Ch. 13, 27, 121)*

Plates 34–36

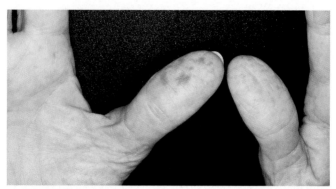

PLATE 34. Acral cyanosis/cryoglobulinemia. *(Ch. 91, 117, 121, 124, 126)*

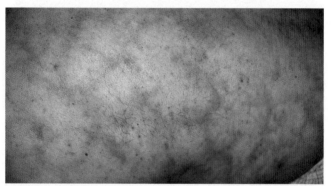

PLATE 35. Livedo reticularis/lupus. *(Ch. 60, 91, 119)*

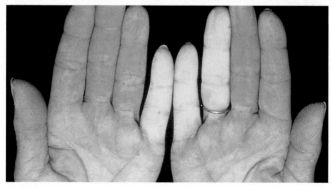

PLATE 36. Raynaud's phenomenon. *(Ch. 1, 5, 11, 19, 36, 54, 71, 80, 87, 90, 91, 93, 117, 123)*

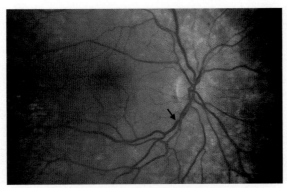

PLATE 37. Hypertensive A-V nicking *(Ch. 23, 60, 117, 143)*

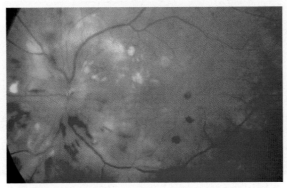

PLATE 38. Accelerated hypertension. *(Ch. 22, 23, 71, 100, 104, 143)*

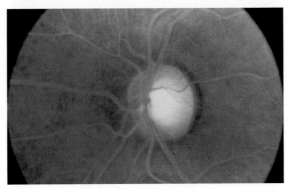

PLATE 39. Lipemia retinalis. *(Ch. 143)*

Plates 40–42

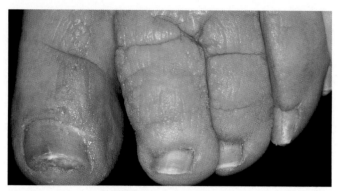

PLATE 40. Lymphedema. *(Ch. 22, 29)*

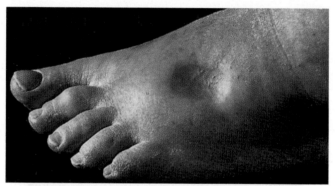

PLATE 41. Pitting edema. *(Ch. 4, 6, 15, 22, 36, 44, 48, 55, 58, 71, 100, 105, 120)*

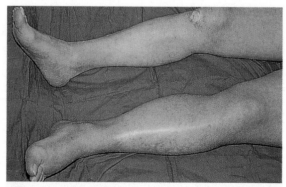

PLATE 42. Deep vein thrombophlebitis. *(Ch. 5, 11, 17, 19, 21, 22, 27, 29, 30, 32, 38, 40, 43, 111)*

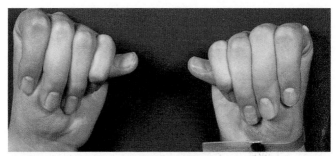

PLATE 43. Thumb sign/Marfan's. *(Ch. 11, 111)*

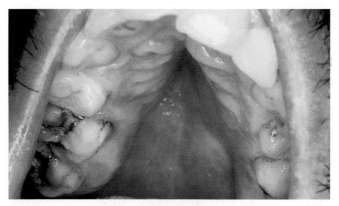

PLATE 44. High-arched palate/Marfan's. *(Ch. 11, 111)*

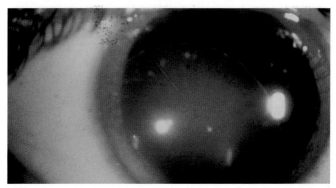

PLATE 45. Lens dislocation/homocystinuria. *(Ch. 11, 111)*

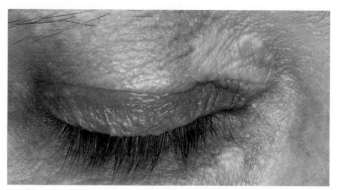

PLATE 46. Xanthelasma palpebrae. *(Ch. 1)*

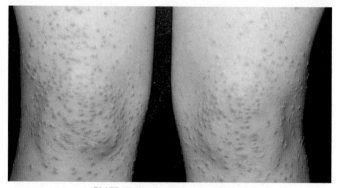

PLATE 47. Eruptive xanthomas. *(Ch. 118)*

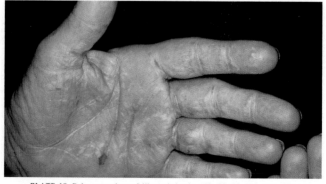

PLATE 48. Palmar xanthoma/biliary cirrhosis. *(Ch. 55, 56, 113, 118, 120)*

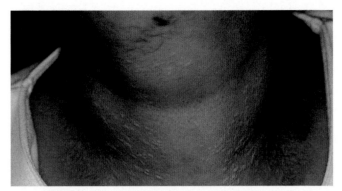

PLATE 49. Plucked-chicken skin/pseudoxanthoma elasticum. *(Ch. 1)*

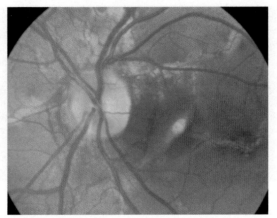

PLATE 50. Angioid streaks/pseudoxanthoma elasticum. *(Ch. 143)*

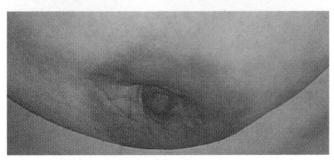

PLATE 51. Nipple retraction/breast cancer. *(Ch. 33, 34, 81)*

Plates 52–54

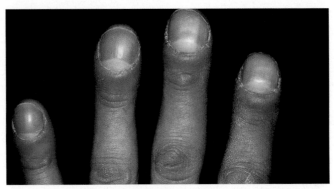

PLATE 52. Clubbing. *(Ch. 20, 35, 36, 42, 43, 49, 87, 126)*

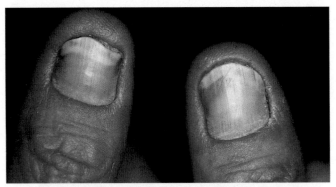

PLATE 53. Yellow nail syndrome. *(Ch. 1, 87)*

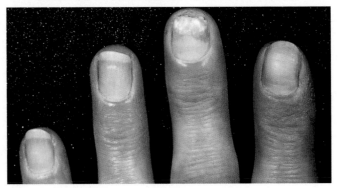

PLATE 54. Candida paronychia. *(Ch. 93)*

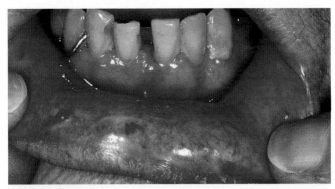

PLATE 55. Hereditary hemorrhagic telangiectasia. *(Ch. 18, 19, 38, 123)*

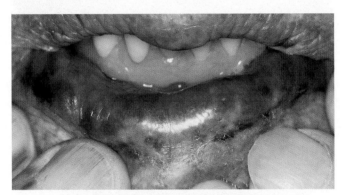

PLATE 56. Buccal lentigines/Peutz-Jeghers. *(Ch. 126)*

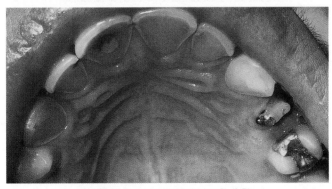

PLATE 57. Enamel erosion/bulimia. *(Ch. 6, 73)*

Plates 58–60

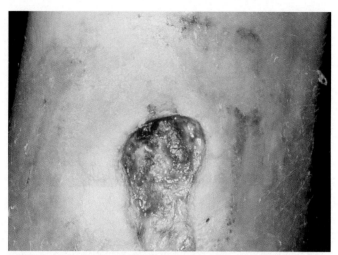

PLATE 58. Pyoderma gangrenosum/ulcerative colitis. *(Ch. 49, 50, 53, 56, 85, 87, 90, 117)*

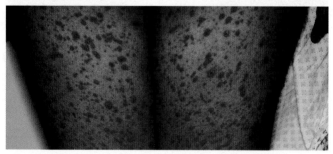

PLATE 59. Dermatitis herpetiformis/sprue. *(Ch. 22, 44, 49, 125)*

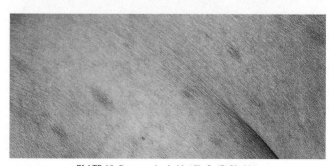

PLATE 60. Rose spot/typhoid. *(Ch. 5, 47, 58, 114)*

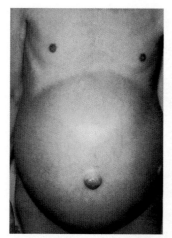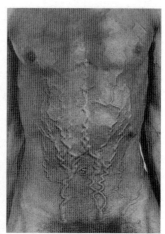

PLATE 61. Ascites. *(Ch. 6, 22, 37, 44, 53, 55, 56, 58, 87, 100, 123)*
PLATE 62. Caput medusa. *(Ch. 22, 30, 44, 55, 58, 100, 123)*

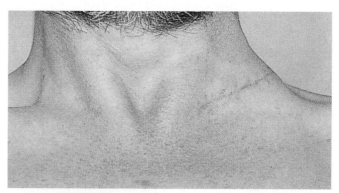

PLATE 63. Virchow's node. *(Ch. 4, 6, 22, 44, 45, 49, 50, 53, 55, 139)*

Plates 64–66

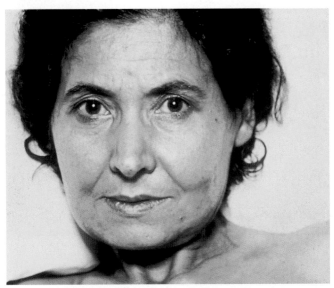

PLATE 64. Jaundice. *(Ch. 1, 6, 12, 22, 55, 56, 57, 58, 120)*

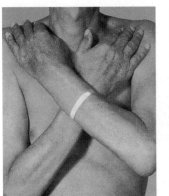 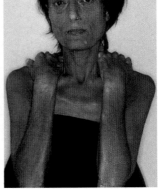

PLATE 65. (Left) Hemochromatosis. *(Ch. 55, 56, 78, 113)*
PLATE 66. (Right) Hyperpigmentation/tuberous xanthoma/primary biliary cirrhosis. *(Ch. 55, 56, 113, 118, 120)*

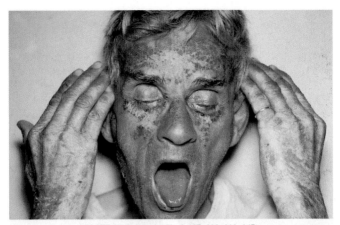

PLATE 67. Pellagra. *(Ch. 6, 107, 113, 119, 147)*

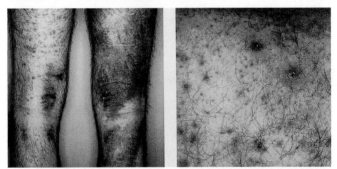

PLATE 68. Perifollicular hemorrhages/ecchymoses/scurvy. *(Ch. 6, 121)*

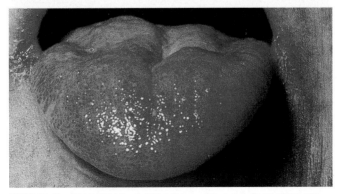

PLATE 69. Glossitis/cheilitis/vitamin B12 deficiency. *(Ch. 1, 3, 6, 12, 25, 97, 99, 100, 101, 107, 140, 147)*

Plates 70–72

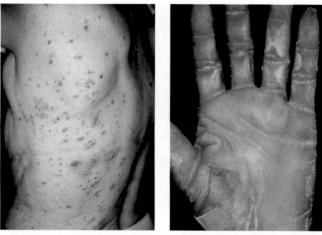

PLATE 70. Inflamed seborrheic keratoses (Leser-Trelat)/gastric cancer *(Ch. 4, 126)*
PLATE 71. Palmar hyperkeratosis/esophageal cancer. *(Ch. 4, 50, 52, 53, 126)*

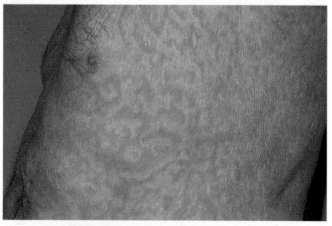

PLATE 72. Erythema gyrata repens. *(Ch. 4, 119, 126)*

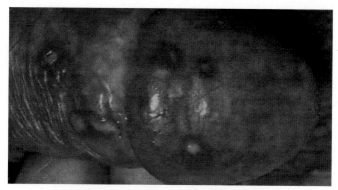

PLATE 73. Genital herpes simplex. *(Ch. 64, 125)*

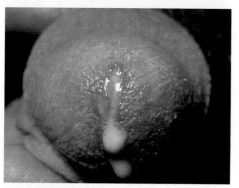

PLATE 74. Gonococcal urethritis. *(Ch. 61)*

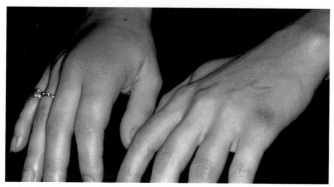

PLATE 75. Gonococcal tenosynovitis. *(Ch. 5, 77, 78, 80, 83, 89, 90, 93, 121, 125)*

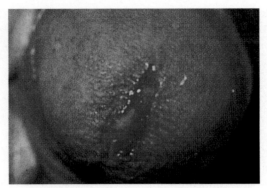

PLATE 76. Chlamydia urethritis. *(Ch. 61)*

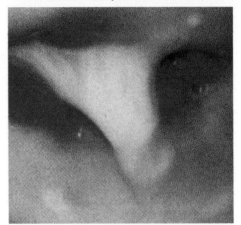

PLATE 77. Mucopurulent cervicitis. *(Ch. 45, 46, 61, 68, 76)*

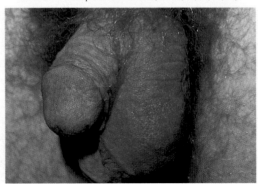

PLATE 78. Epididymitis. *(Ch. 72)*

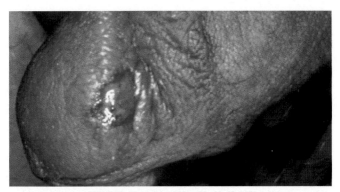

PLATE 79. Chancre/syphilis. *(Ch. 64, 67, 117)*

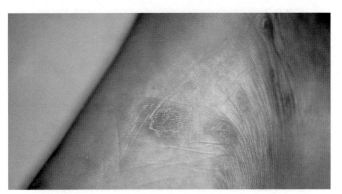

PLATE 80. Copper-penny lesion/secondary syphilis. *(Ch. 1, 5, 7, 83, 114, 122)*

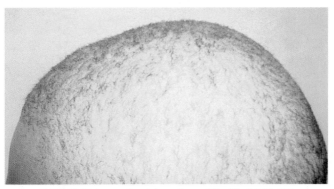

PLATE 81. Moth-eaten alopecia/secondary syphilis. *(Ch. 5, 7, 83, 116)*

Plates 82–84

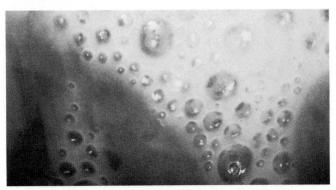

PLATE 82. Frothy vaginal discharge/Trichomonas. *(Ch. 61, 68, 76)*

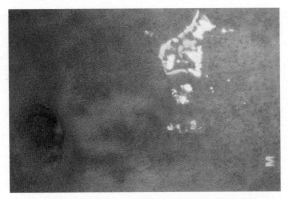

PLATE 83. Strawberry cervix/Trichomonas. *(Ch. 61, 68, 76)*

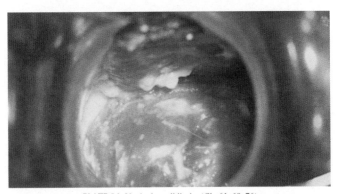

PLATE 84. Vaginal candidiasis. *(Ch. 61, 68, 76)*

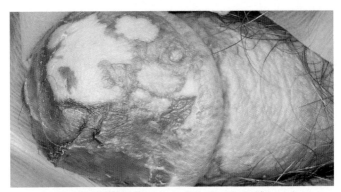

PLATE 85. Genital ulceration/Behçet's. *(Ch. 64, 80)*

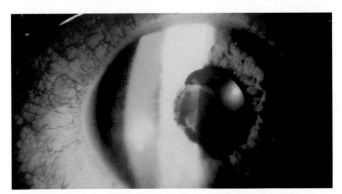

PLATE 86. Iritis/synechiae. *(Ch. 49, 50, 53, 61, 64, 80, 85, 90, 127, 132, 142)*

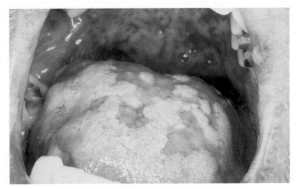

PLATE 87. Oral ulcers/Behçet's. *(Ch. 64, 80, 140)*

Plates 88–90

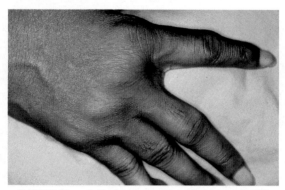

PLATE 88. Rheumatoid arthritis/hand. *(Ch. 7, 42, 58, 80, 90, 93, 133)*

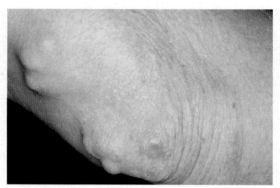

PLATE 89. Rheumatoid nodules. *(Ch. 7, 42, 58, 77, 80, 90, 93, 118)*

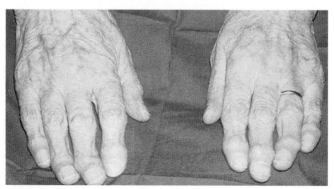

PLATE 90. Heberden's and Bouchard's nodes/osteoarthritis. *(Ch. 78, 82, 84, 85, 90, 93, 99)*

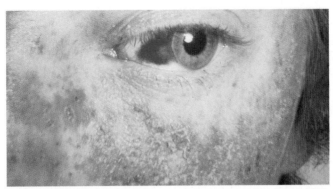

PLATE 91. Malar (butterfly) rash/thrombocytopenia/systemic lupus. *(Ch. 3, 5, 11, 15, 71, 80, 90, 91, 93, 116, 119, 121, 123)*

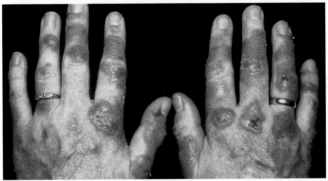

PLATE 92. Systemic lupus/hands. *(Ch. 3, 5, 11, 15, 71, 80, 90, 91, 93, 121, 123)*

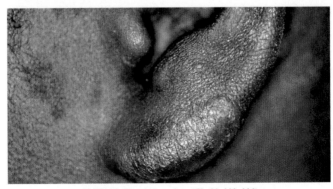

PLATE 93. Discoid lupus/ear. *(Ch. 80, 113, 116)*

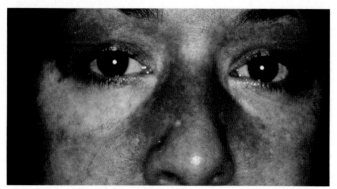

PLATE 94. Heliotrope/dermatomyositis. *(Ch. 1, 3, 80, 123, 126)*

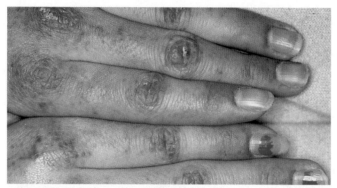

PLATE 95. Gottron's papules/dermatomyositis. *(Ch. 80, 123, 126)*

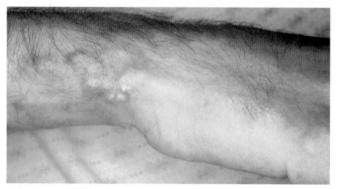

PLATE 96. Calcinosis cutis/dermatomyositis. *(Ch. 80, 118)*

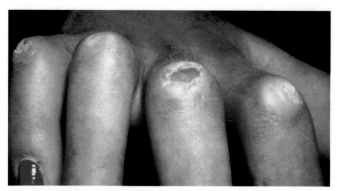

PLATE 97. Scleroderma/hand. *(Ch. 42, 51, 52, 54, 80, 90, 91, 93, 117, 123)*

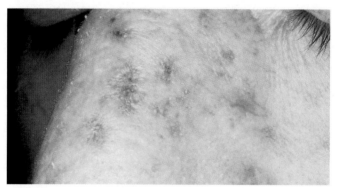

PLATE 98. Mat telangiectasias/CREST. *(Ch. 80, 90, 91)*

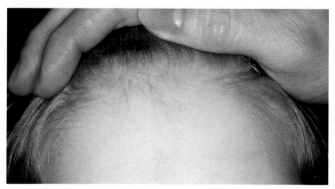

PLATE 99. Coup-de-sabre/linear scleroderma (morphea). *(Ch. 1, 116)*

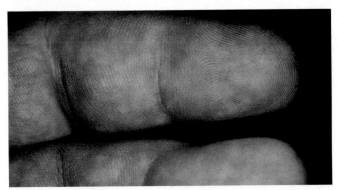

PLATE 100. Tophi/gout. *(Ch. 1, 78, 83, 90, 93, 118)*

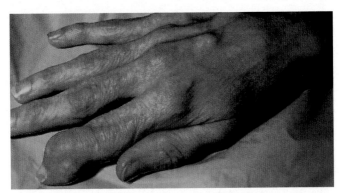

PLATE 101. Arthritis/gout. *(Ch. 78, 90, 93)*

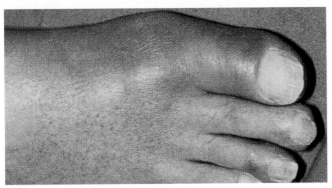

PLATE 102. Podagra/gout. *(Ch. 78, 79, 90)*

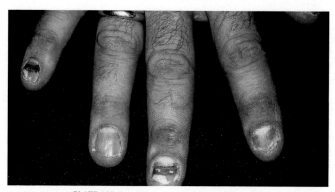

PLATE 103. Psoriasis/nails. *(Ch. 80, 87, 90, 93, 122)*

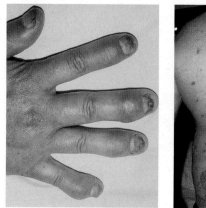
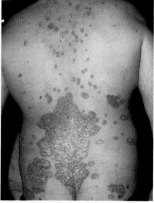

PLATE 104. (Left) Arthritis/psoriasis. *(Ch. 80, 90, 93)*
PLATE 105. (Right) Micaceous plaques/psoriasis. *(Ch. 1, 80, 90, 93, 122, 129)*

Plates 106–108

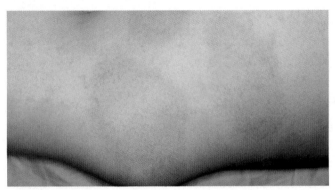

PLATE 106. Erythema migrans/Lyme disease. *(Ch. 5, 14, 77, 78, 80, 90, 108, 119)*

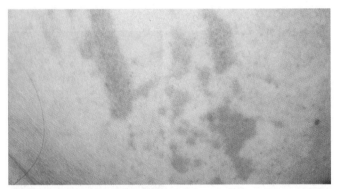

PLATE 107. Evanescent rash/Still's disease. *(Ch. 5, 80, 90)*

PLATE 108. Erythema marginatum/rheumatic fever. *(Ch. 5, 14, 80, 90, 112, 119)*

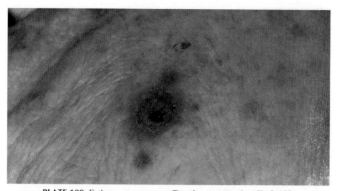

PLATE 109. Ecthyma gangrenosum/Pseudomonas sepsis. *(Ch. 5, 125)*

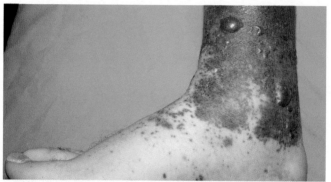

PLATE 110. Palpable purpura/leukocytoclastic vasculitis. *(Ch. 5, 60, 80, 90, 100, 107, 117, 121)*

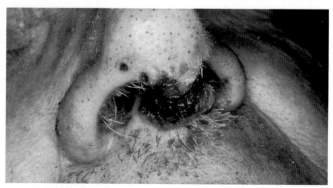

PLATE 111. Nasal ulcer/Wegener's granulomatosis. *(Ch. 38, 65, 130, 138)*

Plates 112–114

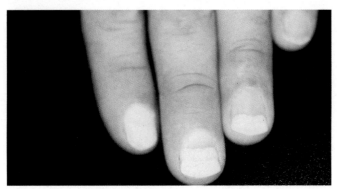

PLATE 112. Leukonychia. *(Ch. 87)*

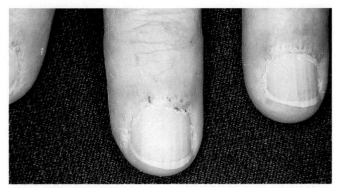

PLATE 113. Nailfold telangiectasias. *(Ch. 80, 87, 90, 91, 93, 123)*

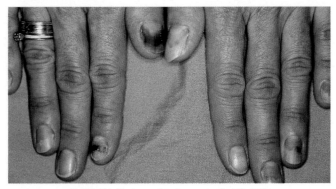

PLATE 114. Blue-green Pseudomonas nails. *(Ch. 1, 87)*

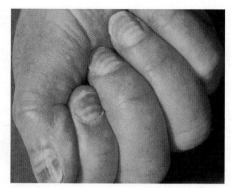

PLATE 115. Transverse leukonychia/chemotherapy cycles. *(Ch. 87)*

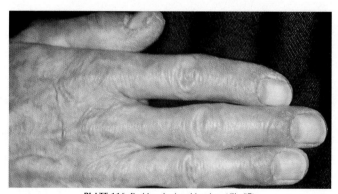

PLATE 116. Red lunulae/azathioprine. *(Ch. 87)*

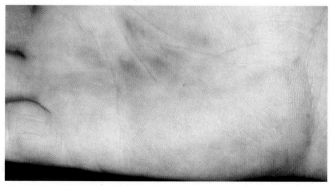

PLATE 117. Acral erythema/chemotherapy. *(Ch. 115)*

Plates 118–120

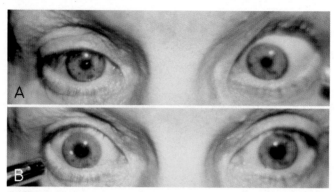

PLATE 118. Argyll-Robertson pupils/neurosyphilis. A. Accomodation; B. Light. *(Ch. 97, 101, 107, 127, 128)*

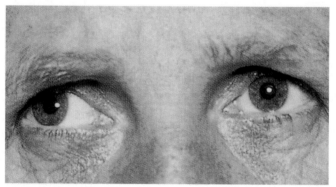

PLATE 119. Internuclear ophthalmoplegia/multiple sclerosis/lateral gaze. *(Ch. 74, 96, 97, 99, 103, 106, 108, 112, 128)*

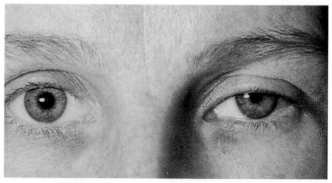

PLATE 120. Horner's syndrome. *(Ch. 104, 108, 127, 141)*

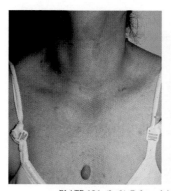

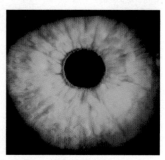

PLATE 121. (Left) Cafe-au-lait/neurofibroma. *(Ch. 113, 118)*
PLATE 122. (Right) Lisch nodules/neurofibromatosis. *(Ch. 113)*

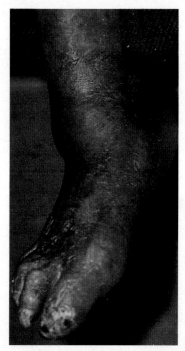

PLATE 123. Charcot joint. *(Ch. 107)*

Plates 124–126

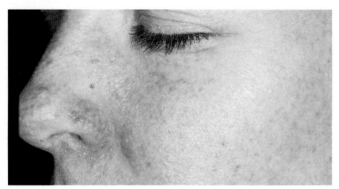

PLATE 124. Adenoma sebaceum/tuberous sclerosis. *(Ch. 113, 118)*

PLATE 125. Ash leaf/tuberous sclerosis. *(Ch. 113)*

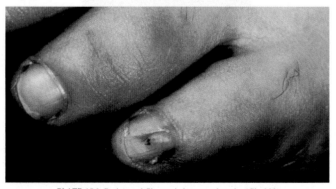

PLATE 126. Periungual fibroma/tuberous sclerosis. *(Ch. 113)*

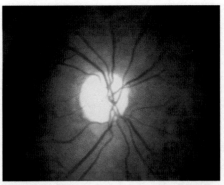

PLATE 127. Optic atrophy. *(Ch. 74, 96, 97, 99, 103, 106, 108, 112, 128, 137, 143)*

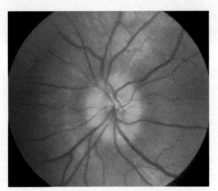

PLATE 128. Inflammatory optic neuritis. *(Ch. 74, 96, 97, 99, 103, 106, 108, 112, 128, 132, 134, 137, 143)*

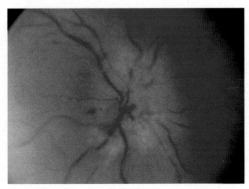

PLATE 129. Papilledema. *(Ch. 2, 23, 57, 104, 137, 143)*

Plates 130–132

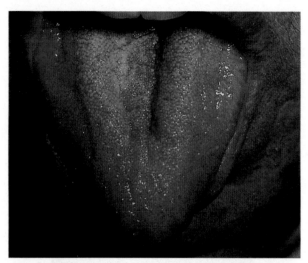

PLATE 130. Trident tongue/myasthenia gravis. *(Ch. 4, 19, 106)*

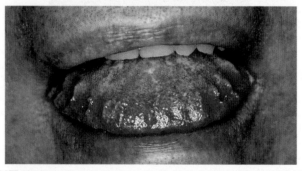

PLATE 131. Macroglossia/amyloidosis. *(Ch. 25, 55, 69, 71, 96, 99, 107, 118, 126, 147)*

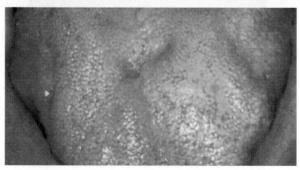

PLATE 132. Scalloped tongue/amyotrophic lateral sclerosis (ALS). *(Ch. 19, 86, 99, 106, 108, 112)*

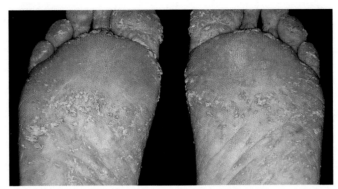

PLATE 133. Arsenical keratosis. *(Ch. 99, 107, 126)*

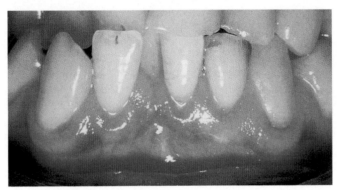

PLATE 134. Lead toxicity/Burton's lines. *(Ch. 12, 50, 99, 100, 107, 128)*

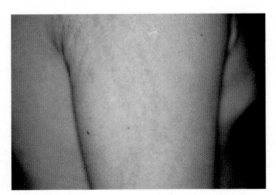

PLATE 135. Linear graft vs. host reaction/bone marrow transplant.

Plates 136–138

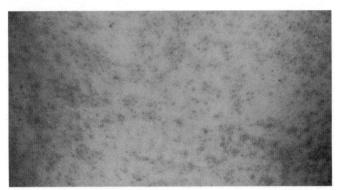

PLATE 136. Atypical measles. *(Ch. 114, 142)*

PLATE 137. Rubella. *(Ch. 90, 114)*

PLATE 138. Reticular erythema/Parvovirus. *(Ch. 90, 114)*

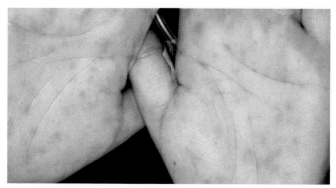

PLATE 139. Rocky Mountain Spotted Fever. *(Ch. 5, 114, 121)*

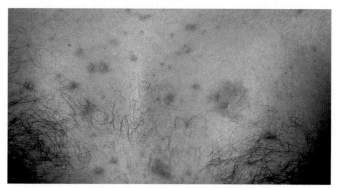

PLATE 140. Varicella (chickenpox). *(Ch. 114, 125)*

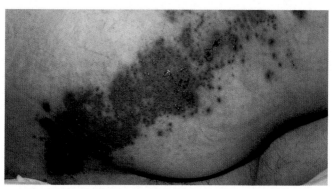

PLATE 141. Dermatomal zoster (shingles). *(Ch. 11, 125)*

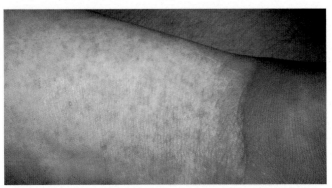

PLATE 142. Scarlet fever/Pastia's lines (flexor crease accentuation). *(Ch. 114, 135, 147)*

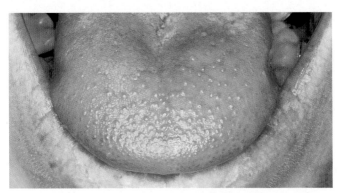

PLATE 143. Strawberry tongue/scarlet fever. *(Ch. 114, 147)*

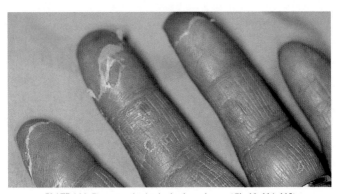

PLATE 144. Desquamation/toxic shock syndrome. *(Ch. 13, 114, 115)*

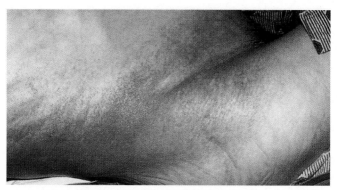

PLATE 145. Gray-Turner's sign. *(Ch. 25, 27, 46)*

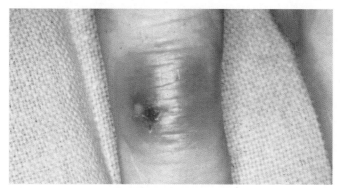

PLATE 146. Tularemia. *(Ch. 5)*

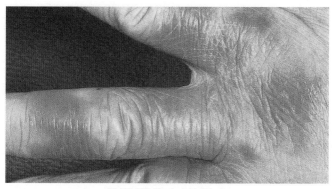

PLATE 147. Erysipeloid. *(Ch. 1)*

Plates 148–150

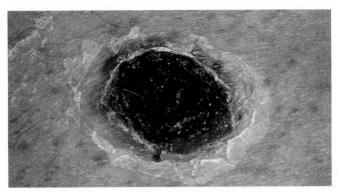

PLATE 148. Anthrax.

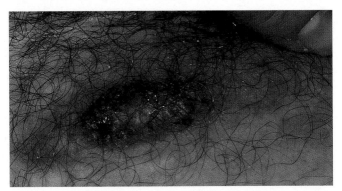

PLATE 149. Brown recluse spider bite. *(Ch. 117)*

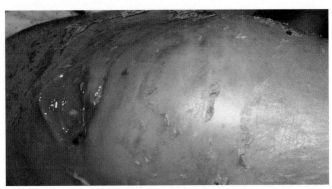

PLATE 150. Necrotizing fasciitis.

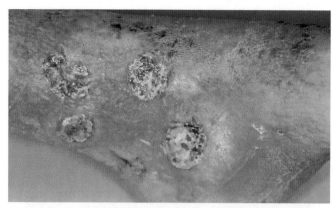

PLATE 151. Venous stasis/ulcer. *(Ch. 22, 29, 117, 122)*

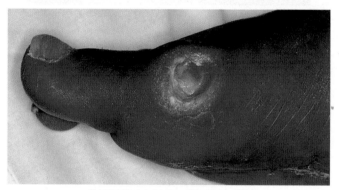

PLATE 152. Arterial ulcer. *(Ch. 17, 19, 117)*

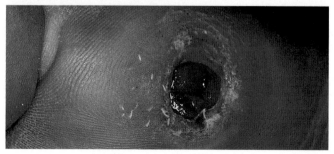

PLATE 153. Neuropathic ulcer. *(Ch. 117)*

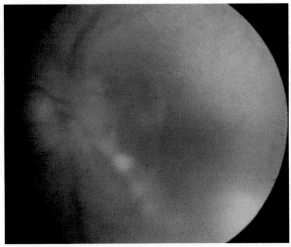

PLATE 154. Fungus balls/Candida. *(Ch. 142)*

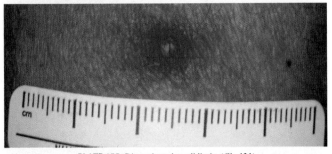

PLATE 155. Disseminated candidiasis. *(Ch. 121)*

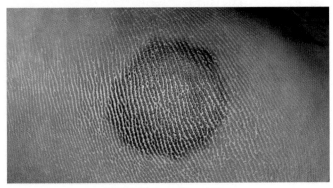

PLATE 156. Aspergillus embolism.

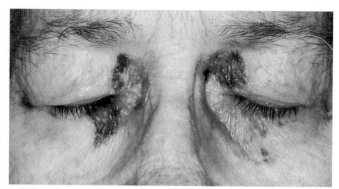

PLATE 157. Amyloidosis/plaques. *(Ch. 1, 25, 55, 69, 71, 99, 107, 118, 121, 126)*

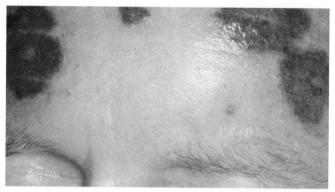

PLATE 158. Sweet's syndrome/leukemia (AML). *(Ch. 4, 55, 118, 126)*

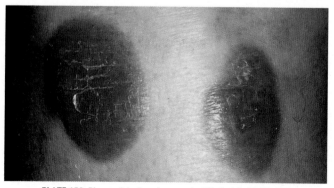

PLATE 159. Plum nodules/lymphoma cutis. *(Ch. 1, 4, 5, 55, 58, 118)*

Plates 160–162

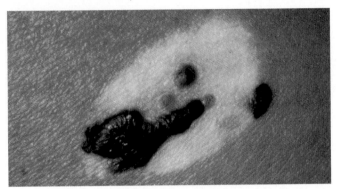

PLATE 160. Melanoma. *(Ch. 1, 118)*

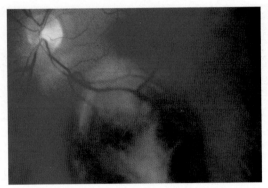

PLATE 161. Choroidal melanoma. *(Ch. 137)*

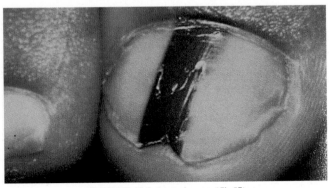

PLATE 162. Nail plate melanoma. *(Ch. 87)*

Plates 163–165

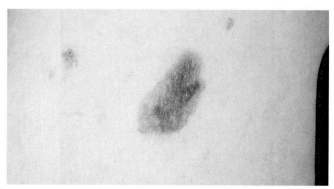

PLATE 163. Dysplastic (atypical) nevus. *(Ch. 118)*

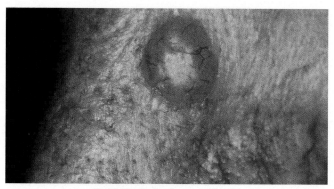

PLATE 164. Basal cell cancer. *(Ch. 118)*

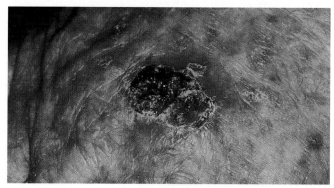

PLATE 165. Squamous cell cancer arising from actinic keratoses. *(Ch. 117, 118)*

Plates 166–168

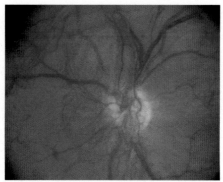

PLATE 166. Diabetic retinopathy/neovascularization. *(Ch. 6, 25, 49, 60, 69, 71, 73, 74, 99, 107, 117, 137, 141, 143)*

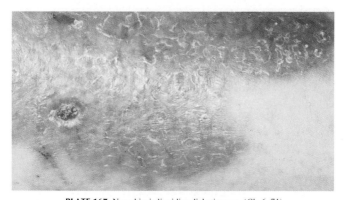

PLATE 167. Necrobiosis lipoidica diabeticorum. *(Ch. 6, 71)*

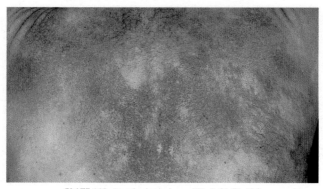

PLATE 168. Acanthosis nigricans. *(Ch. 1, 53, 73, 126)*

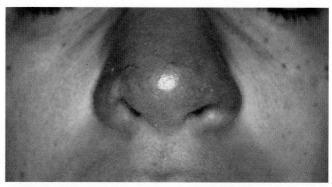

PLATE 169. Lupus pernio/sarcoidosis. *(Ch. 7, 14, 42, 58, 69, 80, 90, 108, 118, 138)*

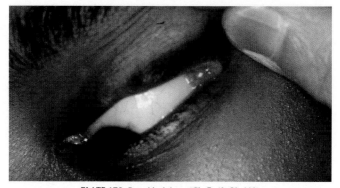

PLATE 170. Sarcoidosis/eye. *(Ch. 7, 42, 58, 118)*

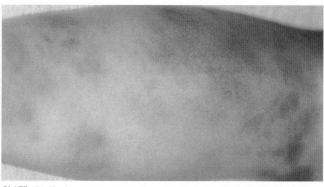

PLATE 171. Erythema nodosum. *(Ch. 7, 14, 42, 47, 49, 50, 53, 58, 69, 80, 90, 108, 118)*

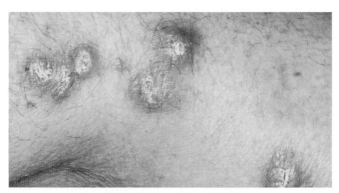

PLATE 172. Sporotrichosis. *(Ch. 7)*

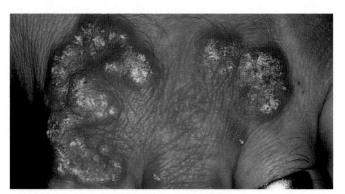

PLATE 173. M. marinum. *(Ch. 7)*

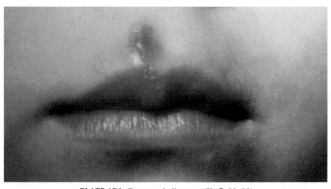

PLATE 174. Cat-scratch disease. *(Ch. 7, 81, 83)*

Plates 175–177

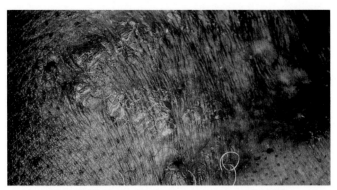

PLATE 175. Lupus vulgaris/cutaneous tuberculosis. *(Ch. 1, 4, 118)*

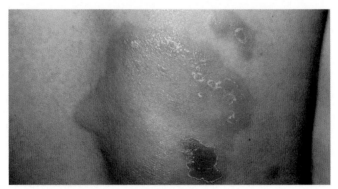

PLATE 176. Leprosy.

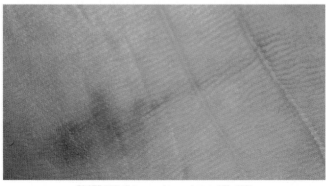

PLATE 177. Cutaneous larva migrans. *(Ch. 119)*

Plates 178–180

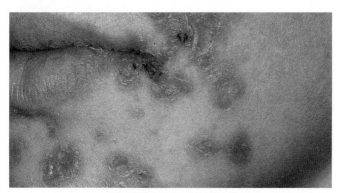

PLATE 178. Impetigo. *(Ch. 60, 140)*

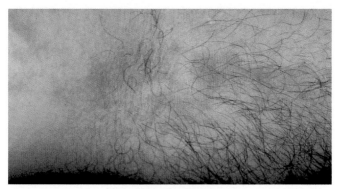

PLATE 179. Lymphangitis. *(Ch. 7)*

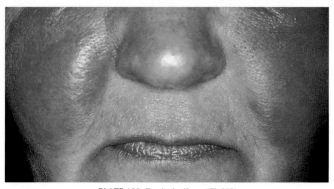

PLATE 180. Erysipelas/face. *(Ch 119)*

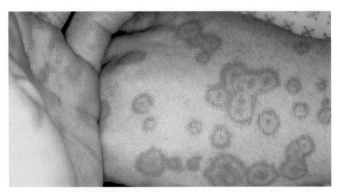

PLATE 181. Erythema multiforme. *(Ch. 5, 7, 60, 114, 119, 125)*

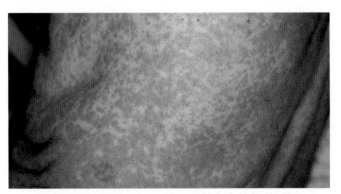

PLATE 182. Morbilliform drug reaction. *(Ch. 5, 7, 27, 60, 71, 104, 114)*

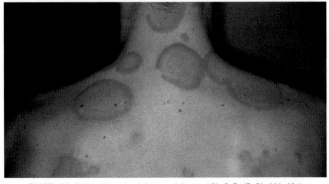

PLATE 183. Polycyclic urticaria/serum sickness. *(Ch. 5, 7, 47, 58, 119, 124)*

Plates 184–186

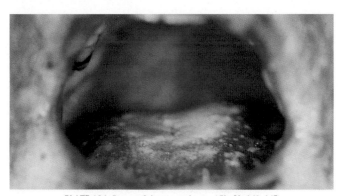

PLATE 184. Stevens-Johnson syndrome. *(Ch. 52, 140, 147)*

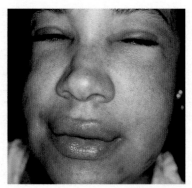

PLATE 185. Angioedema. *(Ch. 27, 32, 43, 96, 124, 136, 141, 147)*

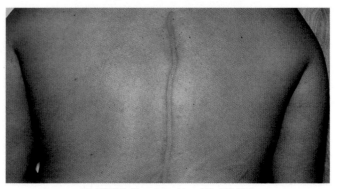

PLATE 186. Dermatographism. *(Ch. 115, 124)*

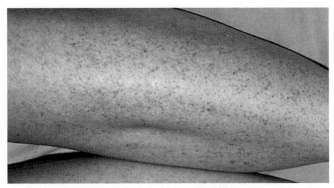

PLATE 187. Idiopathic thrombocytopenic purpura. *(Ch. 75, 121, 130)*

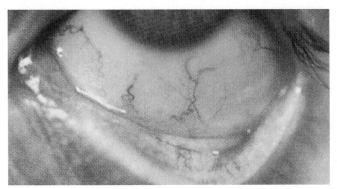

PLATE 188. Conjunctival pallor/anemia. *(Ch. 4, 5, 12, 26, 52, 53, 56, 58, 111)*

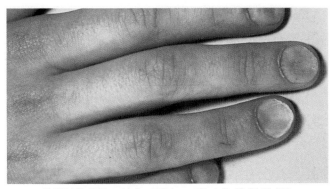

PLATE 189. Koilonychia/iron deficiency. *(Ch. 4, 12, 52, 86, 87, 116)*

Plates 190–192

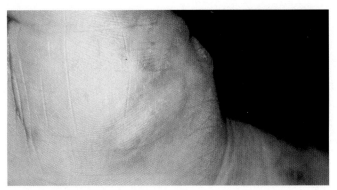

PLATE 190. Coma bullae. *(Ch. 125)*

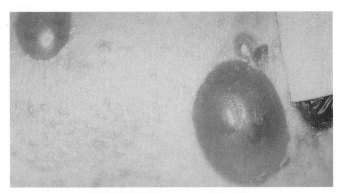

PLATE 191. Bullous pemphigoid. *(Ch. 125)*

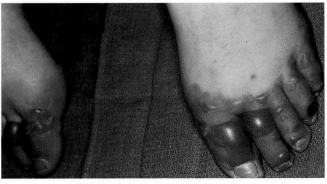

PLATE 192. Hemorrhagic bullae/frostbite. *(Ch. 125)*

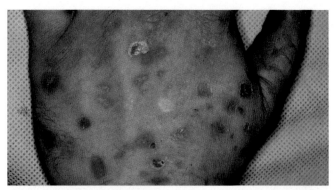

PLATE 193. Porphyria cutanea tarda. *(Ch. 113, 119, 125)*

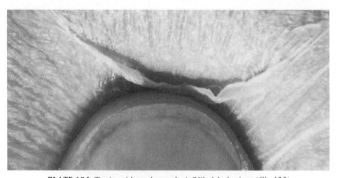

PLATE 194. Toxic epidermal necrolysis/Nikolsky's sign. *(Ch. 125)*

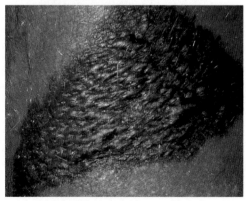

PLATE 195. Warfarin necrosis. *(Ch. 121)*

Plates 196–198

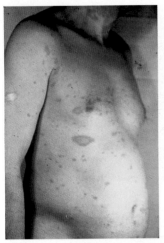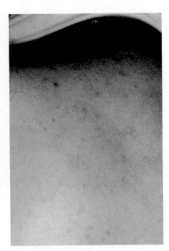

PLATE 196. (Left) Pityriasis rosea. *(Ch. 114, 122)*
PLATE 197. (Right) Tinea versicolor. *(Ch. 113, 122)*

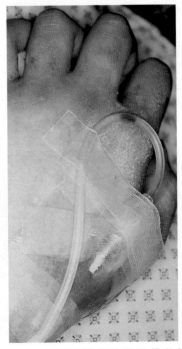

PLATE 198. Uremic frost. *(Ch. 3, 4, 11, 15, 22, 39, 48, 57, 60, 86, 99, 100, 120)*

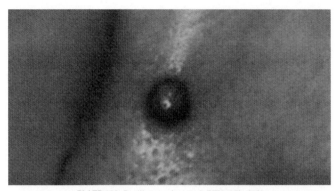

PLATE 199. Bacillary angiomatosis/HIV. *(Ch. 118)*

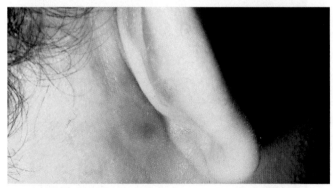

PLATE 200. Kaposi's sarcoma/HIV. *(Ch. 1, 31, 118, 123)*

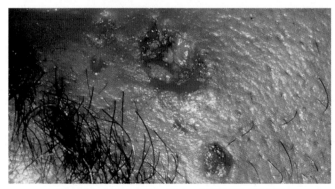

PLATE 201. Disseminated cryptococcosis/HIV. *(Ch. 101, 104)*

Plates 202–204

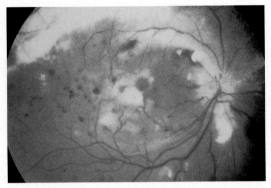

PLATE 202. Cytomegalovirus retinitis/HIV. *(Ch. 1, 137, 143)*

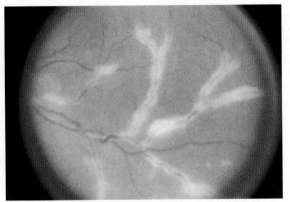

PLATE 203. Frosted branch sheathing/cytomegalovirus/HIV. *(Ch. 137, 143)*

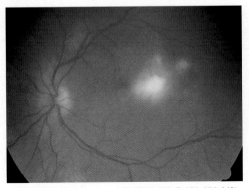

PLATE 204. Toxoplasma retinitis/HIV. *(Ch. 7, 101, 104, 143)*

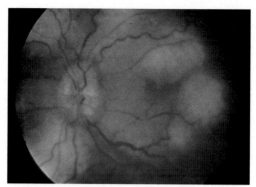

PLATE 205. Pneumocystis choroiditis/HIV. *(Ch. 143)*

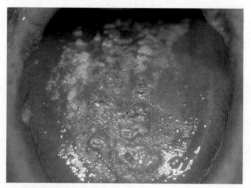

PLATE 206. Thrush/Candida. *(Ch. 7, 52, 54, 144, 147)*

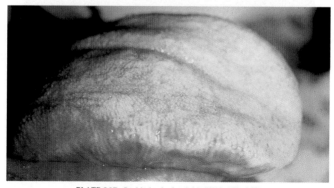

PLATE 207. Oral hairy leukoplakia/HIV. *(Ch. 147)*

Plates 208–210

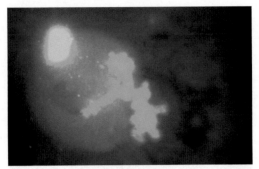

PLATE 208. Corneal dendrites/herpes simplex keratitis. *(Ch. 132, 142)*

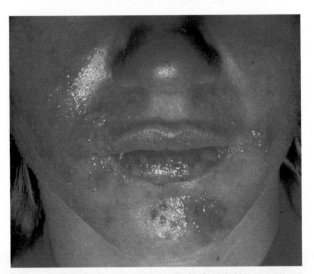

PLATE 209. Herpes labialis. *(Ch. 52, 54, 140, 144)*

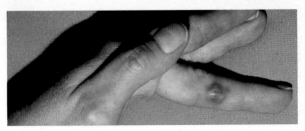

PLATE 210. Herpetic whitlow. *(Ch. 125)*

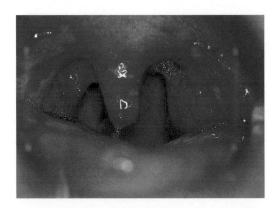

PLATE 211. Herpetic gingivostomatitis. *(Ch. 11, 140, 144)*

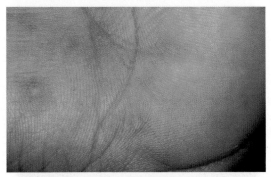

PLATE 212. *Hand*-foot-mouth/Coxsackievirus. *(Ch. 125)*

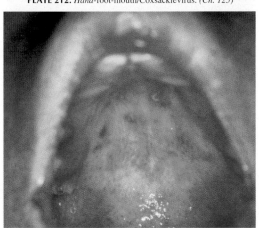

PLATE 213. Hand-foot-*mouth*/Coxsackievirus. *(Ch. 125, 140)*

Plates 214–216

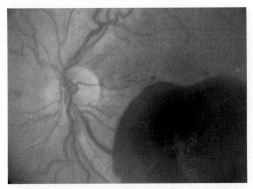

PLATE 214. Retinal hemorrhage. *(Ch. 137, 143)*

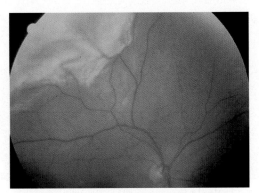

PLATE 215. Retinal detachment. *(Ch. 134, 137, 143)*

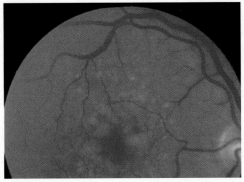

PLATE 216. Drusen/age-related macular degeneration. *(Ch. 137, 143)*

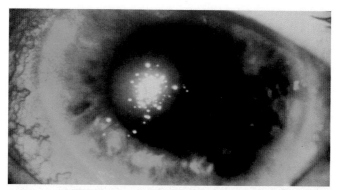

PLATE 217. Acute glaucoma. *(Ch. 104, 127, 132, 137, 142)*

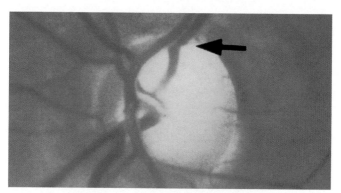

PLATE 218. Cupping/glaucoma. *(Ch. 104, 134, 137, 143)*

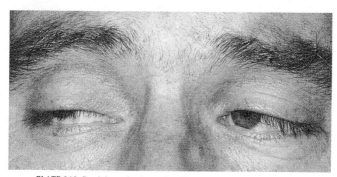

PLATE 219. Ptosis/myasthenia gravis. *(Ch. 3, 4, 19, 36, 52, 106, 128, 141)*

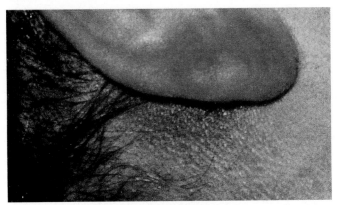

PLATE 220. Battle's sign. *(Ch. 98, 100, 101, 104)*

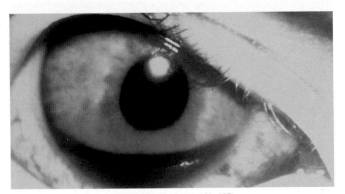

PLATE 221. Hyphema. *(Ch. 127)*

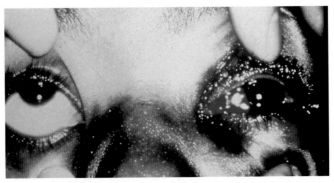

PLATE 222. Orbital blow-out fracture. *(Ch. 127, 128, 132, 133)*

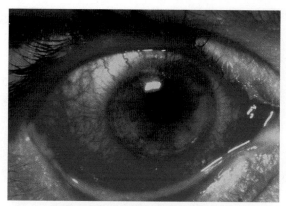

PLATE 223. Bacterial conjunctivitis. *(Ch. 132, 142)*

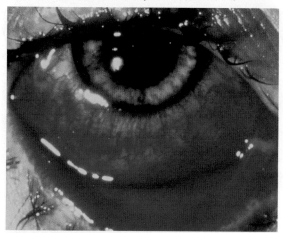

PLATE 224. Viral conjunctivitis. *(Ch. 132, 142)*

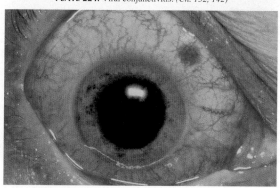

PLATE 225. Allergic conjunctivitis. *(Ch. 132, 142)* **CP-75**

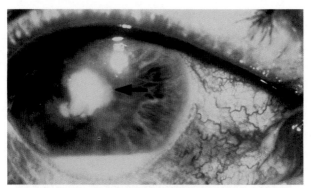

PLATE 226. Corneal ulcer/hypopyon. *(Ch. 142)*

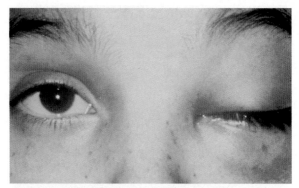

PLATE 227. Orbital cellulitis. *(Ch. 128, 131, 132)*

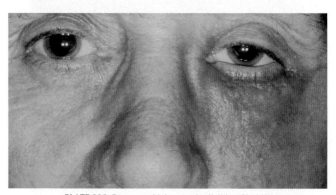

PLATE 228. Dacryocystitis/preseptal cellulitis. *(Ch. 142)*

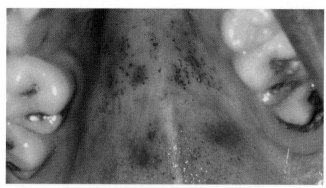

PLATE 229. Palatal petechiae/infectious mononucleosis. *(Ch. 4, 7, 58, 88, 105, 114, 144)*

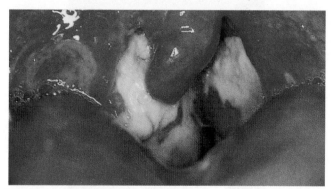

PLATE 230. Tonsillar exudate and hypertrophy/infectious mononucleosis. *(Ch. 4, 7, 58, 88, 105, 114, 139, 144)*

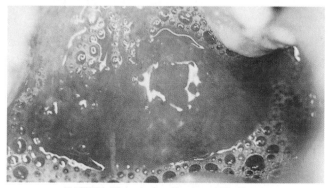

PLATE 231. Trismus/peritonsillar abscess. *(Ch. 43, 144)*

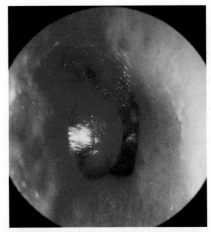

PLATE 232. Bullous myringitis/mycoplasma. *(Ch. 31, 41, 144)*

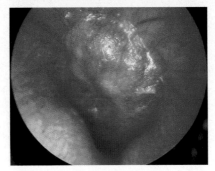

PLATE 233. Otitis media. *(Ch. 104, 129, 135, 146)*

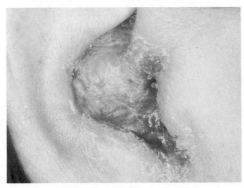

PLATE 234. Otitis externa. *(Ch. 129)*

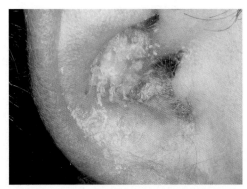

PLATE 235. Herpes zoster oticus/Ramsey-Hunt syndrome. *(Ch. 3, 103, 129)*

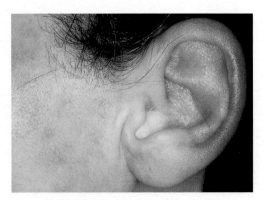

PLATE 236. Relapsing polychondritis. *(Ch. 129)*

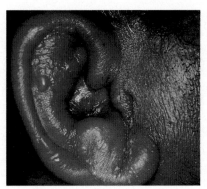

PLATE 237. Erysipelas/ear. *(Ch. 129)*

Plates 238–240

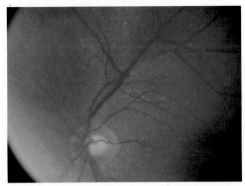

PLATE 238. Amaurosis fugax/retinal arteriolar embolism. *(Ch. 101, 102, 104, 110, 134, 137, 143)*

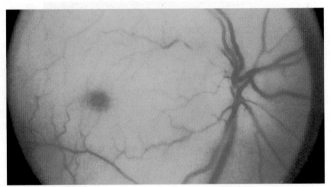

PLATE 239. Central retinal artery occlusion. *(Ch. 137, 143)*

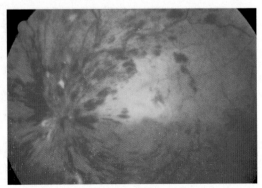

PLATE 240. Central retinal vein occlusion. *(Ch. 137, 143*